D0891993

Cambridge History of Medicine

EDITORS: CHARLES WEBSTER AND CHARLES ROSENBERG

The physician-legislators of France

Charles Webster, ed.   *Health, medicine, and mortality in the sixteenth century*

Ian Maclean   *The Renaissance notion of woman*

Michael MacDonald   *Mystical Bedlam*

Robert E. Kohler   *From medical chemistry to biochemistry*

Walter Pagel   *Joan Baptista Van Helmont*

Nancy Tomes   *A generous confidence*

Roger Cooter   *The cultural meaning of popular science*

Anne Digby   *Madness, morality and medicine*

Guenter B. Risse   *Hospital life in Enlightenment Scotland*

Roy Porter, ed.   *Patients and practitioners*

Ann G. Carmichael   *Plague and the poor in Renaissance Florence*

S. E. D. Shortt   *Victorian lunacy*

Hilary Marland   *Medicine and society in Wakefield and Huddersfield 1780–1870*

Susan Reverby   *Ordered to care*

Russell C. Maulitz   *Morbid appearances*

Matthew Ramsey   *Professional and popular medicine in France, 1770–1830*

John Keown   *Abortion, doctors and the law*

Donald Denoon   *Public health in Papua New Guinea*

Paul Weindling   *Health, race and German politics between National Unification and Nazism, 1870–1945*

William H. Schneider   *Quality and quantity*

The physician-legislators of France

MEDICINE AND POLITICS IN
THE EARLY THIRD REPUBLIC, 1870–1914

Jack D. Ellis

Department of History, University of Delaware

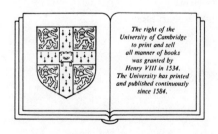

The right of the
University of Cambridge
to print and sell
all manner of books
was granted by
Henry VIII in 1534.
The University has printed
and published continuously
since 1584.

CAMBRIDGE UNIVERSITY PRESS

CAMBRIDGE

NEW YORK   PORT CHESTER   MELBOURNE   SYDNEY

Published by the Press Syndicate of the University of Cambridge
The Pitt Building, Trumpington Street, Cambridge CB2 1RP
40 West 20th Street, New York, NY 10011, USA
10 Stamford Road, Oakleigh, Melbourne 3166, Australia

First published 1990

Printed in the United States of America

Library of Congress Cataloging-in-Publication Data
Ellis, Jack D.
The physician-legislators of France : medicine and politics in the
early Third Republic, 1870–1914 / Jack D. Ellis.
p.   cm. – (Cambridge history of medicine.)
Includes bibliographical references.
ISBN 0-521-38208-4
1. Physicians – France – History – 19th century.   2. Physicians –
France – History – 20th century.   3. Legislators – France –
History – 19th century.   4. Legislators – France – History – 20th
century.   5. Health reformers – France – History – 19th century.
6. Health reformers – France – History – 20th century.   7. France –
History – Third Republic, 1870–1940.   I. Title.   II. Series.
[DNLM: 1. History of Medicine, 19th cent. – France.   2. History of
Medicine, 20th cent. – France.   3. Legislation, Medical – history –
France.   4. Physicians – France.   WZ 70 GF7 E47p]
B505.E44   1990
610'.944 – dc20
DNLM/DLC
for Library of Congress   89-25357
                                                                 CIP

British Library Cataloguing in Publication Data
Ellis, Jack D.
The physician-legislators of France.
1. France. Medicine. Political aspects, history
I. Title
610'.944

ISBN 0-521-38208-4 hard covers

FOR MARGARET AND CLAIRE

CONTENTS

TABLES AND FIGURES

Tables

Figures

ACKNOWLEDGMENTS

This book would not have been possible without the support of numerous institutions. A grant from the Delaware Institute for Medical Education and Research allowed me to begin laying the groundwork for the study, and a subsequent fellowship from the American Council of Learned Societies provided the means for carrying out part of the work in Paris. I express my special thanks to the staffs of the Archives Nationales, the Bibliothèque Nationale, the Bibliothèque de l'Académie Nationale de Médecine (especially to Monique Chapuis, assistant librarian), and the Bibliothèque de la Faculté de Médecine de Paris. The director of the Service des Archives of the last, Catherine Moureaux, went out of her way to help me locate student records of the physician-legislators and was unfailingly cooperative and generous in giving me her time. The same was true for the late Maurice Daroussin, director of the Service des Archives of the National Assembly, and for his counterpart at the Senate, Gilbert l'Yavanc. I am also indebted to the staff of the College of Physicians of Philadelphia, where I was able to use the college's holdings in the nineteenth-century French medical press, and to the staff of the National Library of Medicine, particularly Dorothy Hanks of the History of Medicine division, who helped me obtain copies of medical theses written by the doctors in my group.

Most of all, I express my appreciation to the University of Delaware – to its Center for Advanced Study, where a fellowship for 1983–4 afforded me time to complete a first draft of the manuscript, and to its excellent library, which provided me with both space and resources for research and writing and whose staff assisted me in every way. Special thanks are owed to Joyce A. Storm, Nancy Froysland-Hoerl, Jon Penn, and Cheryl Thompson of the Reference Department. Leila Lyons and Ken Weiss of Academic

Computing Services helped me with the quantitative aspects of the study. Michael Patton, then a graduate student in history, rendered enormous services during the initial stages by helping me identify members of parliament before 1914 who held degrees in medicine. My colleagues in the Department of History were especially supportive in their willingness to share their own expertise and to help me clarify my ideas as the work unfolded. I mention especially the names of George Basalla, Willard A. Fletcher, Edward Lurie, and Stephen Lukashevich, the last of whom read an early draft of the manuscript and provided many helpful suggestions relating to both style and content.

Of the many other individuals who helped along the way, I should like to single out Erwin H. Ackerknecht, who encouraged me in my plans and provided copies of some of his own unpublished essays on the medicopolitician, and the late William Coleman, who likewise provided encouragement and support at the outset of the project. Throughout the research and writing, I have profited greatly from the advice of George Weisz of the Department of Humanities and Social Studies in Medicine at McGill University, who read a draft of the manuscript and provided me with invaluable criticisms and insight. I am grateful also to Charles Rosenberg, editor of the Cambridge History of Medicine series, for his advice and suggestions during the final stages of revision. Naturally, all errors of either fact or interpretation are entirely my own.

Last, I express my most heartfelt thanks to my wife, Diane Marie Ellis. From start to finish, I have benefited from her counsel, encouragement, and enthusiasm, not to mention her own considerable knowledge of modern literature and history. It is a pleasure to acknowledge her contributions, without which this book could not have been finished.

INTRODUCTION

During the 1889 campaign for parliament in the district of Morlaix, department of Finistère, a monarchist newspaper expressed bewilderment over the popularity of the republican candidate, Dr. Jean Clech, noting that his stuttering rendered him a clumsy orator who, in any case, had never exhibited any qualifications for the past of deputy: "In the old days it was said: Let each do his job and the cows will be well tended. The republicans have changed all that. Doctors of all kinds leave their patients and their clients, wishing to save agriculture." Voicing the same sentiments was a resident of Lanmeur, where Clech had been mayor for ten years:

> We people of the commune of Lanmeur have a lot to complain about; our doctor wants to leave us to go to Paris to the Chamber of Deputies. What would a doctor be able to do up there? If it is to treat the sick, it seems to me that in Paris there are celebrities of a renown superior to that of our modest country doctor (I take nothing away from the abilities of Mr. Clech – they are certainly sufficient for rural maladies which, lacking all the refinements of well-being and civilization in the capital, also lack all the vices and evils). But if, good Lord, it is to occupy himself with the country's affairs, I must say that our doctor is not quite up to handling what's required for that.

Noting that three other medical men in Finistère were also in the running, the writer remarked that if every department were in the same situation and if every physician-candidate were elected, there would be nearly four hundred doctors in the Chamber of Deputies: "Is France to be considered an insane asylum?" he asked.[1]

The elections in Finistère, in which Dr. Clech went on to win an easy first-ballot victory, were typical of local politics under the Third Republic, despite complaints that medical men had invaded all branches of public life and that parliament, as the saying went, had become "an assembly of assistant veterinarians." Between

1871 and 1914, a total of 358 physicians won election as deputies or senators. They were most prominent on the republican Left, denoting a common ideological tendency among physicians of that era that contrasts with the political conservatism of medicine in our own times. Second only to lawyers among the liberal professions in parliament, doctors exercised an influence over the political life of France that was out of proportion to their numbers in society.

For most practitioners, such a phenomenon was only natural. "The medicine of today," wrote one provincial doctor in 1897, "is the crossroads of all the sciences: Through hygiene, it touches on politics; through the latest physiological research, it borders on philosophy; through the pity it exhibits in regard to all human miseries, it becomes a religion."[2] The medical press had been hammering away at this theme since the birth of the Republic, reminding readers that the healing arts had long transcended individual therapy and that it was the doctor who directed local hygiene and welfare, ran the country's insane asylums, dominated its scientific societies, and implemented its social laws. Medicine, declared *L'Union médicale,* was the social science par excellence: "It is not our fault if this terrain borders on that of politics and sociology."[3]

Modern historians have come to recognize the importance of medicine as a political activity, one whose progress has rarely been dictated by events in the laboratory alone.[4] The France of the early Third Republic offers a useful framework for observing the interplay between medicine and politics and the reciprocating social forces that govern the development of each. Despite the horrors of battlefield surgery during the war with Prussia, the prestige of medicine grew steadily in the years after 1870. The ideas of Louis Pasteur and Joseph Lister vindicated themselves in the decline of hospital mortality rates and in the success of new animal and human vaccines. An understanding of the role of microorganisms in the transmission of cholera and typhoid fever spurred the building of modern sewer systems and the tapping of pure water sources. Here, and in other areas, new and comprehensive theories of public health threatened the rights of local governments, weakened old notions of individual liberty and property rights, and furthered the intervention of the state in economic life. At the same time, the social movement of the late nineteenth century sought to extend the benefits of progress to the very young and the very old, to the indigent sick, and to men and women who labored in unhealthy mines and factories. Welfare programs created new bureaucracies, which relied on the medical judgments of physicians and often on their administrative and political talents.

Although Molière's image of the physician as a quack and cynic died hard in France, the prestige of medical men was visible in many ways. At the local level, the doctor began to supplant the priest in status and influence, indicating a shift in social perceptions that had begun before 1870 and that was often mirrored in popular literature. Local politics reflected the trend. Doctors were present on almost every municipal council in the nation and served as mayors of hundreds of villages, towns, and cities, including Lyon, Marseille, Bordeaux, Limoges, Reims, Amiens, and Toulouse. They often headed the Municipal Council of Paris and as a group formed 8.6 percent of its membership between 1870 and 1914. The same patterns applied to the *conseils généraux,* or departmental legislatures. Indeed, by the 1890s, medical men made up between 12 and 14 percent of their membership, at a time when the total number of doctors stood at only 12,000. The second-class practitioners known as *officiers de santé* formed an additional 2,500. Remnants of the Napoleonic reorganization of medicine, they had been declining in number since mid-century and were much less active in politics than were regular medical doctors.

The prestige of doctors in national life is best measured by their presence in parliament. When judged by their numbers in the population, they tended to have higher rates of success than did men of law, at least if the latter are defined in a very broad sense. In 1891, for example, the total membership of all judicial professions in France stood at 40,695, which meant that the 174 jurists who sat in the legislature of that period represented just 0.42 percent of all jurists.[5] If one counts only the most characteristic parliamentary type – the *avocat*-deputy – in relation to the total number of *avocats,* the figure rises to 1.36 percent. Physicians were second, constituting 0.57 percent of all doctors of medicine. This outranked all other professions, including engineers and architects (0.15%) and primary and secondary schoolteachers (0.01%).

The distribution of parliamentary membership by occupation reflected these patterns. In 1871, lawyers (*avocats, avoués*), magistrates, and notaries accounted for 227 of all deputies, or about a

Table I.1. *Numbers and percentages of doctors in legislative assemblies*

Legislative assembly	Number of doctors	Percentage in assembly	Total number of doctors in France
1876–7	43	8.0	10,743
1877–81	60	11.4	
1881–5	65	12.0	11,643
1885–9	55	9.6	
1889–93	58	10.3	12,407
1893–8	71	12.5	
1898–1902	63	11.0	15,415
1902–6	65	11.3	
1906–10	65	11.3	18,211
1910–14	65	11.2	

third of the total. This proportion remained fairly constant in each of the ten legislatures of the post–1876 period and on occasions went even higher. Nearly 41 percent of the deputies in the Chamber of 1881–5 had degrees in law; for that of 1906–10, the figure stood at just over 37 percent. Jurists, as Yves-Henri Gaudemet has noted, held a "quasi monopoly" over the politics of the Third Republic.[6]

Doctors followed next among the liberal professions, usually constituting between 10 and 12 percent of each legislature. Their actual numbers and percentages break down as shown in Table I.1. The Senate, chosen by a limited suffrage, had a total of 125 doctors over the period as a whole, of whom 52 had served first in the lower house. Of these, the majority (59 percent) was elected for one nine-year term, 33 percent for two terms, and 8 percent for three terms. The proportion of physician-deputies that went on to win seats in the Senate (19.2 percent) was almost identical to that for all deputies.

In addition, thirteen physicians served as cabinet ministers. Three of them, all radicals, were of special importance in the history of the Third Republic: Paul Bert, who, before his death from cholera in 1886 helped ensure passage of lay educational laws; Emile Combes, who as prime minister helped bring about separation of church and state in 1905; and Georges Clemenceau, who had practiced medicine among the poor of Montmartre during his youth and served as prime minister between 1906 and 1909 and again during World War I. These are just the most famous of a type that Erwin H. Ackerknecht once described as the "medico-politician."[7] One could mention also Théophile Roussel, author of the law of 1874 on wet nursing; Victor Cornil, professor on the Paris medical faculty, who contributed to almost all laws on medicine and public health; François-Vincent Raspail, champion of social medicine and one of the founders of cellular pathology; Alfred Naquet, author of the divorce law of 1883; and D. M. Bourneville, editor of *Le Progrès médical,* who led the campaign to expel the nursing orders from the hospitals. Among the socialist leaders holding medical degrees were Edouard Vaillant, Paul Brousse, Paul Lafargue, Siméon Flaissières, and Victor Augagneur.

In addition, parliament contained thirty-six pharmacists, whose appearance in politics signified an extensive influence at the local level, and eleven doctors of veterinary medicine. Members of both groups were active in the fight against epizootic diseases and in the crusade for pure food and drink laws. A dozen or so other deputies and senators had backgrounds in physiology or chemistry, including Charles Chamberland, one of Pasteur's most famous collaborators, and Marcellin Berthelot, a pioneer in chemical studies on organic synthesis.

This visibility of doctors in the political assemblies of France had few counterparts in other societies. Although German medical men had been active in the revolutions of 1848 and in the nationalist movements that had preceded them, they had largely disappeared as a force in politics with the weakening of middle-class parties of the Left under Otto von Bismarck. In 1887, the Reichstag contained only 10 doctors and in 1902 only 6. Austria's parliament by that point had 15, that of Hungary, 5. In England, the House of Commons contained 11, most of them Irish. Canadian physician-legislators were a little more in evidence, the Senate having 9 and the House of Commons, 15. By contrast, the United States had only 2, both in the Senate. Despite the earlier prominence of a few, such as Benjamin Rush, the American medico-political tradition remained weak. Of 1,040 state governors holding office between 1870 and 1956, only 13 held degrees in medicine.[8]

Many more politically active doctors could be found in rural societies lying beyond the primary zones of economic modernization. In 1905, Italy's parliament contained thirty doctors, that of Spain twenty-two, and of Portugal, eleven. In Italy, as in Iberia, medical men tended to be associated with advanced political ideas. The same was true for Turkey and for Russia, where practitioners of "zemstvo medicine" helped foster hygienic improvements at the local level and by the turn of the century had emerged as a national force for social reform. Similar examples can be found in other countries, ranging from José Rigal of Manila, in the Philippines, executed for his resistance to the Spaniards, to Sun Yat-sen, in China. In Latin America, doctors had played a political role since the liberation movements of the early nineteenth century. Typical was the young surgeon Juan B. Justo, leader of the socialist party of Argentina, who translated *Das Kapital* into Spanish. The continuity of this leftist tradition is evidenced in modern times by the careers of Salvadore Allende (Chile) and even Che Guevara (Cuba).[9]

It was in France, however, that a medicopolitical tradition was manifested most strongly and most consistently. Its origin can be traced to the intellectual and demographic forces that had begun to transform French society during the late eighteenth century. A growing desire to prolong life promoted a greater awareness of corporal well-being and weakened old assumptions regarding the inevitability of sickness as part of the divine order. An emerging bourgeois sensibility concerning the tragedy of infant deaths reflected these trends, as did a new consciousness among the elderly who, as Philippe Ariès has noted, no longer accepted at the close of their productive lives the social death that preceded physiological death. Although improvements in diet and in the material conditions of life contributed more to the fall in death rates after 1760 than did medicine, doctors of that era were already asserting a competence that transcended old therapies.

As social hygienists, these doctors stressed that preventive medicine was the key to improving the happiness and well-being of humanity. The claims of *la médecine preservatrice* had enormous political implications, for in extending diagnosis from the bodily to the social organism, doctors sought to make all institutions the legitimate objects of medical inquiry and authority. Many insisted that health was a basic right of the citizen and that the state had an obligation to aid the sick and disinherited, a doctrine that the philosophers of that era termed *philanthropie* and that during the 1790s was subsumed under the revolutionary catchword of *frater-*

nité. Such ideas fit well into the doctors' professional aspirations, for they appeared to promise a medical role in the formulation of all policies that touched on the physical well-being of citizens. The doctor, as the hygienist Jean Noel Hallé wrote, was to become "the counsel and spiritual guide to the legislator."[10]

Educated and articulate, physicians took an active part in the local assemblies that in 1789 prepared the grievances of the Third Estate.[11] Afterwards, 22 medical men won election to the Estates-General, which increased to 28 in the Legislative Assembly and to 49 in the Constitutional Convention of 1793, the most radical legislature of the epoch. Altogether, a total of 123 medical men sat in the assemblies of the revolutionary and Napoleonic periods.[12] There were firebrands and terrorists among them, from Jean-Baptiste Bô of Aveyron to Jean-Paul Marat, the bloodthirsty editor of *L'Ami du peuple.* More typical, however, were the moderate, small-town doctors and surgeons coming from the rural center, west, and southwest, along with a few professors and medical reformers of the cities. Among the latter were Jacques Tenon, crusader for hospital reform, and Jean Gallot, long identified with the public health work of the Royal Society of Medicine. Even better remembered is Joseph-Ignace Guillotin, professor of anatomy on the Paris faculty, whose arguments on behalf of decapitation for capital crimes (by means of an instrument that he had not invented but that, to his dismay, soon bore his name) sprang from his desire to create a humane method of execution. An intelligent and hardworking man who had long campaigned for public health in Paris, Guillotin's main efforts while in office centered on issues of hygiene, assistance, and medical reform, as was true for most other physician-deputies.[13]

Between 1815 and 1848, the number of doctors in national political life declined. The Restoration Chamber had just fourteen, and the various legislatures of the July Monarchy had only thirty-eight, over half of whom belonged to the Left opposition. The reason for their absence was their inability to pay the requisite electoral tax. In 1827, the taxes paid by the average member of the Chamber of Deputies represented an annual income of twenty thousand francs a year, beyond the capacities of most physicians. The lowering of the tax requirements after the revolution of 1830 doubled the number of deputies from the professions, but doctors still found it hard to qualify. Their situation was more favorable within the departmental *conseils généraux*. By 1848, doctors constituted 6.7 percent of the membership of these assemblies, as compared with 27 percent for lawyers and notaries. Included were a number of wealthy practitioners, but the majority fell far below other members in their annual incomes. About 35 percent, for example, earned five thousand francs or less, whereas an additional 21 percent earned between five thousand and ten thousand francs.[14]

Although excluded from the legislatures of the pre-1848 period, doctors were involved in numerous other political activities. Membership lists of secret societies, for instance, show great numbers who participated in conspiratorial activities, ranging from Philippe Buchez, a founder of the French *carbonari,* to Pierre Caffe of Saumur, condemned to death in 1821. Doctors also appeared among the advocates of schemes to cure the ills of early industrial society. The plans of the utopian visionary Charles Fourier for model communities – the *phalanstères* – were especially attractive because of their emphasis on preventive medicine (each community was to have a physician, who would be paid in proportion to the health of its members). Jean Maitron's massive *Dictionnaire biographique du mouvement ouvrier français* includes seventy-two major entries for doctors on the Left between 1789 and 1864; of these, fifty-five called themselves republicans or socialists, terms that often meant the same thing.[15] It is true that one could find doctors in all political camps; yet the idea of *la République* held a strong attraction. It symbolized the career open to talents, universal suffrage, and the possibility of participation in public life. It also promised to spread the values of science and lay education and to wage war against the ignorance and religious credulity that nourished the power of illegal practitioners among the lower social orders. The latter formed the potential basis for medical power in French society but had long remained indifferent to hygiene and hostile to the claims of scientific medicine.[16]

The revolutions of 1848 saw physicians reappear among the political vanguard of the nation. Jules Guérin, editor of *La Gazette médicale de Paris,* argued that the doctor was obligated to become involved in public affairs, for only he understood the defects of social organization and the means by which to improve the physical and moral condition of the lower classes.[17] Physicians who ran for parliament that year repeated these themes in numerous ways, reminding voters that they had lived among the people and knew their grievances firsthand and that they themselves had suffered from class inequality.[18] The subsequent Constituent Assembly contained 52 doctors, the Legislative Assembly of the following year, 42. Ten of these fell victim to the repression following Louis Napoleon's coup d'état in December 1851. The degree to which physicians as a group were perceived as a threat to the new regime can be seen in the lists of those who were arrested or deported: Of 1,671 professional men, 325 were doctors, and 225 were lawyers.[19]

During the years that followed, doctors again faded as a force in national politics. Only twelve sat in the Corps législatif during the Second Empire and only four in the Senate. They did, however, remain active at the local level, accounting in 1870 for 7 percent of the departmental *conseils généraux*.[20] In the cities, the doctors' influence can be seen in their emergence as a political force soon after the outbreak of war with Prussia in 1870. They appeared in numerous branches of administration in Paris, for example, and several served with distinction as mayors of the twenty arrondissements. At first, most were radical republicans, but as the siege wore on these were eclipsed by more militant practitioners who identified with the revolutionary Left. The latter soon came to dominate the political life of the poorer quarters, and as the war came to an end, they appeared on numerous candidate lists for elections to the National Assembly in February 1871.[21] Throughout the country as a whole, thirty-three medical men won seats to the new legislature, the majority of them small-town practitioners.

Thus, by 1870 a tradition of medical involvement in politics had long existed in France and had manifested itself most strongly during those brief interludes when universal male suffrage had temporarily erased the barriers of wealth. It was the birth of the Third Republic, however, that allowed doctors to achieve a sustained influence at the local and national levels. During the years that followed, they scored enormous successes in expanding the range of their political activities, at the same time presenting to voters a similarity in outlook, goals, and behavior that would have no parallels in the post-1919 era. Most important, they exercised an unprecedented influence over the affairs of parliament and over most of the new social laws it passed. As Theodore Zeldin remarked in 1973, the rise to power of the French medical corps stands as one of the most striking features of modern political history.[22]

This book will try to answer the most important questions related to this phenomenon. Who were the doctors in parliament, and what is known about their reasons for entering politics? Had they studied medicine only as a general preparation for occupations elsewhere, or were they professional failures who chose politics as a substitute career? To what extent was their decision to enter public life prompted by the difficulties that they encountered in the practice of medicine, from low fees and professional over-crowding in the cities to the competition of the *curés,* nursing orders, and assorted charlatans who flourished with impunity in the countryside? Were they all atheists, materialists, and freemasons intent on spreading the dogmas of science among the peasants, as the Right charged? Having achieved political power, did they use it to promote any special ends as a corporate group, whether the cause of public health or the economic interests of the medical profession?

Especially important is knowing whether the doctors' political commitment was the natural and logical extension of their medical commitment and whether the interaction between their professional and social concerns produced a distinct medicopolitical behavior and ideology. Many doctors stressed that their medical work among peasants and workers had first stirred their social consciousness and had given to them special insights into the relationships between disease and social institutions. Others spoke of *la médecine sacerdoce* – the priesthood of medicine – and in their calls for political reforms that would improve the physical condition of the people, they echoed the 1848 dictum of the famous German pathologist Rudolf Virchow that "medicine is a social science, and politics nothing but medicine on a grand scale."[23]

The evidence presented here will show beyond doubt that medicine had a direct bearing on the decision of the physician-legislators to enter politics and that it played a large part in their tendency to identify with the republican Left. It will also show that far from being professional failures, the majority were successful practitioners whose political triumphs rested on their status as part of the local elites and on their medical work among the people. Like other members of the middle and lower-middle classes, most were attuned in their social vision to the country lawyers, notaries, civil servants, teachers, and small producers whom Léon Gambetta hailed in 1872 as the *couches nouvelles* of the Republic. Like them, many had found their paths blocked by the aristocracy of birth and wealth and viewed the Republic as best suited to their own aspirations. Nevertheless, each profession has its own perspective on politics, which has been shaped by the circumstances of its historical evolution and by its particular training, skills, and theoretical values. Each has distinctive forms of social experience and opportunity, and each seeks to advance its power and authority along different routes.[24]

My analysis thus stresses the political consciousness that accompanied medical recruitment, training, and practice in France. This consciousness evolved along many levels, starting with the social origins of doctors and with the quest for upward mobility among the lower-middle classes from which most of them came. It is visible also in the materialist dogmas that characterized teaching at the Paris faculty and in the kinds of values that students acquired during their hospital training among the poor. Young men studying law or engineering had rather different experiences, for it was not only their more privileged backgrounds that produced conservative political attitudes but also the nature of their training itself, which, as Christophe Charle has observed for the administrative elites, produced a similarity of views based on notions of social order, unity, and stability.[25] Similar points have been made by Thomas R. Osborne for graduates of the Ecole libre des sciences politiques and by Terry Shinn for those of the Ecole polytechnique, whose central values tended to be elitist, authoritarian, and conformist.[26]

Most critical of all were the problems that doctors faced in the practice of their craft, which the physician-deputy of Drôme, Antoine Chevandier, described in 1880 as "professional questions, connected to large public interests."[27] Although state control of medical education in France had brought a degree of unity and coherence to the profession that was lacking in other countries, doctors still worked in conditions of isolation, insecurity, and dependency, far from having attained what modern sociologists have deemed essential to true professionalization.[28] In certain regions, such as the south and the southwest, a fairly strong medical culture had grown up, but even here medical men were faced with persistent opposition, ranging from the clergy and folk healers to the nursing orders, which in turn constituted only one segment of what Jacques Léonard has described as a pervasive medical subculture dominated by women. Often allied with these in opposing the extension of scientific medicine, with all the secular values that this implied, were clerical and monarchist municipal governments, which harbored a special distrust for medical men because of their association with the masses. It is thus to local conditions and to the ways in which these affected the doctors' professional autonomy that we must look in searching out the immediate causes for their plunge into public affairs. Two points should be kept in mind.

First, the introduction of universal manhood suffrage after 1870 intensified the clash of local political factions, each of which used the powers of patronage to reward friends and to punish enemies. In matters that concerned doctors, the power of municipal governments over hospitals, public health, and welfare politicized some of the most vulnerable areas of their professional life, often leaving them defenseless against the whims of local bosses and administrators. Even those practitioners in rural communes whose popularity and landowning status gave them a degree of immunity were subject to pressures from rival groups and their electoral committees; the latter well understood the vote-getting power of the country doctor, who was often an agriculturalist of note and whose area of practice roughly corresponded to the single-member districts that prevailed in most elections of the period.

Second, far from viewing political activism as an abdication of their role, many physicians welcomed it as a means of furthering efforts to enhance medical power and authority. The campaign toward this end was being waged long before the birth of the Third Republic and had taken a variety of forms, as will be seen in our doctors' early careers. Like other groups during the initial and vulnerable stages of professional growth, French practitioners had developed numerous traits that were to serve them well in the age of mass suffrage, including a sense of mission, an exaltation of service, and a tendency to magnify their social contributions and the range of their nontechnical skills, all of which were necessary to overcome their own fragile resources as healers.[29] This equating of professional aspirations with the public good was important to doctors in all countries and appears to have given them an advantage over competing social forces.[30]

Because the careers of the physician-legislators cannot be understood apart from the ideological struggles of the post-1870 period, I have tried to integrate the political history of medicine in France with what might be called a medical history of its politics. Part I of the book examines the doctors' social and geographical origins, the types of professional training that they received, and the ways in which medical practice first thrust them into the local political limelight. Besides answering questions that are central to both medical and political history, I have tried to cast additional light on the evolution of socioprofessional elites. Modern research has elucidated a variety of types, ranging from businessmen and educators to prefects, diplomats, magistrates, state engineers, and other *fonctionnaires*.[31] Of special interest have been the political characteristics that define various groupings, a point of added importance in the case of France, where there existed a mutual dependency between the free professions and the state bureaucracy and where professional training lay in the hands of centralized educational institutions.[32] On the political elites themselves, there are several studies, including those by Thomas D. Beck and by Patrick-Bernard Higonnet, both dealing with the first half of the century, and, at the local level, by André-Jean Tudesq and by the team of Louis Girard, Antoine Proust, and R. Gossez.[33] The most extensive investigation of parliamentary membership under the Third Republic is that by the French scholar Mattei Dogan.[34] Besides Gaudemet's work on the jurists who held seats there, Jean Estèbe has provided a detailed analysis of the social backgrounds of all those who held cabinet positions between 1871 and 1914.[35]

At the outset of my work, my plan had been to focus on the origins and local careers of the physician-legislators and, where parliament was concerned, to limit myself to an analysis of their political affiliations and voting records. These goals were achieved, but in the process it became clear that more was required in order to complete the story. For one of the most conspicuous features of the doctors' rise to local prominence had been the successful pressing of their claims of superior knowledge in the realm of health and welfare, which they supported by reference to their scientific learning and their experiences among the people. Only by considering their parliamentary labors in detail, therefore, did it become possible to comprehend fully their particular social vision. As Chapter 3 shows, doctors who sat in parliament bore a striking resemblance to what modern political scientists have described as programmatic legislators – that is, those whose foray into public life emanates from a desire to modify their physical and social environments and who exhibit the pragmatism and sense of detail that are required for problem solving.

Part II of the book thus shifts the focus to parliament and to those specific issues of public policy that most captured the attention of doctors. It includes a look at their efforts to reform their own profession, a task that most regarded as an essential first step toward the realization of public health goals. Although a number of them proved helpful to the drive to secure professional ends, they did not and could not consider themselves to be the deputies and senators of the medical corps. What emerges from their labors, rather, is a preoccupation with problems that they regarded as being critical to the future of the nation. Of these, the majority touched on areas of their professional competence, ranging from infant mortality, cholera epidemics, and unsanitary housing to alcoholism, insane asylums, and rural medical assistance.

These and similar issues, I might add, dominated the agenda of the hygienic crusade throughout Europe as a whole. As Claire Salomon-Bayet has shown, they lay at the heart of efforts to shift the bacteriological revolution from a scientific to a political plane, and it was a process that involved medical men at every stage. In England, doctors served as the vanguard for sanitary reform, from the hundreds of state medical officers of health in the towns to the handful of physician-MPs who sat on the Parliamentary Bills Committee of the British Medical Association. The same was true in Germany, both in the poor-law medical services of the states and in the Reich Health Office, established in 1876. Examples abounded elsewhere, from Austria and Italy to Holland and Sweden. As Jeanne L. Brand has argued, the resistance of the organized profession to the extension of state authority in health and welfare during the twentieth century should not obscure the earlier contributions of doctors in this regard.[36]

As heirs to a rich legacy of hygienic activism that had flowered before 1850, the physician-legislators of the Third Republic were in a strong position to influence the fortunes of public health legislation. The final chapters will describe their achievements in this regard, along with their failures and the causes of their inability to move the country more speedily along the road to hygienic security, as was happening in England and Germany. As we shall see, that failure denoted not only the frailty of hygienic administration in France but also a larger unwillingness by the regime's leadership to address the nation's social needs.

Despite their visibility in French political life, the physician-legislators have never been the subject of a serious historical study. Indeed, until recent years little had been done on the social and political history of the French medical profession in general. The most exhaustive work to appear thus far is that of Jacques Léonard, whose monumental thesis on doctors in the western departments during the nineteenth century has explored the social role of medical practitioners and provided rich information on the political activities of the medical corps as a whole. A subsequent work, *La Médecine entre les savoirs et les pouvoirs,* published in 1981, incorporates further detail and interpretation of these themes.[37] I should also mention in this regard the work of George Weisz on the medical elites.[38] Others who have contributed to a better understanding of medical development in France are George D. Sussman, on professional overcrowding; William Coleman, on medical reformers of the industrial era; Matthew Ramsey, on illegal practice; Robert A. Nye, on the politics of insanity; and, for an earlier era, Toby Gelfand, on Paris surgeons during the late eighteenth century.[39] More recently, Martha L. Hildreth has offered a detailed look at the role of doctors in the move for professional reform and social assistance at the end of the nineteenth century.[40]

A collective biography of the kind I offer here posed many challenges, not the least of which was the initial identification of all doctors who held seats in parliament between 1871 and 1914. The first step was to search the two standard biographical dictionaries: that of Adolphe Robert and Gaston Cougny, dealing with the period to 1889, and that of the more reliable Jean Jolly, containing entries on all deputies and senators between 1889 and 1940. These were supplemented with contemporary publications on specific legislatures.[41] Thereafter, I tried to gain additional information from a variety of primary sources: from birth certificates in the archives of the National Assembly; student records in the archives of the Faculty of Medicine of Paris; campaign biographies contained in the *Professions de foi* of candidates in the Archives nationales; personnel files for those who held positions on the medical

faculties; obituaries in the medical press; and, for the most prominent figures, the *éloges* of the Academy of Medicine. This information, coded and transferred to data sheets, was run on SPSS
(Statistical Program for the Social Sciences). Although I did not
neglect the political activities of pharmacists and other health
professionals, my computer analysis centers on the 358 individuals
holding doctorates in medicine. Variables included numerous
pieces of information, from place and date of birth to father's
occupation; medical school attended; area, type, and duration of
practice; membership in medical and other societies; local political
activities; party labels; and so on. Unless otherwise noted, it is
this source on which my tables are based and on which much of
the biographical information is derived. For those who wish additional information or who seek to learn more about a particular
individual, specific citations in the footnotes and bibliography will
serve as a convenient starting place.

PART I

At the local level

1

The social formation of the physician–legislators

Physicians of the Third Republic sometimes claimed that medicine had endowed them with a neutral perspective on human affairs. As with other professional men, however, their beliefs reflected the values and assumptions of their own milieu and social class, and nowhere was this more evident than among those who succeeded in politics. The voice of rural and bourgeois France echoed in most of their pronouncements on public policy; it was often loudest on issues in which ideology and medical opinion intersected, from marriage and the family to deviance, abortion, and the place of women. Our first task, then, is to examine those forces that shaped the attitudes of the physician–legislators. In this chapter, we will focus on their social backgrounds and medical training.

REGIONAL AND FAMILY ORIGINS

Above all, the successful doctor in politics was a man of the soil. Breton or Provençal, Savoyard or Lorrainer, each took pride in his *pays natal,* frequently exemplifying the personality traits with which it was associated in the popular mind. Over 96 percent of these physician–legislators had spent their formative years in the department of their birth, and it was usually the same department, often the same arrondissement, in which they established their practices and ran for political office. Table 1.1 illustrates the regional distribution of these areas.[1]

Although France was still an agricultural society when most of the doctors came of age (the median year of birth was 1843), the departments of origin were typically those having strong rural majorities. Many were located in the most backward zones of the country when judged according to literacy rates, population

Table 1.1. *Region of physician-legislators' birth*

Region of birth	%
North	6.1
East	13.1
Paris region and the Center	13.7
West	12.8
Southwest	15.9
Massif Central	14.0
Lyon region, Savoy, and Dauphiné	11.7
Mediterranean region	10.3
Overseas colonies	2.0

growth, and economic modernization. Only 3.4 percent were natives of Paris, for example, and most of these belonged to families whose roots and property holdings lay in the provinces. The single agrarian department of Yonne claimed a comparable share, as did several others of rural Bourgogne and the center plains. Here one found few cities or regional markets, and the rates of population growth, farm income, and illiteracy fell below the national average.[2] The same was true for the Massif Central, one of the poorest places in France. Over 10 percent of the doctors came from a single grouping of five departments in this region, one of which, Haute-Vienne, was tied with the Seine and Yonne for second place. In first place, as the home of 3.6 percent, was Dordogne, 90 percent rural during the 1840s and, like other parts of Aquitaine and the southwest, marked by small plots, sharecropping, and tenant farming.

Similar trends prevailed elsewhere. The Lyon region, hub of a thriving manufacturing life under the July Monarchy, was the birthplace of only a few physician–legislators. The picture shifts as one moves to the more remote agricultural departments of the east and southeast – to Ain in lower Bourgogne, to Jura, Haute-Saône, and Doubs in Franche-Comté, to Isère and Drôme in ancient Dauphiné, to the Alps and Savoy. Just over 12 percent originated in these regions, whose forests and snowy mountain hamlets masked a brutal poverty. In the east, the more populated departments of Alsace and Lorraine produced less than half that proportion. The same was true for the northern industrial districts,

Table 1.2. *Populations of physician-legislators' locale of origin*

Locale of origin	%
Rural communes, villages, and towns under 2,000	41.8
Towns, 2,000–6,000	23.2
Towns, 6,000–20,000	13.3
Cities, 20,00–50,000	7.4
Cities, 50,000–100,000	3.4
Cities over 100,000	7.1
Urban communes, over 2,000	3.7

including the Somme, Nord, and Pas-de-Calais; in any case, most of the northerners in our group hailed from the small farming towns. Lille was the birthplace of only three, Amiens of two.

Clearly, the physician-legislators of the Third Republic were not the products of the cities that had traditionally attracted medical men. Only 20 percent were born in cities that served as the *chefs-lieux* of their home departments, and 14 percent in those that served as the *chefs-lieux* of arrondissements. Around 30 percent, on the other hand, grew up in the small market towns that functioned as the *chefs-lieux* of cantons and 35 percent in towns or villages that had no administrative status of any kind. Table 1.2 shows the distribution of home-town populations.

What is the explanation for these patterns? Although only a minority of our doctors originated in the cities, there existed for certain parts of the country a rough parallel between the place of origin and the regional distribution of all physicians. In 1847, France had an estimated 11,177 doctors and 7,532 health officers in a population of just over 35 million. On average, that amounted to 1 practitioner per 1,898 people or, if doctors alone are counted, 1 per 3,184. But the figures are misleading. Bas-Languedoc in the south had 1 doctor per 1,885 inhabitants, whereas Brittany in the west had only 1 per 5,736. The industrial north, Lorraine and parts of Alsace, the bulk of the Massif Central, and scattered pockets in the Rhône plains and the Alps were also poor in doctors. Aside from Paris, which claimed 13 percent of all physicians,[3] the most favored regions were found in the south and southwest – especially Languedoc, Provence, Gironde, and Aquitaine, where doctors had long been active in civic life and where an abundance of medical families and schools testified to the presence of a strong medical culture.[4]

Of related importance, in the Midi and in other regions sharing its social characteristics, were the aspirations of rural property owners and small-town bourgeoisie. These people saw the liberal professions as a way to advance their sons and to enhance their prospects for a good marriage. Poor families had no such possibilities for upward mobility, as they could not afford even the cost of the requisite secondary education. Working-class boys who wanted to enter medicine usually pursued the less-expensive degree of health officer, which explains the dominance of the second-class practitioner in the northern industrial districts.[5] The young men belonging to the commercial and industrial classes tended to follow the business careers of their fathers or, if they wished to enter a profession, to study law, which was more prestigious than medicine and which formed the traditional gateway to positions in government.[6]

Such patterns were still in evidence at the birth of the Third Republic and could be seen in the regional concentrations of medical students as well as doctors. Comparing these with the birth-places of our doctors reveals similar proportions for the north, east, southwest, Mediterranean, and (if Paris is removed from consideration) the Center. Exceptions include the Massif Central and parts of Savoy, Dauphiné, and the Alps, which, though weak in their ratios of doctors to population, were rich in physician-legislators. In such exceptionally backward areas – even when their total numbers in society were relatively small – physicians were still able to achieve ascendancy by their leadership in agriculture and their role as the local representatives of science and culture, points that will be developed in later chapters.[7]

What is known about the fathers of our doctors? Although some were men of modest wealth and influence, the majority were the products of the villages and market towns, many of them country practitioners or small-scale artisans and shopkeepers. Table 1.3 is based on 292 known cases.[8]

Birth certificates formed the main sources for determining these groupings. Naturally, the occupational designations found there provide only a clue to the father's true wealth and status, which varied within each profession. In addition, many individuals had

Table 1.3. *Distribution of occupations among physician-legislators' fathers*

Occupation[a]	%
Commercial and industrial bourgeoisie	2.7
Professionals	39.0
High	
Doctors of medicine (19.2)	
Notaries, lawyers (6.8)	
Army officers (1.7)	
Low	
Pharmacists (2.7)	
Primary school teachers (2.4)	
Health officers (1.8)	
Protestant pastors (1.4)	
Military surgeons (1.0)	
Principals of *collèges* (1.0)	
Others (1.0)	
Petite bourgeoisie	30.5
Shopkeepers, merchants (11.3)	
Artisans (10.3)	
Clerical employees (4.8)	
Low civil service (3.1)	
Police (1.0)	
Landowners (*propriétaires*)	18.1
Peasant farmers	5.5
Industrial workers	1.7
Others (unskilled rural, orphan, illegitimate)	2.4

[a]Numbers in parentheses are percentages.

more than one occupational identity, especially if they were land-owners. One thus finds such terms as *médecin et propriétaire* or *propriétaire-commis au forge*. The term *propriétaire* itself illustrates the imprecision of all such terms; no doubt, it meant an owner of land, but this may have ranged from a few acres to a large estate.[9]

The professions constituted the largest single category within our group, of which doctors were the most numerous. If health officers, military surgeons, and pharmacists are added, the proportion for medical men rises to a fourth of the known cases. Their number illustrates the importance of family tradition in the son's choice of occupation. For example, on leaving the *lycée* at Nantes

in 1858, Clemenceau decided to study medicine, as he recalled
later, "without hesitation. My father had been a doctor, my grandfather, my great-grandfather."[10] Only one among the sons of doctors is known to have followed another career; that was François
Fesq, later deputy for Cantal, who studied literature at the Ecole
normale supérieure but then switched to medicine and ended up
practicing at Aurillac, just as his father had done. The exception
points up another characteristic: when the son's choice of a profession differed from that of his father's it was at least equal if not
superior to it in prestige. Thus, the sons of medical doctors rarely
became veterinarians or health officers, though the sons of the
latter often aspired to become doctors. This explains the low number of lawyers among the fathers of the physician-legislators, for
as already noted, law had a higher social ranking than did medicine.

The fathers who belonged to the medical professions included
many obscure country doctors, but this was by no means true of
them all. Great numbers had managed to carve out places for
themselves among the local elites. The father of Victor Cornil,
one of the most distinguished physician-legislators of the Third
Republic, held the post of hospital doctor at Cusset in Allier, where
he was also mayor and inspector of thermal establishments. The
father of Antoine Blatin, deputy for Puy-de-Dôme, was a property
owner at Clérmont-Ferrand and member of a medical family that
had provided the city with five of its mayors since the fifteenth
century. Medical dynasties of this kind were fairly common.[11] In
fact, some of the fathers presided over powerful medicopolitical
families that had already produced mayors, municipal councillors,
conseillers généraux, and members of parliament. An example is the
Calès family at Villefranche, which had been providing representatives to political assemblies since the French Revolution.

One finds other notables outside the medical profession. In law,
there was Félix Liouville, whose son taught on the Paris medical
faculty and served as deputy for Meuse under the Third Republic.
Although their roots lay in Lorraine, the Liouvilles were an established family in the capital, where the father had served as
president of the Paris bar. In the provinces, prominent legal families included that of Emile Goy, senator for Haute-Savoie, whose
great-grandfather had sat in the Constituent Assembly in 1792,
and of Lucien Penières, deputy for Corrèze, whose grandfather
had sat in the Convention. Among other professional men was a

sprinkling of army officers, primary school teachers, principals of *collèges communaux,* and at least one "man of letters." One also finds an occasional Protestant pastor, including the father of Siméon Flaissières, the first socialist mayor of Marseille, and the father of the Pozzi brothers – Adrien and Samuel – the first a professor of clinical surgery at Reims and the second a leading gynecological surgeon of the pre-1914 era.

Less well known are the fathers grouped under the heading of petite bourgeoisie, most of whom lived in small towns. For merchants and shopkeepers, the terms that appear most frequently on the birth certificates are those of *marchand* and *commerçant,* though sometimes there is also a reference to specific products, such as spices or candles. An additional group (around 4% of the total) used the term *négociant;* although this generally implied greater wealth than did either of the other two terms, most of those in our group were modest men of affairs. The artisans included an assortment of occupations, from butchers and bakers to blacksmiths, printers, tailors, carpenters, tanners, and harness makers. Although some probably owned their own establishments and could thus be considered shopkeepers, one finds in this grouping the most striking examples of poverty, as in the case of the future prime minister Emile Combes.[12] Rounding out the petit-bourgeois category were clerks, salaried workers, bookkeepers, and commercial employees. The rest were local tax collectors, customs officials, and policemen.

The last category was that of the landed occupations. If landowners and small peasant farmers are combined, their proportion rises to almost 24 percent of the total. The terms used on the birth certificates were those of *propriétaire* (17%), *cultivateur* (3%), *rentier* (1%), and *fermier* or a combination of this with one of the other terms (2%). Some of these people are known to have owned sizable estates, but this does not appear to have been true for the majority. Although they were by no means impoverished, most were farmers of only modest agricultural wealth who worked their own land. They showed their heaviest concentration in the rural communes of the Center and southwest.

We can draw several conclusions from this survey of social origins. The first is the similarity between the backgrounds of our doctors and those of the medical profession as a whole. In 1865, only 22 percent of the fathers of students who were enrolled in the medical faculties lived off property or capital. Wealthy merchants, industrialists, and high-level civil servants made up an even smaller proportion, very close to those seen in Table 1.3. By contrast, around 21 percent were themselves medical men. Shopkeepers, artisans, employees, and primary school teachers accounted for 32 percent, and agrarian workers an additional 11 percent.[13] Just as striking is the modesty of these backgrounds in relation to those of other socioprofessional elites. Thirty-five percent of the fathers of law students, for examples, lived off property or capital, whereas only 20 percent were identified with the lower-middle class. The tendency was even more pronounced among engineers. At the Ecole polytechnique, 32 percent of the students' fathers lived off property or capital, and an additional 38 percent belonged to the business and administrative elites. The popular classes constituted a mere 13 percent, a pattern that Christophe Charle has shown to have been true for the upper ranks of the bureaucracy in general.[14]

Finally, although the families of many future physician-legislators formed part of the local elites, as a group they had a less privileged status than did those of other political elites of the Third Republic. Estèbe's analysis of the backgrounds of cabinet ministers between 1871 and 1914, for example, shows that 35 percent came from the ranks of large-scale property owners, *rentiers,* industrialists, and upper-level bureaucrats, along with an additional 38 percent from the liberal professions, primarily law.[15] Even the overall social composition of the Chamber, when compared with that of its medical members, showed a much smaller petit-bourgeois representation, despite the steady growth of this element under the early Republic. In this regard, physicians showed few changes over time, in that the proportion of those who sprang from the popular classes remained at roughly the same high levels from one legislature to another. As for how these backgrounds affected their political thinking, a cross tabulation of father's occupation by ideology shows such a similarity of distributions as to confirm the essential sameness of their backgrounds. Put another way, sons of country doctors or small-town notaries had about the same leftist propensities as did the sons of clerks, tradesmen, artisans, and even rural *propriétaires.*

We have so far stressed only the role of the father. But in some instances, a medical tradition emanated from the mother's side of the family, as in the case of Charles Robin of Ain. Among many artisan and shopkeeping families, women worked alongside their husbands or, like the mother of Gustave Chopinet of Seine-et-Marne, who was a seamstress, practiced their own occupations. At times, one perceives what must have been a powerful influence exerted by those who had to struggle in order to advance their sons. For instance, the mother of the famous surgeon and senator Léon Labbé became the guiding force in the boy's education after the death of her husband, a notary's clerk in rural Orne. At the *lycée* of Caen, young Labbé decided on a military career, but his mother forced him to drop his plans and to enroll in the preparatory school of medicine there. His was not the only example. Several of the medical theses written by our doctors acknowledge the mother's sacrifices in this regard.

The question of money was a serious matter, for in many families the decision to support a son through medical school affected everyone. "I could name families who wore themselves out and often ended up in ruin in order to allow their sons to study for the doctorate," Xavier Blanc, senator of Hautes-Alpes, told his colleagues in 1892. He added that even those pursuing the degree of health officer often used up their own patrimony and that of their brothers and sisters.[16] In the 1830s, a family spent at least twelve thousand francs for the doctorate, six times what the training of a health officer required. Paul Bert put the total at fifteen thousand francs in the 1870s, and Charles Richet, a professor on the Paris faculty, estimated it at almost twice that amount in 1908.[17] One gains a better appreciation of these costs in realizing that the salaries of industrial workers during the last decade of the Second Empire ran between nine hundred and twelve hundred francs a year, comparable to what many modest provincial bakers, printers, masons, and tailors earned.

The sacrifices began with secondary schooling. Our doctors, like others in the liberal professions, attended the state *lycées* or municipal *collèges*. The classical program dominated in both types and prepared one for the prized *baccalauréat ès-lettres,* which was the ticket for admission into a faculty and into most positions of social leadership. During the 1860s, annual costs for boarding and tuition averaged 739 francs for the former and 649 francs for the latter.[18] Fees were cheaper for day students, especially in the municipal schools, but many rural communities had neither a *lycée* nor a *collège*. What most characterized life in these institutions was strict discipline and rigorous drills in rhetoric, philosophy, mathematics, ancient history, and Latin. Little in the curriculum prepared students for medical study, particularly in the experimental sciences.

Among those physician–legislators for whom the secondary schools are known, *lycées* accounted for around 66 percent, *collèges* for 20 percent, and private schools for 14 percent. The average age on completing the *baccalauréat ès-lettres* was 18.4 years, which was typical for medical students, as was the percentage of *lycée* graduates among them.[19] Only a handful attended the elite secondary schools of Paris, and those who did so belonged to families that maintained a residence there. About half our samples, on the other hand, studied at big-city provincial schools, including a dozen or so who attended the *grands lycées* located in the seats of the academies at Bordeaux, Clérmont-Ferrand, Grenoble, and Marseilles. Most were boarders, the sons of landowners and professionals who could afford the fees. Aside from a handful who attended private schools and Catholic *petits séminaires*, the rest studied in small-town *lycées* and *collèges*.

Besides family pressures, the forces that steered young men toward medicine at this point in their lives was the subject of much speculation. In 1880, Edouard Charton's *Dictionnaire des professions,* one of the best-known career guides of the period, described the motives of medical students in this way: "Family convenience, unforeseen circumstances, the constantly increasing overcrowding of other careers, have propelled them along this path, and it is by exclusion, especially, and without the least enthusiasm, that the majority are inscribed on the registers of the faculty."[20] *Le Concours médical* was saying the same thing as late as 1900, arguing that medicine, along with the notarial profession, was the only one that allowed a country boy to return to the home of his parents, where he could live cheaply until he found a woman with a dowry and where, unlike the notary or the lawyer, he did not always have to purchase a clientele.[21] Still, the obstacles could be formidable: prolonged expense, fatigue, exposure to typhoid or diphtheria in the teaching wards, the *piqûre anatomique* during dissections. Idealism cannot be excluded altogether; many young men shared the excitement surrounding the sciences and believed that the doctor was destined to be a leader in the reform of society.

That was true for many in our group as well, among whom one can detect a variety of career goals.

Around 14 percent, for example, appear to have pursued medicine as a part of broader interests that did not involve plans to practice. The length and difficulties of study, however, made medicine less appealing than law for those who wished simply to continue their general education. In fact, several physician-legislators began their careers as law students, and a few even earned the licentiate in law before turning to medicine.[22] Next came those for whom medical study served as an adjunct to their scientific interests. Adolphe Wurtz, later dean of the Paris medical faculty, was performing chemistry experiments at home at age seventeen, much to the dismay of his father, who wanted him to follow in his own footsteps as a Lutheran pastor. Instead, young Wurtz enrolled in the medical faculty of Strasbourg. One of his later students in Paris, Alfred Naquet, got his licentiate in physical science in 1857 and his doctorate in medicine three years later. Until his political activities got him into trouble, Naquet taught organic chemistry on the Paris faculty, where, according to a note in his dossier from Dean Wurtz, he displayed "a great ardor and rare aptitude for science."[23] Naquet's contemporary, Paul Bert, first earned his licentiate in law, then followed it with one in the natural sciences, and only later got a degree in medicine. Finally, just under 3 percent of our group held degrees in both medicine and pharmacy.

For others, medicine formed part of their general interest in agriculture. Though often forgotten today, the natural links between the two were of special importance in an agrarian society. Albert Viger, three-time minister of agriculture, credited his own expertise to medicine, which had equipped him to deal with problems in livestock breeding, animal nutrition and disease, artificial fertilizers, and the application of organic chemistry to such farm industries as brewing, sugar refining, and distilling.[24] Beyond these advantages, many rural property owners regarded a career in medicine as offering their sons prestige and the possibility of enhancing family estates through favorable marriages. About 7 percent in our group were to gain reputations as *médecins-agriculteurs,* but a far greater number were involved in the life of the soil. Many were the sons of *propriétaires* and well-to-do professional men, the latter including several doctors who practiced medicine only rarely. One thinks of such landed families as those of Mathurin Legal-Lasalle in Côtes-du-Nord or Paulin Cannac in Aveyron.

Lastly, several individuals entered medicine for their own private reasons, including a few who had disastrous starts in other fields. Eugène Turgis, a stonecutter's son from Calvados, had been a schoolteacher in Caen before his republican opinions got him into trouble with local Bonapartist officials. Emile Javal, a graduate of the Ecole des mines, and, like his father, destined for a career in business, turned to medicine in an effort to find a cure for strabismus, which afflicted his sister. Emile Combes, though intending to follow an ecclesiastical career, decided to abandon it because he fell in love with the daughter of an influential family at Pons, where he was teaching. The marriage contract stipulated that the couple was to live near the bride's parents, and as Combes has recorded in his memoirs, medicine provided him with the independence and income he needed.[25]

MEDICAL STUDY IN THE PROVINCES AND IN PARIS

Just as the motives for entering medicine varied among the doctors, so did the methods of attaining their goal. For sons of the poorest parents, military service provided the most accessible route. At one time, the army had freely recruited its doctors and trained them in military hospitals, but the flaws of this system – best illustrated by the disasters of the Crimean War – led to the creation of the School of Military Health Service in Strasbourg. Young men who had completed part of their medical study in a preparatory school or faculty could be admitted here by competitive examination, though the training was done at the civilian faculty of Strasbourg. Upon earning their degrees, they spent ten months at the teaching hospital of Val-de-Grâce in Paris, after which they were obliged to serve at least ten years in the military. About 4 percent of our group chose this route, of which the majority originated from the eastern departments (the traditional recruiting ground for army doctors) and studied at Strasbourg. An additional 2.5 percent, mostly from coastal departments, entered the navy, which had medical schools at Rochefort, Toulon, and Brest. After two years of training, students usually served in the colonies or on board warships, in many cases earning their degrees at a regular

Table 1.4. *Medical faculty from which physician-legislators received degrees*

Faculty	%
Paris	79.8
Montpellier	11.3
Strasbourg	3.5
Nancy	0.6
Bordeaux	0.6
Lille	1.2
Lyon	2.3
Toulouse	0.3
Foreign schools	0.6

faculty only after years of service. In both groups, the typical student had a petit-bourgeois origin.

Most aspiring doctors chose more conventional paths. They could enroll in a faculty, or they could begin their work in one of twenty-two preparatory schools of medicine and pharmacy. These were closer to home, which relieved parents of both the expense of Paris and the worry over the temptations it offered. Although many preparatory schools were little more than teaching branches of municipal hospitals, all granted degrees for the title of health officer, herbalist, second-class pharmacist, and midwife.[26] Candidates for the doctorate were allowed to take up to two years of work there (extended to three after 1878) before completing their work at a faculty. Among 207 cases for whom the information is known, about 35 percent began their studies in a preparatory school. Usually, this was the one nearest their home departments, with those at Lyon, Clérmont-Ferrand, Bordeaux, and Toulouse attracting the largest numbers.

Most, however went directly to a faculty, usually Paris. Table 1.4 shows their distribution. Although Strasbourg served the needs of army doctors, a few others in our group had earned degrees there as well. As for Montpellier, its days of glory had long passed, and by the birth of the Third Republic, Paris was attracting nearly ten times the number of students. The dean at Montpellier, Etienne Bouisson, himself a deputy during the 1870s, complained that this was so only because Paris was a center of amusement and pleasure. In fact, Montpellier's problems went much deeper, among the worst of which was the faculty's absorption in doctrinal quarrels, which gave the school a reputation for producing the "intellectual doctor" rather than the solid practitioner. Such quarrels centered on philosophical vitalism, an elusive notion that saw the physical organism as containing a vital life force, separate from body or soul and transcending physiochemical laws.[27]

Almost all physician-legislators who took their degrees at Montpellier were southerners. Otherwise, their backgrounds varied little from those attending other faculties. Differences emerge only at the level of training, for despite the sameness of the curriculum, students at Montpellier suffered several disadvantages. The professors there were not as prominent as those in Paris. Nor was the school strong in the experimental sciences. The city itself offered only modest hospital resources, inferior even to those of the preparatory schools at Lyon and Bordeaux. For many of those who earned Montpellier degrees, the most significant clinical experiences had come in the hospitals of other cities during their study at preparatory schools.[28]

Three-fourths of the Montpellier graduates went into active practice. The degree to which the school's philosophical outlook actually influenced them is difficult to gauge. Occasionally, their medical theses mirror vitalist ideas, and some contain religious sentiments that appear less frequently in those of the Paris school. But one must be cautious. The Montpellier graduates did include a slightly lower percentage of political radicals than did the Paris graduates, but with the exception of Bouisson, one finds few instances in their later speeches and writings in which vitalist assumptions seem to have had much importance, certainly not in rendering their political outlook more conservative. In fact, several of the best-known doctors on the socialist Left were products of Montpellier, including Flaissières, François Isoard, Ernest Ferroul, and Paul Brousse.

Whatever its flaws, study in the provinces provided the possibility of close bonds between teachers and students, which was far from being the case in Paris. "Those among you who are doctors cannot recall without a certain terror that first year of medicine we made some thirty years ago," Antoine Gadaud of Dordogne remarked to the Senate in 1894, "We arrived from the provinces without guide, without counsel; we went and signed up for our courses, and that was that. We had absolutely no relationship with our professors, whom we did not know."[29] His reaction was common. In order to register for the first of sixteen course *inscriptions,* the student had only to appear before the secretary of the faculty with a diploma in letters, a birth certificate, and a good-conduct statement signed by the local mayor. In return, the student was given a list of courses and told to consult the catalogue for the names of the professors teaching them.

What followed proved to be a disappointment. In Paris, professors spent most of their time in research and private practice or in attending to their duties within the hospital hierarchy. They were, as Bert once said, "unknown to their students, except for a few among the elite whom they admit like royalty to their private circle for personal reasons."[30] The most useful courses, particularly those featuring pathological and anatomical exhibits, were so crowded that only a few could profit from them. Others were largely theoretical, the professors taking care to cultivate their eloquence and oratorical skills. The absence of practical instruction made first-year studies in chemistry, physics, and natural history a frustrating experience, and students often stopped coming to class after the first few weeks. As Gadaud recalled: "Nothing in us was drawn to these courses because we found them cold and because we had heard the same kinds of things in the *lycées* without being any better educated for all that. . . . A profound boredom set in among the young students, this *taedium discendi* that we know and that very few escaped."[31]

After the first-year courses in the basic sciences, the second and third years were to be spent in anatomy, histology, physiology, dissections, internal and external pathology, and clinical medicine and surgery. *Fin d'année* examinations concluded each of the first three years. Then came more work in pathology, surgical medicine, therapeutics, obstetrics, pharmacology, materia medica, hygiene, and forensic medicine. The final requirements included five doctoral examinations, on all the material covered since the first year, and a thesis. This was the curriculum that applied to about 80 percent of the doctors in parliament. It lasted until 1878, at which time the *fin d'année* examinations were abolished and the five examinations were distributed over the whole period of study.

In theory, one could finish the program in four years, but most students needed at least seven.[32] For the physician-legislators, the average age on completing the degree was 26.3 years. In those cases for which the dates of both the degree in letters and that in medicine are known, the average number of years that elapsed was 7.9. Only 2.5 percent of the students graduated within 4 years and just 4.7 percent in 5 years. Another 4.7 percent did not finish until their early thirties, having been in medical school for 10 years or more.

The uselessness of the lectures drove many students to futile efforts at self-instruction using study guides and handbooks, but the best realized that their only hope lay in the hospitals. Here, in fact, was the foundation of French medical education, symbolized by the system of bedside instruction that had once attracted students from all over the world. In 1870, Paris had twenty-six hospitals and hospices: Besides the nursing orders, their personnel included physicians and surgeons, demonstrators in anatomy known as *prosecteurs,* externs and interns in medicine and surgery, pharmacists, and pharmacy interns. All students had to undergo a period of hospital training, an obligation known as the *stage* that had been expanded in 1862 from one to two years. It began during the third year, but conflicts between the faculty, which fell under the Ministry of Public Education, and the hospitals, which were owned and administered by the city, meant that the *stage* was often a waste of time. Added to this was the excessive numbers of students who packed the wards, only to receive the most perfunctory instruction. Naquet described the experience in this way: "It consists in following a doctor who, at each bed, prescribes a potion or pills, without saying why, often without even pronouncing the name of the disease."[33]

The best students chose to follow the *concours* for hospital positions, a competitive examination that placed a premium on memory and rhetoric. It helped to have the patronage of a faculty member, for although hospital posts fell under the jurisdiction of municipal authorities, the professors formed part of the examination boards and were not loath to indulge their rivalries at the expense of the students. The initial test was for externships, which brought no pay but which one had to pass in order to become an intern. Interns received room and board at the hospitals and were paid a salary of up to seven hundred francs in the third year. They were able to work with a professor in a particular field and were on call during his absence. The advantages were immense, whether one wished to go into private practice or to pursue the *concours* up to a teaching post. Only a few dozen were chosen each year, however, and the competition was tough.

In all, 30 percent of the Paris students in our group served as externs and 16 percent as interns. As one would expect, the latter were the ones who scored highest on examinations and who won prizes and medals for their work. They included a strong concentration of individuals destined for careers in surgery, several of them exceptionally talented and ambitious men who would marry wealth and whose professional fame would open many political doors. As students, their status can be seen in the bonds they were able to forge with particular professors of distinction. Among the latter was Léon Gosselin, surgeon at the Hôpital Beaujon (in those cases for which the thesis director of our doctors in known, he ranked first); Paul Broca, renowned for his studies of the brain; and Aristide Verneuil, who took over the chair of clinical surgery in 1868. Like Broca, Verneuil was part of a tiny coterie on the faculty that fought to introduce the microscope into medical studies. His followers included numerous gifted students who would later have parliamentary careers, most notably Théophile Reymond, Gabriel Maunoury, Samuel Pozzi, Léon Labbé, and Victor Cornil. Among other professors, one should mention the neurologist Jean Martin Charcot, who had an enthusiastic following at the hospice of Salpêtrière during the 1860s. Several interns in our group based their theses on his ideas, of whom the most brilliant was D. M. Bourneville, renowned in later years for his work on mental illness. He once recalled that Charcot's bearing had been marked by "a severity, often in the extreme," but that the young were intensely loyal to him, even when the master's "mania for the thermometer" (still not in general use) made them the object of jokes among other interns.[34]

The best students used every opportunity to advance their education abroad. Young Cornil went to Berlin to work on cellular pathology with the great Virchow, whom he always regarded as his finest teacher. Henry Liouville set off in 1864 to study clinical laboratories in Germany, at the same time visiting Danish and Austro-Prussian ambulance services involved in the war that year in Schleswig. Although few members of the faculty shared their enthusiasm, other students were fascinated by Lister's application of Pasteurian ideas to surgery. Maunoury, for instance, studied with Lister at Edinburgh and followed this up with observations

in German and Austrian hospitals. Returning to Chartres, he transformed the operating rooms of the Hôtel-Dieu into "a veritable
temple to the new doctrines" and became one of the first to spread
the doctrine of antisepsis to the provinces. Pozzi made similar
travels, as did Ambroise Monprofit, who later applied Listerian
principles to his surgical services at Angers.[35]

Why the very brightest should seek to hone their skills beyond
the frontiers is not hard to understand. Cornil, who later pictured
the Paris faculty as having "dozed a little" in sleeping off its former
glory, found it strange at the time that some of his teachers should
urge him to seek models in the old authors. Then there was the
reaction of his examining committee to his own research:

> When I passed my doctoral thesis in 1864 on the histology of nephritis
> [i.e., Bright's disease], one of my judges, very kindly in other respects,
> said to me, "You have written an infinitely meritorious work, sir, but
> what the devil good does it serve? Have you found under your micro-
> scope the means of curing albuminuria?"
>
> It was only too easy to respond that it was necessary to know the
> structure of the kidney in order to understand what happens when it is
> inflamed. That is the basis of our knowledge on this point. One certainly
> does not cure a victim of nephritis by examining urinary sediments under
> a microscope, but one makes a more correct diagnosis that helps in
> finding a medication. Another of my judges, a professor much loved by
> us all, argued with me in this way: "Sir, you speak in your essay of the
> multiplication, the proliferation, of cells. Have you ever seen any? For
> my part, I've tried many times without any result." He gave me the
> method he had used in order to do so; it was so hilarious that it was
> impossible to answer without making fun of him. The excellent man
> triumphed by my silence.[36]

For less-motivated students, the necessity of self-direction usually spelled trouble at examination time. Ours were no exception,
although relative to students as a whole they performed fairly well
in this regard. By the late 1860s, around 45 percent of all medical
students were interrupting their studies for periods ranging from
two to ten years. The reasons for the high failure rates varied, but
Bert believed the main one to be the students' responsibility for
directing their own work.[37] Individual dossiers at the Paris faculty
include examination ratings for 164 in our group (the scores used
most often were *refusé, satisfait, bien satisfait, très satisfait,* and *ex-
trêmement*). If we weigh the relative value of these scores, along

with that of any prizes or other honors that the students received, we arrive at the following approximate academic record for them: poor or fair, 11.6 percent; average, 50.6 percent; above average, 32.8 percent; and superior, 5.5 percent. A number who managed to give passable performances, however, did so only after years of effort. Twelve percent failed to pass the first time around on one or more of the *fin d'année* tests. Twenty-one percent failed the first time on one or more doctoral examinations. The worst performance was that of Joseph Janin, future deputy of Isère, who failed the first of his doctoral examinations four times between July 1885 and October 1886, finally earning a weak pass in July 1887. He flunked the second examination three times, and the fourth and fifth examinations once each, receiving his degree only in 1892.

That such a record was all some could show after years of living in Paris often reflected the city's many distractions. Few had the self-discipline of Odilon Lannelongue who, he tells us, realized the dangers of his own fun-loving *méridional* nature and, in accordance with a vow to his father, regulated his time in detail, spending each morning in the hospitals and, above all, avoiding the life of the cafés.[38] But not everyone had parents who could afford to send a hundred francs a month, as his did. Sons of artisans or shopkeepers sometimes had to work as tutors or laboratory assistants in order to meet the high cost of living in the capital. On the other hand, those assured of an income frequently indulged themselves, regarding academic life as a final rite of passage before entering respectable society. The less frivolous traveled abroad, though not with the seriousness of Cornil or Maunoury. Ferdinand Villard, future senator of Creuse, interrupted his studies for eight months in 1868 in order to visit Greece, Syria, Palestine, and Egypt. His purpose was to study the hygiene of other cultures, but his travels led him to the cafés of Cairo, where he had to fend off an Arab seductress while observing among the patrons "the curious effects" of hashish, a plant he believed to hold therapeutic qualities and to which he devoted his thesis.[39] Some dabbled in the arts or tried their hands at literature and journalism. After coming to Paris, Clément Clament of Dordogne, later to serve thirty-four years as a deputy, completed two novels, a biography of Sarah Bernhardt, and a guide to Paris for young men. It took him twelve years to get a degree.

Young provincials in Paris could easily fall into the maelstrom of politics, which often spilled over into the amphitheaters of the school. Among the oldest in our group were a few who, as students, had participated in the revolution of 1830. Several others were part of the opposition to Louis Philippe, including Armand Testelin and Henri Courturier, both advocates of Charles Fourier's cooperative theories. There are no known cases of any having been involved in the revolutionary violence of 1848. Antigovernment activities were also minimal during the authoritarian phase of the Second Empire that followed; Cornil later recalled that resistance was limited to support for the handful of Paris deputies who sat in parliament.[40] This changed during the post-1859 liberal era, despite government efforts to hold the line. Clemenceau was one of several to serve time at the Mazas prison for his political activities. Another troublemaker was Emile Villeneuve, a doctor's son from Basses-Pyrénées and one of three brothers involved in a series of antigovernment plots. He, Clemenceau, and the Parisian Léonce Levraud (himself condemned in 1867 to a year in jail for belonging to a secret society) numbered among the student followers of the legendary Auguste Blanqui. They were also the instigators of an attempt in 1865 to form a "fraternal association of students in medicine."

A glance at the percentages studying in Paris under successive regimes sheds light on the political climates to which the doctors were exposed. Pre-1848 figures are small – 1.4 percent for the Restoration and 11.3 percent for the July Monarchy – but among these were several elder statesmen of the Third Republic, all but five of them republicans for whom the romanticism and utopianism of the 1840s had been powerful influences. A few had gone on to win seats in the legislatures of 1848–9, including Laussedat, Testelin, Rampont-Lechin, Jean-Baptiste Chavoix, Bernard Lavergne, and Théophile Roussel. Thirty-nine percent studied between 1848 and 1870, a period in which hatred for Bonapartism and brooding over the fate of the Second Republic marked the mood of Parisian youth. By then, science and the new dogmas of positivism and materialism were beginning to replace the romantic idealism of an earlier age. Among the new generation were such radical republicans as Bert, Blatin, Bourneville, Clemenceau, Combes, Félix Frébault, Georges Martin, Naquet, and Jean Turigny. The largest group, close to half the total, was composed of those who got their training during the first two decades of the Third Republic. Except for a few who were involved in the early battles to consolidate the regime, these showed a much smaller incidence of student activism.

Few, however, could escape the ideological trappings of medical instruction in the capital. Just as Montpellier had its vitalism, so Paris had its philosophical materialism, a doctrine rooted in the sensualist theories of the late eighteenth century and developed by the Ideologues of the early nineteenth. At its most extreme, it denied the reality of the soul and other supernatural phenomena, arguing that human consciousness was a product of the physical senses and hence a part of the human biological makeup. Its stress on the sovereignty of the experimental method and the necessity to ascertain facts also accorded well with the teachings of Auguste Comte, although in a letter to *Le Temps* in 1868, Dean Wurtz denied that Paris medicine owed any allegiance to positivism.[41]

Wurtz's letter had come in response to complaints in the Senate, which was debating the merits of a petition accusing the Paris faculty of teaching atheism and materialism to the young. Senate conservatives had denounced Comte's subversive influence, contending that his ideas dominated the faculty and citing as proof several theses written in a positivist and materialist vein. Among the critics were the cardinals Donnet and Bonnechose, who argued that materialist teachings had subverted the religious faith of medical students and that few could resist their influence, as the professors who taught them also sat on examination boards.[42] Who were the guilty? Those mentioned most frequently were Auguste Axenfeld, Broca, Germain Sée, Charles Robin, and Alfred Vulpian, an assessment with which few on the Left would have disagreed. In fact, one materialist writer proudly singled out eleven titled professors on the faculty as being "pure atheists" and materialists; most of the rest, he said, were either agnostics or deists.[43] Robin's case leaves little doubt. A founder of the Society of Biology and a close friend of Comte's, he viewed positivism as providing a philosophical unity to all science. His *Dictionnaire de médecine,* coauthored with Emile Littré and published in 1855, was so popular that it became known as the "breviary" of medical students. This was especially upsetting to the Right, whose spokesmen in the Senate quoted Robin's definition of the soul ("an ensemble of brain functions") and thought ("the contractibility of the muscles") as evidence for their charges.

The professors whom conservatives singled out for attack worked with numerous students from our group, and their names appear as thesis committee presidents for about a fifth of the known cases.[44] Robin himself directed the theses of Bert, Cazeneuve, Combes, Villeneuve, and Clemenceau, the last of whom defended Robin's theories on spontaneous generation.[45] Villeneuve's thesis, entitled an "Essay on the Philosophic History of Medicine in Antiquity," was an attack on the regressive influence of religion on medical progress. In the same vein was the thesis by Albert Theulier, directed by Germain Sée, which ridiculed miracles in medicine and argued that purported cases of supernatural cures were the result of fraud or the workings of known physical laws.[46]

How deep an impact positivism and materialism had on the majority of our students is more difficult to determine. One does find a few of them in that later circle of physicians who were active proponents of Comtean doctrines, as in the case of Ernest Delbet, president of the Society of Sociology of Paris. Others were equally outspoken, including Cornil, who called himself "a positivist in philosophy like Littré" and extolled physics and chemistry as the best means of learning philosophy.[47] For most, however, the influence was far less systematic, absorbed as part of the philosophical biases that informed their training and expressed in a variety of intellectual attitudes that they brought to medical practice. As we shall see later, a materialist and positivist outlook harmonized well with the efforts of rural practitioners to advance their own scientific authority against the claims of the church, even among those who had little interest in formal questions of philosophy.

Besides positivism and materialism, one can detect many other intellectual influences that affected the content of medical learning in the capital. The doctoral theses provide some of the best insights in this regard, despite the numbers that were ground out in haste and that, as Combes later observed, owed whatever merit they contained "to a few clinical or laboratory observations in which the hand and spirit of the professor show themselves in easily recognizable form."[48] The extreme modesty of some of these efforts confirms the point. One author stressed that his attempt to explain infant encephalitis was intended purely for "personal instruction." Another, endeavoring to show how the physical ailments of Edmond and Jules de Goncourt had affected their literary portrayals of sickness, could conclude only that the two brothers expressed "an intellectual diathesis toward neurosis, a melancholy of jaded spirits."[49] Among the handful with any scientific merit were Roussel's work on pellagra (1842), Labbé's on genitourinary fistulas (1861), Bert's on the transplantation of animal tissues (1863), Cornil's on nephritis (1864), Javal's on strabismus (1868), Pozzi's on pelvic-rectal fistulas (1873), Cazeneuve's on the chemistry of the blood (1876), and Laurent Amodru's on the transudation of liquids in serous membranes (1879). As for the rest, their real interest lies in the insights that they provide into the intellectual assumptions of their young authors. Table 1.5 breaks them down by topic.

For some, choice of a topic was dictated by personal reasons. Delbet's 1854 thesis examined the causes of persistent vomiting among pregnant women, which three years earlier had killed his sister.[50] Among others, the thesis offered a chance to celebrate some feature of their home regions, especially if these boasted thermal or mineral waters. Former army or navy doctors frequently dealt with their experiences while in uniform. Jean Le Borgne, a medical officer on board *La Somme* during the 1860s, provided a medical topography of the islands and peoples of the Pacific. Gustave Gauthier, a graduate of the school at Brest and later senator for Haute-Saône, detailed his experiences at the French military hospital in Canton. He painted a bleak portrait of Chinese hygiene and was appalled by the widespread use of opium, though curious enough to try it himself, suggesting that "three to six pipes full" were sufficient to achieve a "delicious semi-sleep."[51]

The largest category of topics fell in the area of general medicine. These focused on a range of human woes – stroke, anemia, ulcers, tumors, fistulas, gangrene, scurvy, goiters, hernias, fractures, rheumatism, sciatica, cirrhosis of the liver, and even acne. Both etiology and diagnosis usually reflected prePasteurian assumptions. Thus, the causes of disease are seen as "infectious miasmas," "brusque variations of the temperature," "the action of vitiated blood on the tissues of the organs," "physical constitution and temperament," and heredity, whose role as the source of human maladies is often cited. Only one author, Combes, rejected the

Table 1.5. *Thesis topics of physician-legislators who were Paris graduates*

Topic[a]	%
General medicine	35.3
Surgery	7.6
Specialties	31.5
Obstetrics (5.7)	
Pediatrics (5.7)	
Ophthalmology (5.3)	
Gynecology (3.8)	
Neurology (3.8)	
Mental disease (3.4)	
Forensic medicine (1.5)	
Others (2.3)	
Public health, contagious diseases	15.6
Tuberculosis (3.4)	
Typhoid (3.4)	
Sexually transmitted diseases (1.9)	
Smallpox (1.5)	
Scarlet fever (0.8)	
Hospital infection (0.8)	
Specific epidemics (0.8)	
Other diseases (3.0)	
Medical sciences	5.3
Medical philosophy, history	2.3
Military medical experiences	1.9

[a]Numbers in parentheses are percentages.

idea, arguing that it "substitutes an incomprehensible unknown cause for the action of multiple forces whose role hygiene is beginning to unravel little by little."[52]

Most theses accepted contagionist ideas, which several authors could attest to from experience. Claude Ducher, an ex-navy surgeon who had served on board a frigate during the Crimean War, described how the spread of typhoid had devastated the French army and how, even in the hospitals of Paris, it was a common sight "to see individuals who were admitted for a different affliction subsequently come down with typhoid fever after being bedded in wards where it was present." In regard to smallpox, the majority appear to have accepted Edward Jenner's vaccine as an effective safeguard, although some raised the possibility of transmitting syphilis through the vaccination of newborns. Few were certain regarding the contagiousness of tuberculosis, although one, Louis Dubuisson of Finistère, who experimented by injecting animals with tuberculous substances, concluded that the resulting animal deaths had proved the possibility of developing a vaccine against the disease.[53]

Suggested therapies followed the prevailing orthodoxies of the era, whether bleeding, purging, expectorants, evacuants, emetics, cauterization, friction, antiphlogistics, or (for sexually transmitted diseases) mercury. Testelin, who wrote on an epidemic of influenza he had observed in the Nord in 1837, reported that purgatives and bleeding were best, as they calmed the patient and reduced inflammation. Alexis Chavanne, who described a rare form of puerperal fever he had seen as an intern at Lyon in 1850, suggested cauterizing infected areas with chlorohydric acid. Casimir-Laurent Michou thought pulmonary congestion in typhoid was best cured by "position, antiphlogistics, evacuants, friction, and diminution of external pressure." For ulcerations of the uterus, Joseph Soye recommended bleeding, purging, and cauterization with silver nitrate. Maximilien Lesage touted the virtues of cod-liver oil and digitalis for pregnant women suffering from scarlet fever.[54] A few were skeptical of all such cures. Joseph André's 1853 study of strokes concluded that electric shocks and *nux vomica* were useless: "As to blistering agents, setons, and cauterization, these methods are aptly suited to make patients suffer, but their effectiveness seems to me to be quite doubtful." Paul Bourgeois of the Vendée regarded diet and abstinence as antidotes for most disorders, whereas Emile Rey of Lot considered diet plus exercise to be the best defense against tuberculosis, cancer, scurvy, and insanity.[55]

Only occasionally do these works touch on any medical aspects of sexuality. It is rare even to see the kinds of remarks contained in the 1870 thesis of Georges Martin, who condemned masturbation as an unnatural act "that puts the imagination in a state of tension it cannot support without doing violent damage to the intelligence and to the whole cerebrospinal system."[56] Sexual matters were treated with the utmost delicacy in the hospitals as well. This exaggerated sense of modesty affected what most aspiring doctors were able to learn about obstetrics, a field dominated by midwives whose training facilities at Port-Royal were closed to students. The faculty itself possessed just one obstetrical clinic, to which access was possible only after passing the third doctoral examination. Even then, one was allowed to examine just three women a week, and only between eight in the morning and ten at night. This meant that a medical student was often unable to attend the delivery of a woman he had assisted during labor. Such a system, one critic complained in 1881, allowed many students to pass their examinations and to set up practice "without ever having been obliged during their studies to attend a single birth."[57]

It is not surprising that student theses in obstetrics dealt mainly with theory. One, for example, provided the reader with only an introduction and bibliography of works concerning the dangers women faced in childbirth – in order, he said, to give beginners like himself an understanding of the subject.[58] Such ignorance, it might be added, did not prevent our young authors from expounding at length on the physical and emotional makeup of women, stressing in particular the delicacy of women's physical and psychological structure, which was seen as being responsible for a variety of feminine ills.[59]

Almost all students believed in the merits of breast feeding. Charles Le Bretton, a native of Finistère and former navy surgeon, was typical in bemoaning the ignorance of young mothers in Brittany, who thought breast feeding ruined one's beauty (the women of Greece and Rome breast-fed their babies, he said) and who still swaddled their infants. Jean Garrigat's 1864 essay focused on the same issues in infant nutrition that his father had dealt with in a thesis written thirty years earlier; the son, however, rejected his father's description of breast feeding as a by-product of Jean-Jacques Rousseau's romanticized view of peasants, and he disagreed with his belief that poor health and female passions – the "two principal vices" of women – made mother's milk unhealthy. Nevertheless, the younger Garrigat acknowledged a relationship between maternal temperament and infant health, arguing that if a wet nurse were absolutely necessary, she should be of high moral character and "sweet, affectionate, [and] good."[60]

Such works often expressed deep concern over infant deaths in the hospitals of Paris. The young Maurice Bourrillon, a native of Lozère, wrote his thesis on a murderous epidemic of infant diarrhea he had witnessed in 1879. Although he was unable to pinpoint the cause, which he thought ranged from hereditary digestive disorders to the chemical decomposition of the mother's milk (the result of "lively emotional sensations, sickness, resumption of the menstrual cycle, obesity"), he was absolutely sure of one thing: Bottle-fed infants suffered the most deadly cases of diarrhea.[61] Bourrillon's experiences illustrate an important element in the professional training of doctors, which was their early exposure to the most tangible manifestations of poverty, ignorance, and oppression.

For some, such experiences were first acquired in those cities where they did their preparatory training, whether in routine hospital work or in combating epidemics, for which several were decorated. Those who had grown up in medical families had often seen the social face of disease at an even earlier age. As a boy, Lucien Guillemaut accompanied his father on his rounds at Louhans, where a diphtheria epidemic had broken out in 1862. The hardest hit of the victims, he recalled later, were children of the rural poor, all of them poorly clothed and fed. Most deplorable was their housing, which was the reason the disease spread quickly from village to village:

In many houses, the flooring is badly tiled or not at all; more than once I have seen water used for domestic purposes transformed into mud in one of the corners of the room and become thus a cause of humidity and insalubrity. Ordinarily, one room serves simultaneously as the kitchen, dining room, and bedroom for the whole family; and often, during the day, the hens abandon the poultry yard and the pigs their sties and invade these places. . . .

At night, when the family is poor and numerous, there is an overcrowding that one cannot imagine. Sick or not, the children sleep several in a bed; one thus often sees them all sick at the same time. . . . The father, the mother, [and] a little girl ordinarily occupy the head of the bed; at the foot, and pointed in the opposite direction, are often still other small children.[62]

For most members of our group, however, it was the Paris hospitals that served as the first real introduction to physical and economic misery. Crowding their wards and corridors were the masses of urban poor, refugees from the filth and squalor of slums where smallpox, cholera, and tuberculosis took their greatest toll. Pierre Lesoeuf, later deputy for Seine-Inférieure, long remembered these scenes, having been there during the 1850s as an extern at Sainte-Eugénie and an intern at Salpêtrière. What struck him most was the vast number of incurable patients, mostly victims of tuberculosis, who "solicited admission to the hospitals, which could not be denied them, but who could not be kept long, as they would have taken up all the beds and hence the places for those with curable afflictions."[63] By his time, conditions in the wards had greatly improved, the death rate standing at about one in eleven, down from one in six some thirty years earlier. Still, hospitals continued to symbolize suffering and death. Nöel Pascal, editor of *Le Mouvement médical,* defined a hospital in 1869 as "the best place to put a sick person in order to kill him."[64] When Brouardel was appointed to the staff of Maternité the same year, he faced an epidemic of puerperal fever that was killing a third of the newborns and nearly half the mothers.[65]

The impact of the hospitals can be seen in the training of many future doctors in parliament, starting with Roussel, who became one of the most active social reformers of the early Republic. Serving as an intern at Saint-Louis during the 1840s, Roussel repeatedly encountered patients who had worked in the match industry, and his curiosity led him to identify white phosphorous as the cause for their sickness and to call for its ban. It was here also that he chanced upon a case of pellagra and set out to study it in detail, first in his thesis and then in subsequent works. He was able to show that this affliction, though known as *mal de la rosa* in the Asturias and by other names in parts of southern France and Italy, constituted a single disease. Though the niacin deficiencies causing pellagra were not fully understood until later, his work represented an important step forward, because instead of faulting the physical and moral degeneration of its victims, as some had done, he called attention to the absence of balanced nutrition among the rural poor.[66]

There were others. Ernest Lafont, future deputy of Basses-Pyrénées, studied the effects of lead poisoning among patients at Charité, focusing his attention on the tremors that were associated with this affliction and that many doctors had confused with alcoholism. Lafont showed instead that these could be identified with specific professions that worked with lead.[67] Félix Ducoudray, offspring of a wealthy family in rural Nièvre, based his thesis on his internship at the Hôpital des Enfants, where he studied the relationship between infant feeding and rickets, a bone deficiency.

He soon came to realize that the problem went beyond medicine, especially when he discovered that the mortality rates for children on welfare ran as high as 50 percent. Although Ducoudray argued that breast feeding constituted the best defense against the disease, he refused to place all the blame on women. Many had to work in order to support their families, he said, a fact often forgotten by extreme proponents of natural feeding, who saw in women only a womb and a bottle. Moreover, the state itself bore much responsibility for its failure to implement preventive measures, including the surveillance of wet nurses. Ducoudray concluded with a plea for more hospices and nurseries in the industrial districts and for the creation of homes for unwed mothers, who could remain there up to ten months if they were willing to breast-feed their infants.[68]

Dr. Henri Henrot, mayor of Reims, believed that the early hospital experience was decisive in the development of a social and political consciousness among physicians. Himself a member of a medical family that had long been active in local politics, he made the point eloquently during a speech to the incoming class at the preparatory school at Reims in 1890:

From your first year, while your friends in other faculties remain attached to their books, you have already entered into the real world. You have to master your own nature in order to carry out repugnant research and to probe into the man who has just died in order to find the secret of his disease.

All that excites, all that calms, all that impassions human beings, you have experienced; death, suffering, disease, and despair have in their turn stirred your heart. At an age when so many others know only joys and delights, you have no choice but to give up something of yourself to your patients in hearing the cries of the wounded, the laments of the dying, or the shrieks of the insane. Though you have not yet reached adulthood, experience has already ripened your character: You have been the confidant, the protector, and the consoler for these unfortunate people for whom you often represent the only family.

From your first step in this life, you come to know humanity. . . . You ask yourself with growing anxiety whether all these maladies that cause the physical and moral degeneration of men, women, and children are truly necessary in modern society, and you ask yourself whether there is not a cure to prevent these unfortunate people from falling so fast and so far. At this point, you are conscious of the social role that you are called upon to play. . . . As a hygienist, you realize that you have a duty to make a supreme effort to stop the development of diseases that can be prevented.[69]

Thus far, our analysis has stressed several themes that aid in understanding the subsequent political careers of the physician-legislators. Their rural and small-town origins were perfectly suited to the agrarian, localistic mentality that characterized deputies and senators under the Third Republic. In addition, their professional training, especially as it related to their hospital experience, suggests that their intellectual and social formation was different from that of other young professionals and that their later attitudes cannot be explained solely by reference to their membership in a particular social class. We will now shift our attention to the physician-legislators' entry into active practice. We will see how their training continued to influence them and how the practice of their craft strengthened their political awareness and inclined them toward involvement in the affairs of their communities.

2

Early medical careers

Although the average doctor in our group spent close to twenty-three years in practice before entering parliament, his involvement in politics usually began the moment he nailed up his shingle. In this chapter, I will explain the reasons for this phenomenon as they relate to the general conditions of medical practice in post-1870 France. In the next chapter, I will show more specific ways in which the doctors first found themselves involved in public life. In either case, it is essential to keep in mind their dual identity as members of a social class and a profession. As we shall see, many began their careers having certain advantages in wealth and status that other practitioners did not have, which enabled them to bear the costs of a political career and provided greater independence in coping with challenges to their authority. We will begin by describing their various types and the place each of these occupied within the professional hierarchy.

PROFESSIONAL IDENTITY AND SOCIAL STATUS

Physician–legislators were seldom at a loss for words on the subject of their own humble station in life. Armand Gauthier of Aude, twice a cabinet minister, remarked to the Senate in 1904 that only two doctors in the upper house were truly distinguished in medicine, that the rest, including himself, represented the "proletarians" of the profession.[1] Some contemporaries went further, claiming that only the poorest went into politics and that most had been professional failures who chose public life as a substitute career. Bouisson of Montpellier, though himself a deputy, once described politically active doctors as men without patients who "swell the category of the *déclassés,* often throwing themselves into opposition politics as if in search of a remedy for their lack of success."[2] Later, in his famous essay on the "intellectual proletariat" of France, Henry Bérenger repeated this theme, characterizing doctors in politics as the "least favored" of the medical corps.[3]

The argument had a certain logic, as each new legislature seemed to contain still more individuals who held medical degrees but who identified little with the profession. The press called them *les sociologues* and *les évadés de la médecine,* and they were of three types. The first was the small group for whom medical study had served as a general education. They were a varied lot, ranging from the agronomist Albert Le Play to the statistician Léon Vacher. The second consisted of a few wealthy landowners and agriculturalists who, since earning their doctorates, had rarely if ever laid hands on a sick person. The third was made up of Parisian deputies, many of whom resided in poor districts of the city and who, at certain points in their careers, bore a resemblance to the legendary *médecin de quartier.* Here was a popular figure of working-class lore, the hero of porters and greengrocers whom Balzac had immortalized in the person of Dr. Poulain.[4] The majority had practiced for only brief periods, usually early in their careers, and included many well-known radicals and socialists. Paul Brousse established himself in the impoverished Epinettes Quarter of the seventeenth arrondissement during the early 1880s, at the same time that Clemenceau was running a part-time clinic in working-class Montmartre. In suburban Clichy, Emile Villeneuve practiced briefly before winning election as mayor in 1875; in later years, it was the socialist Adrien Meslier who built a reputation there as physician to the poor.

Did these typify the physician–legislators as a whole? Clearly, the answer is no, as they accounted for so few of the total. Only 3 percent could be termed true *sociologues,* in the sense that their careers involved no form of activity in the field of medicine. To these should be added 4 percent from the ranks of agriculturalists and urban radicals who practiced only sporadically. Medicine was thus a full-time occupation for close to 93 percent, if we count professors, administrators of asylums and clinics, and former army and navy doctors. Fifty-eight percent of the professors had private practices or hospital posts, and 70 percent of the army and navy doctors created civilian clienteles after retiring from service. In all, 87 percent of the members of our group had engaged in private

Table 2.1. *Primary professional identity of physician-legislators*

Identity[a]	%
Médecins de campagne	41.1
Rural communes, towns under 2,000 (19.7)	
Towns, 2,000–6,000 (21.4)	
Médecins-agriculteurs	6.7
Communes, towns under 6,000 (4.8)	
Towns over 6,000 (1.9)	
Small-town doctors	23.6
Towns, 6,000–20,000 (15.2)	
Towns, 20,000–50,000 (8.4)	
Urban practitioners	13.2
Cities, 50,000–100,000 (2.5)	
Cities over 100,000 (10.7)	
Professors	8.6
Paris (3.6)	
Provincial cities (5.0)	
Asylum administrators, directors of clinics	3.1
Paris (0.6)	
Provincial cities (2.5)	
Nonpractitioners	3.1
(Missing cases = 4)	

[a] Numbers in parentheses are percentages.

practice over extended periods of their lives before entering parliament.

Of these, general medicine characterized the practices of close to 80 percent. Less than 7 percent became surgeons (at least of any distinction), and another 8 percent cultivated specialties varying from ophthalmology to hydrotherapy. The most prevalent type was the rural and small-town doctor, which is not surprising in light of their origins and the fact that nearly 70 percent established practices in their home departments (and 61% in their home arrondissements). Although most individuals embodied features of more than one practitioner type, I have grouped them in Table 2.1 according to their most prominent professional traits.

Most of those practicing in a department other than that of their birth were professors or former military doctors, plus a few who had settled in neighboring districts as the result of marriage ties.

Table 2.2. *Region of practice of physician-legislators*

Region	Physician-legislators, 1870–1914 (%)	All doctors, 1893[a] (%)
North	5.4	6.5
East	11.7	8.9
Paris region and the Center	18.3	29.3
West	13.8	17.7
Southwest	11.4	13.4
Massif Central	12.9	5.4
Lyon region, Savoy, and Dauphiné	12.0	7.6
Mediterranean region	10.8	10.7
Overseas colonies	3.3	NA

[a]Figures on region of practice for all doctors in 1893 from *Annuaire statistique de la France*, 1892–93–94, pp. 32–33.

Because the majority practiced where they were born, most areas maintained an equilibrium between their percentages as region of birth and region of practice (see Table 2.2). Although these distributions tended to reflect those of all doctors, exceptions occurred in the Massif Central and in certain isolated stretches of Bourgogne, Jura, the Alps, and Savoy, where the proportion of physician-legislators was higher. The pattern was reversed in the industrial north, Normandy, the Gironde, and Paris, the capital itself being home to 9.9 percent, as opposed to 19.4 percent for all doctors. Excluding Paris, only 11 percent lived in cities of fifty thousand and over; in 1893, the figure for all physicians was 28 percent.[5]

Not only had those in parliament been active in medicine, but their status as property owners also distinguished them from the poorest members of the profession. It is difficult to determine precisely their wealth, which included earnings from medical practice, land, dowries, and inheritance. Few private papers are available, and standard biographical dictionaries are largely silent on this score.[6] Still, enough is known to suggest that far from typifying the medical proletariat, these doctors had enjoyed considerable status as practitioners and *propriétaires* before entering politics.

Almost by definition, members of parliament formed an elite, if for no other reason than they had the money needed in order to win a seat. This was especially true for those with larger ambitions: according to Estèbe, the average cabinet minister before 1914 had a net worth of 455,000 francs, which translated into an annual income of between 35,000 and 50,000 francs a year.[7] In most cases, membership in parliament followed service in local assemblies, which also tended to be dominated by men of wealth. It is true that the incomes of doctors belonging to these bodies fell below those of other professionals; in the *conseils généraux* of 1870, for example, only 15 percent had incomes of 20,000 francs or more a year, which is less than half the proportion among the lawyers who were members.[8] Yet, these doctors were still better off than most of their fellow practitioners. The journalist Marcel Baudouin, writing on the membership of *conseils généraux* during the 1890s, observed that only the wealthiest could afford to belong to them and that most physicians were "not financially secure enough to confront the hazards of politics without running the risk of losing their modest clienteles."[9]

A seat in parliament posed even greater strains. Aside from the expense of entertaining visiting constituents, deputies and senators had to maintain two residences, and rents in the capital were high. It was a doctor, Auguste Baudon of Oise, who in 1906 presented the case to the Chamber for raising salaries from nine thousand to fifteen thousand francs. He noted that the cost of living had doubled since 1849, when the sum of nine thousand was first established, and lamented the increasing expense of keeping in touch with constituents.[10] Campaign spending consumed the greatest amounts, averaging, according to some estimates, between ten thousand and twenty thousand francs per election. Publication costs alone were formidable, as illustrated in the case of Léon Joubert, a physician and *châtelain* of Indre-et-Loire, who had 100,000 posters printed for just one campaign. Local committees assumed only part of the debt. The 1898 campaign of Eugène Dufour in Isère cost six thousand francs, of which the doctor paid five thousand from his own pocket.[11] Could a modest practice have supported such expense? Those who tried soon found the answer. A prominent Paris doctor later recalled being visited by a physician-deputy who was seeking help in building a small practice on the side. "Since I became a deputy," the latter said, "I have lost my clientele; half my little town opposes me, and I pass my time running errands for the other half. With the nine thousand francs I receive from the Chamber, I can hardly meet the expenses of my rent and food."[12]

Certainly, it may have been possible for a few prominent specialists and professors to support a career in politics from their earnings, and occasionally one encounters a country doctor like Pierre Merlou, the ambitious deputy of the Yonne who made himself an expert on money matters (later becoming minister of finance) and who, according to *La Chronique médical,* earned between 20,000 and 25,000 francs a year in his practice at Saint-Sauveur.[13] But that was the exception. "You can rest assured," Dr. Dubuisson of Finistère told the Chamber in 1909, "that the income of the immense majority of doctors in France does not surpass 5,000 francs a year."[14]

Dubuisson's estimate was close to the mark. An 1881 poll by *Le Concours médical* showed that French doctors had an average annual income of 6,341 francs, which, after a loss of 1,500 in uncollected fees, fell below 5,000. Even this varied by region, going from 8,500 in the north and center to 4,500 in the southeast and southwest.[15] A second poll in 1901 showed a few gains – now only 34 percent of those surveyed (as opposed to 44% in 1881) indicated that their receipts were inadequate to cover expenses – but the journal still considered the economic outlook of doctors to be bleak.[16]

It was here that a good marriage revealed its importance, for, as one observer remarked in 1872, to marry a woman without a dowry "is as cruel today as it was in the time of Molière."[17] This, it might be added, was true for the parliamentary elites in general, for a good marriage served as one of the most important stepping-stones on the path to political office.[18] This pattern can be seen in the lives of many in our group. Edmé Bourgoin, earning five hundred francs a year as an *agrégé* in the late 1860s, assured his future by his marriage to the daughter of a wealthy phosphate manufacturer of the Ardennes. Cornil married the daughter of Paul Caffe, a Parisian ophthalmologist and editor of the *Journal des connaissances médicales pratiques,* a post to which Cornil succeeded on the death of his father-in-law. Similar patterns prevailed among many lesser lights who succeeded in attaching themselves to old provincial families. Jules Donnet of Haute-Vienne married into the Daniel-Lamazière family, his father-in-law having been a deputy to the Legislative Assembly of 1849. Louis Devins of Haute-Loire married the daughter of Marspoil de Lamothe, a land-holder of Brioude and himself tied to the family of Antoine Rongier de Flagheac, a *conventionnel* of 1793. The physician-deputy Laurent Amodru was one of the luckiest: He married into the family of Aristide Boucucaut, founder of a profitable chain of discount stores in Paris.

These were only a few of the examples, as a glance at the various professional types in our group shows. Let us consider each in turn, starting with the professors. Of these, 39 percent belonged to the Paris faculty, 30 percent to provincial faculties, and 24 percent to the preparatory schools. A few had appointments elsewhere, including Bert at the Sorbonne and Bourgoin at the superior School of Pharmacy.

The professors occupied the apex of the medical hierarchy, and this was especially true of the Parisians. They accounted for 75 percent of those in our group who held the coveted rank of *membre titulaire* in the Academy of Medicine, for 71 percent who belonged to the Academy of Sciences, and for 57 percent who sat on the Consultative Committee of Public Hygiene. They also produced 70 percent of those who held the post of hospital physician or surgeon in the capital and over 50 percent of those belonging to the Society of Biology and the Society of Anatomy. Their names are among the most influential of the physician-legislators, from titled professors like Cornil and Lannelongue to *agrégés* like Liouville and Jean de Lanessan.

These individuals ranked high in society, and their lives betokened both material comfort and a fascination with the life of the mind. Refined in tastes and sensibilities, many were collectors of paintings and rare books, and a few were even serious artists in their own right. Pozzi, whose facilities at the Hôpital Broca featured murals by his friends in the world of art, specialized in ancient jewelry and coins. Cornil, a dabbler in painting and etching, was drawn to rare books, his private library containing everything from a copy of the Protestant Bible of Geneva to a first edition of Rousseau's *Confessions*. Some, it is true, had been born into comfortable surroundings, but for many this was not the case. Lannelongue, for one, was always quick to remind others that he was "of the people" and that his father had been an obscure health officer for fifty-five years.

Lannelongue represents one of the most dazzling success stories. A Gascon, short and stocky with a prominent nose and close-cropped hair and beard, his granite features were softened only by his southern accent, sense of humor, and unbounded generosity. He owned a country château in his native Gers, where he ran for office and where, at Castéra-Verduzan, his birthplace, he built the Musée Lannelongue, containing reproductions of paintings and sculptures he had seen in his world travels. His yearly contributions to worthy causes surpassed the incomes of many practitioners, whose plight he recognized by frequent donations to the AGMF – a gift of two thousand francs in 1889 to the pension fund, for example, and another of five thousand francs to the fund for widows and orphans on the occasion of his reelection to the presidency of this association in 1897.[19]

What was the source of Lannelongue's wealth? Certainly not his income from teaching. In his time, professorial salaries ranged between twelve thousand and fifteen thousand francs at the Paris faculty and between six thousand and twelve thousand at provincial ones. Charles Robin's salary had been fixed at thirteen thousand francs on his appointment to the chair of histology in 1862, and it remained at this level until he entered the Senate fourteen years later, at which time it was reduced by nine thousand, the equivalent of his parliamentary pay. Pozzi, named professor of clinical gynecology in 1901, received thirteen thousand francs a year, which was raised to fifteen thousand in 1911. Lannelongue's faculty dossier shows what he himself earned during his ascent through the ranks: As *aide d'anatomie* between 1865 and 1868, his salary stood at one thousand francs; as *prosecteur* at the School of Practice between 1868 and 1871, at twelve hundred; and as *agrégé* between 1871 and 1880 at three thousand and later at four thousand. On his appointment as professor of external pathology in 1884, it rose to twelve thousand.[20] In the meantime, he had won the post of hospital surgeon, which brought with it a small additional salary. But this hardly mattered to Lannelongue, who never even needed to create a private clientele. His secret, as an admirer said of him, was that he had learned that in order to succeed "one must know how to utilize all forces compatible with honor." By that he meant his marriage in the 1870s to the vicomtesse de Marsay, a widow and member of the wealthy Rémusat family of Paris.[21]

Although they earned less than titled professors did, many *agrégés* also married well and, in the case of such well-known Paris surgeons as Armand Després, Jean Peyrot, and Léon Labbé, probably derived substantial earnings from private practice (some estimates placed the income of surgeons at their level as high as sixty thousand francs a year). Labbé, a château owner in rural Normandy, certainly was among the best, having earned his degree in 1861 and risen to the top in three years. His ascent had been marked by several notable events, which included the public thrashing of a clumsy assistant and, on another occasion, the successful removal of a fork from a man's stomach.[22]

We should mention several others who, though not members of the faculty, were of such stature in the profession as to merit a place among the Parisian notables. One was Javal, whose wealth had freed him from the necessity of building a private clientele. Instead, he devoted his time to research on strabismus, color blindness, and myopia. Ironically, in 1885, the year of his election as deputy, he himself was stricken with glaucoma and within seven years was blind. Nevertheless, he continued to collect Japanese prints and illustrated books and, indomitable to the last, could often be seen peddling a tandem bicycle behind a servant on his way to the Academy of Medicine.[23] Even more prominent was Roussel, who, like Javal, eschewed private practice for research and was also active in the Academy of Medicine. Roussel spent his time about equally between Paris and Lozère, where he owned a château and enjoyed sufficient wealth by the end of his life to donate fifty thousand francs toward a new town hall.[24]

Others of note were Théophile David, who helped found the Ecole dentaire in 1879; Claude Chauveau, a saddler's son from Côte-d'Or who became a leading European authority in otolaryngology; and Etienne Goujon, a native of Ain (and very rich through marriage), who directed a private *maison de santé* that catered to mental patients from wealthy families. Emile Chautemps, whose family holdings lay in Haute-Savoie, had a successful practice in the capital, as did Gabriel Delarue, who on his death in 1905 managed to outdo even Roussel by leaving a sum of 800,000 francs to his hometown of Gannat.[25]

The professors of provincial schools included several individuals who had made their mark in medicine and local society. Joyeux-Laffuie, who taught anatomy at the science faculty of Caen, oversaw his family holdings near Poitiers, where he ran for parliament.[26] At Reims, there was Alfred Thomas, who in 1878 resigned his academic post in order to devote himself full time to his farm at Montfournois, in the Marne, which the *comice agricole* of Reims cited as "the best maintained in the canton of Verzy." Already the possessor of the "silver medal of the bovine species," Dr. Thomas was commended "for his good care of herds, for harvests as fine as they are varied, and finally for important plantings of vines and cherry trees."[27] Bouisson of Montpellier was one of the wealthiest: On his death in 1884, he left 115,000 francs to the school for scholarships and a library, and when his widow died, she willed it an additional 1.5 million, which included the Château de Grammont outside the city, with one hundred hectares planted in vines.[28]

Other provincials who had managed to achieve a degree of fame were the surgeons Augagneur of Lyon, Adrien Pozzi of Reims, and Monprofit of Angers. Lille had some of the most original, including the anatomist Charles Debierre, known for his books on craniology. Here also were two of the best-known natural historians in the country – Alfred Giard, a leading advocate of Darwinian theories, and the zoologist Théodore Barrois, who came from a wealthy family of cotton-mill owners and had married the granddaughter of Frédéric Kulmann, a magnate in the chemical industry. Along with his duties at the faculty and at the Pasteur Institute of Lille, Barrois sat on the governing board of the Lens Mining Company and was a member of the central committee of the Coal Mine Owners' Trade Association.[29]

Other than professors, only a few in our group represented the medical elites of the large provincial cities. The best known was Testelin of Lille, who made his reputation as an eye surgeon and had won fame during the 1840s as a leader of the cooperative movement.[30] Other examples were Marius Isoard, part-time professor of anatomy at the Ecole des beaux-arts in Marseille, and his son François, who was a hospital administrator. Although prominent in the life of city, both maintained ties in the adjacent Basses-Alpes, where they owned vineyards. One could mention also a small number who specialized in mental disease, which included a handful of alienists who worked as administrators of provincial asylums while continuing to oversee property holdings located in their home departments.

Physician-legislators from the big cities made up only a fourth of the total. Next came those known as *les médecins des petits centres,* who practiced in smaller departmental and arrondissement *chefs-lieux.* Among the brightest, one occasionally hears a note of bitterness regarding their isolation,[31] but small-town doctors still enjoyed numerous advantages when compared with their country *confrères.* Patients were close at hand, and if a local medical society existed, one could build professional friendships. The towns also offered a variety of medical posts, the most desirable being that of physician in a hospital or hospice. The salary was modest (some *médecins d'hôpital* earned as little as one hundred francs a year), and the same was true for other posts in the bureaucracy, such as that of epidemics doctor, *lycée* doctor, or *médecin des enfants assistés.* Yet, these were prized also for reasons of status and the prestige they brought to an individual's own practice. According to *Le Concours médical,* in 1889 around a fifth of all doctors held hospital titles, and nearly 50 percent held one or more salaried public posts. The journal estimated these to be worth, on average, one thousand francs a year for their holders.[32]

Undoubtedly, some physicians coveted medical posts as a means of supplementing their incomes, as appears to have been the case for several in our group. At Arlanc, in Puy-de-Dôme, the future deputy Jean-Pierre Sabaterie, appointed hospice physician and assistant to the justice of the peace in 1886, served over the next few years as *médecin-inspecteur des enfants du premier âge,* president of the commission to inspect pharmacies, physician for an association of shoemakers, and doctor for several mutual-aid societies. Though mayor of the town by 1898, he continued to describe himself as an *enfant du peuple* who had long known "the harsh stages of the strenuous life of the day laborer."[33] Or there was the case of Eugène Haynaut, who worked as a private physician for the Compagnie du Nord and for several mutual-aid societies at Béthune in Pas-de-Calais. Haynaut was so strapped for money after his election in 1889 that he set out building a new practice in Paris, dispensing his card to concierges in different quarters of the city.[34] A few others made extra money as consulting physicians for railroads and insurance companies.[35]

These cases were hardly typical, however. The small number known to have held salaried positions of any kind suggests a certain financial ease on the part of most. Less than a sixth, for example, had held hospital posts, and most of these were professors. Moreover, the few who did hold salaried positions could hardly be described as belonging to the medical proletariat. An example was Théophile Souchu-Servinière at Laval in Mayenne, elected to the Chamber in 1876, who held posts in the hospital, the prison, the *lycée,* and the *école normale.* Another was Maurice Bourrillon, inspector of mineral waters in Lozère, who came from a well-to-do family in Mende, where his grandfather had founded the first wool spinning-mill.

Although many doctors utilized public posts as a springboard to local political office, this was not the typical pattern for those who succeeded in going on to parliament. Most had built solid practices and were seen as men of substance within their communities, which often elected them mayor. Others led dual careers as town doctors and gentlemen farmers, overseeing fields, vineyards, orchards, and herds on their country estates. An example was Amédée Girard of Puy-de-Dôme, offspring of an old family in Riom, who donated money for schools, roads, and monuments. The source of his wealth was land, and like others, he was careful to note his popular roots: "I am a child of the people like my father, like my grandfather," he said in his 1893 campaign for parliament; "If I possess anything, I owe it to my labor and to my economies."[36] At Falaise, in Calvados, Dr. Turgis served as president of the local society of agriculture and was also mayor, chief physician of the town hospital, and vice-president of the *conseil général.* Eugène Dufour, who built a model farm next to the asylum he directed near Grenoble, was secretary of the local society of agriculture, the largest in the department.

This emphasis on agriculture becomes even more pronounced as we move to our last category – the country doctors. They fall into two groups. The first was those living in communities of two thousand to six thousand inhabitants, whom I have included here because even though they practiced in small population centers, they usually had extensive rural clienteles. The second was those in towns, villages, and rural communes having fewer than two thousand inhabitants. Together, these accounted for 137 physician-legislators, or about 38 percent of the total. If we add those *médecins-agriculteurs* living in rural districts, along with a scattering of former army and navy doctors, the proportion rises to 46 percent. Almost all were native to the area of practice, their regional strengths being greatest in the south, the west, and the southwest.

What was the country doctor of that era like? He conjures up a certain image, like Balzac's legendary Benassis. He is seen as humble and idealistic, a man whose own lot was not vastly superior to that of the peasants he treated. "It is only by prodigious economies that the family of a doctor can honorably hold his rank in the small posts of the countryside," one wrote in 1911. Another said: "We have to live in part on the vegetables of a garden that I cultivate myself, with the aid of my wife and maid. The doctor without fortune is a wretched man who lives a very painful life."[37] We must remember, however, that doctors who stayed in the countryside rather than migrating to the cities often did so because they enjoyed a secure place there, much like those living in a coastal canton of the west whom one practitioner described as having "each his own fief, his own berth."[38] Without question, there were some in our group whose lives had not been easy. According to Bourgeois of the Vendée,

I have known that life of the country doctor who doesn't always live in grand style, who, day and night, at all hours, in all weather, in rain or in snow, on foot or on horseback, traverses the countryside, offering to everyone his care and consolations, and, sometimes, like our ancestor Ambroise Paré, dressing wounds and, God willing, healing the sick who become and remain his friends.[39]

Gustave Ravier, physician in Cher, wrote of himself, "I have lived with the cultivator. . . . I was more a physician to agriculturalists than a châteaux doctor."[40] Others practiced extensively among rural populations and gained fame as *médecins des pauvres*. The term was applied to around 10 percent, but it described the practices of many more.

Yet, few typified the poor of the profession. Indeed, to practice free of charge implied the kind of financial ease that characterized most of those who had reputations as physicians to the poor. On the death of one of them, Théophile Collinot, who practiced near Auxerre, the president of the Senate remarked that the doctor had been a "child of his own labors" who owned a fortune.[41] Louis Mathey of Saône-et-Loire, who won a decoration for his medical philanthropy, was an agriculturalist of note and member of an esteemed local family that produced several deputies and senators. A *médecin des pauvres* named Auguste Mallet, who practiced at Bagnols in Gard, devoted much of his time to research on silkworm breeding, which included study trips to Asia. Such types hardly fit the picture of medical legend.

On balance, the country doctors as a group appear to have been at least comfortable property owners who had made good marriages or whose parents had managed to leave them a modest legacy.[42] The degree to which they represented the rural elites can be seen in the fact that 70 percent of them were local mayors and 64 percent members of *conseils généraux,* of which several served as president or vice-president. The variety and abundance of the country doctors' activities in agricultural life are striking: as authors of books and pamphlets on animal science, soil analysis, and food fraud; as chairmen of farmers' unions, horseshow committees, and agricultural fairs; and as officers of agrarian credit organizations and cooperatives.

So active were some doctors that they were known as *médecins-agriculteurs.* The term was applied to just under 7 percent but fit many others as well. Winegrowers were prominent. Examples include Maurice Roy of Charente-Inférieure, who belonged to the Society of Viticulturists of France; Justin Cot, a member of the Central Society of Agriculture of his native Hérault, who wrote extensively on winegrowing issues; and Emile Rey, author of *L'Agriculture progressive dans le Lot* (1906), who focused his attention on the problem of phylloxera. About a third never practiced medicine, or did so rarely, instead offering their services free to the poor in a spirit of philanthropy. Of the rest, most had treated patients at some point in their careers, but the extent of this varied. Dr. Léon Legludic practiced sporadically and always free of charge for fifty-five years at Sablé-sur-Sarthe, where he served as mayor, member of the departmental agricultural society, and president of the farmers' union.[43]

We gain a better understanding of the doctors' economic standing by considering their role in organizations devoted to improving the living standards of the profession. Just over 54 percent belonged to the AGMF, which was comparable with the percentage for physicians as a whole.[44] Membership was especially strong among the urban elites, for whom the defense of less-privileged doctors was a noble endeavor. Their names appeared often among contributors to various charitable funds of the organization, and several held positions in its administrative hierarchy: Cornil as a member of the General Council, Larrey as a vice-president, and Lannelongue as president (he was elected to the post in 1892 and again in 1897). These and others (Robin, Wurtz, Javal, Roussel, and Pozzi) belonged to the Société centrale, the largest of the affiliate groups, encompassing the Seine and surrounding areas. In general, those whose fathers belonged to the more modest petit-bourgeois trades showed the weakest inclination to join, whereas those with the strongest inclination were the sons of professional men, mainly doctors. In regional terms, membership levels tended to reflect the strength of local affiliates.[45]

Jacques Léonard has observed that local AGMF leadership had a *"connotation élitaire"* and that its officers came from the ranks of hospital physicians, professors, mayors, and *conseillers généraux.* This is borne out by our cases, among whom 18 percent had served as local AGMF officers, half of them as presidents or vice-presidents. Many presided over the societies of their home departments while serving in parliament: Of 102 AGMF members in the Senate and Chamber during the 1880s, for example, 16 were local presidents or vice-presidents, most having been elected to these posts before entering parliament. Of them, all but one was elected after 1870, the point at which affiliates had finally been allowed to select their own leaders.[46]

Although the AGMF had long proclaimed "assistance, moralization, and protection" to be its goals, by 1880 it had managed to accomplish little in the battle against illegal practice. Many militant practitioners were thus drawn to the idea of professional unions, or syndicates, which could pursue quacks in court and establish common fees. In 1879, Auguste Cézilly, editor of *Le Concours médical,* founded the Civil society of *Le Concours médical,* whose purpose was "the study and implementation of all works considered useful to the medical profession." At the same time, he began laying the groundwork for the syndicates, the first of which appeared in 1881. Within three years, there were a total of seventy-four, claiming around 3,500 members. Despite a court ruling in 1885 that the recent legalization of trade unions did not apply to the liberal professions, medical syndicates continued to function until gaining recognition in 1892. Afterwards, the pace of growth resumed and by 1906 encompassed about 44 percent of

Table 2.3. *Physician-legislators and professional associations*

	Percentage in AGMF	Percentage in Civil Society of *Le Concours médical*	Percentage in medical syndicates
Country doctors	55.3	26.2	16.4
Médecins-agriculteurs	68.4	18.2	13.6
Small-town doctors	53.8	13.0	10.5
Big-city doctors	47.5	21.2	7.7
Professors	63.6	4.2	8.3

the medical corps. By then, membership in the Civil Society of *Le Concours médical* stood at some 4,500.[47]

Only 12 percent of the physician-legislators belonged to the syndicates at any point in their careers. Of these, two-thirds were rural and small-town doctors, and it is possible that some of them ranked near the bottom of the economic ladder when compared with the physician-legislators as a whole. As with the AGMF, however, one is struck less by the poverty of this group than by the status of its members. Two-thirds came from professional and landowning families, and many were already figures of local distinction by the time they joined. Of known activists in the movement during the years 1879 to 1885, for example, 56 percent had served as mayors or *conseillers généraux*.

Membership in the Civil Society of *Le Concours médical* showed roughly the same patterns and included a number of physician-deputies and senators who wished to express their support for less fortunate colleagues. Again, of those who joined before beginning their careers in parliament, most were local mayors and *conseillers généraux*, several of them having considerable landed wealth. The names of only a few appear among membership lists of the Civil Society's various *"oeuvres,"* or insurance schemes, which had been created for poorer doctors.

Over half of the physician-legislators who were associated with medical syndicalism belonged also to the AGMF. Table 2.3 compares their membership in the AGMF, the Civil Society, and the medical syndicates.

By and large, therefore, those physicians who rose to political prominence under the Third Republic represented neither the medical proletariat nor the misfits of the profession. On the contrary, most had been successful doctors, certainly better off than the rank and file of their colleagues. Their status as professional men, combined with their role as property owners and agriculturalists, allowed them to carve out a place for themselves among the local elites, while offsetting the economic threat posed by a host of antimedical forces, especially in rural areas. Having described the social basis for their influence, I will now examine its professional dimensions.

THE POLITICAL SETTING OF MEDICAL PRACTICE

"If, at one and the same time, you think you're capable of being a physician, surgeon, midwife, dentist, bone setter, pharmacist, herbalist, a bit of a veterinarian and, if need be, a go-between in a horse swap, then by all means go out and set yourself up in practice in the countryside."[48] That was the advice of an old practitioner to the young in 1888, and it echoed the sentiments of countless men of experience. The surgeon Armand Trousseau once remarked that the doctor needed less *savoir* than *savoir-faire* in dealing with patients, the truth of which was hammered home by the medical journalist Julien Noir in 1902:

One asks of him how to make a poultice, how to place leeches, how to prepare a decoction; he is asked to specify the quantity of water for bathing and its temperature and the duration of the bath, and he has to demonstrate the method of making the bed of a sick person, to explain to a young mother the method of swaddling a newborn baby and to insist on cleaning the bottle and numerous other small things, which, certainly, no one has taught him how to do in the faculties or the hospitals.[49]

Such was the first shock experienced by the novice. Coming next was the realization of his own helplessness. Patients rarely seemed to exhibit any symptoms he had studied, and even when he was sure of his diagnosis, he was seldom confident about the cure. Many therapies were useless, differing little from those of earlier times when patients had been bled and clystered, purged and sweated, and subjected to harsh regimens of diet, drugs, and cold baths. The second half of the century did see the decline of bleeding, the sovereign remedy for inflammatory diseases. Still, the spirit of routine lingered long: "Far from all scientific activity, which revives and stimulates," wrote one doctor in 1872, "a person becomes content with an acquired, undisputed situation. He has a few formulas that are always the same, and at the end of ten or twelve years, he has added nothing to his scientific baggage."[50]

In truth, the life of the *médecin de campagne* could be grueling. Victor Lourties, who practiced in rural Landes for fifteen years before entering the Senate, later recalled having served a total of twenty communes in his vicinity, often visiting up to twelve of them a day. That was not unusual. Before the automobile, the doctor's daily range varied anywhere from seven kilometers in the north to eleven in the mountains of the Center.[51] Being isolated in this way meant having to deal with difficult cases alone or, at best, with the help of a farm hand or member of the family. An amputation, a tracheotomy, even the lancing of an abscess posed risks of infection, although many authorities viewed hospital surgery as even more dangerous.[52] On top of this, every practitioner had experienced the frustration of being called in too late on a case and having to endure the subsequent blame. But then, calling the doctor was not usually the first recourse of the sick. A practitioner in Brittany complained in the 1890s that "when the poor (that is to say, the majority) are stricken with disease, they go to bed and patiently await death or recuperation."[53] Or they might try one of many home remedies, for each region had its own syrups, plasters, and herbs. Failing this, there was always the priest or one of the sisters or matrons:

The *curé* charges nothing for his counsels. The sister asks nothing, whether for her tea, her sugar, her laudanum. The old matron is content to savor the good effects produced by her herbs. If a peasant falls from his loft and dislocates his shoulder or breaks a leg, one never thinks about a doctor. There's a bone setter in almost every village.[54]

What were the infirmities that our doctors encountered most often in the rural society of that era? Looking back presents a depressing tableau, a reminder of the days not far distant when almost everyone bore the traces of one physical defect or another – a clubfoot, a hunched back, a harelip, or a goiter. "Our farmers have nothing in common with the peasants of the operetta, well clothed and living off fresh vegetables and poultry," Dr. Sireyjol told the Chamber in 1910.[55] In the countryside, as in the cities, each occupation had its own risks, beyond the common mishaps of farm life. Woodcutters fell from trees or sliced open their feet. Hog butchers chopped off fingers and thumbs. Loosely clothed women and children working alongside the new mechanical mowers had arms and feet mangled. The proximity of people to animals posed a constant threat. Farmhands who bedded down in the stables were exposed to an army of parasites and herpetic infections, typified by those eruptions on hands and chest known in Auvergne as *anders,* in Languedoc as *brillants.* More deadly to human life were anthrax, rabies, and bovine tuberculosis.[56]

Peasant life had its seasonal complaints – bronchitis and pneumonia in winter, dysentery and miliary fever in summer and fall – but most dreaded were epidemic diseases whose visitations could carry away whole villages. Prime Minister René Waldeck-Rousseau noted in the Senate in 1900 that of a total of 200 local epidemics over the previous two years, 151 had broken out in rural communes having populations of between 500 and 1,000.[57] It is easy to understand why. Contamination of drinking water had long been the scourge of the countryside, whether in the public fountains of mountain villages or in the wells and cisterns that served people living on the plains. Cornil once told the Senate of a cluster of wells in Normandy that, over a twenty-year period, and without having once been reported to authorities, had caused six cholera epidemics and eleven deaths.[58] An even greater menace lay in what Paul Bert called the "permanent epidemics" of smallpox, typhoid fever, and diphtheria. The Consultative Committee of Hygiene reported that during 1886 alone, in towns of 10,000 and above, smallpox claimed the lives of 3,289 people, typhoid fever of 4,834, and diphtheria of 4,838. The report added that these figures did not reflect the whole tragedy, especially in the case of diphtheria, which hit the villages hardest and often killed greater proportions of their inhabitants than was true of the towns.[59]

In the countryside, as in the towns, sickness reflected more than simple biological accidents. There was the special vulnerability of the very young, from newborns who survived only a few days to those who died from neglect or abuse. Old age was a form of sickness. Dr. Georges Martin, a senator and specialist in legislative issues affecting the elderly, observed in 1886 that although old people were occasionally looked after by the people of their villages, they faced a bleak future once their productive forces were used up: "You all know that in our rural areas the elderly are obliged on certain days to drag themselves laboriously to the village with a sack on their backs and to go and ask for the bread that sustains them from the public welfare physician." Dr. Bourgeois of the Vendée echoed his sentiments: "Something I have seen everywhere and know well is the misery of the aged in our rural areas, who are absolutely alone in the world. I know this for a fact, having been a doctor for thirty years."[60]

Hygienic conditions in rural France would have seemed a ready market for the doctor's skills, but such was not the case. From the outset, he found himself beset by powerful forces vying for the same clientele, and the inadequacies of his own curative resources rendered his position vulnerable and made any pretense to monopoly ring hollow. Even his most persuasive methods, such as smallpox vaccination, met heavy opposition, and the same resistance continued long after bacteriological ideas had begun to prove their worth. It was thus natural for doctors to blame their problems on the ignorance of rural dwellers. A practitioner at Saint-Brieuc wrote in 1881: "Let us say that the peasants lead a very primitive life, that they are ignorant, credulous, and naive; their greatest and only distraction in winter, so to speak, is in the evening when each relates a tale in which fairies and witches abound."[61]

The evidence was everywhere. Quacks abounded in the towns and villages, from bone setters and magnetizers to urine samplers, nostrum peddlers, and empirics of every description. "They traverse our public squares and streets, show up at all the fairs, all the markets, and in full view and to the sound of drums, they exploit human stupidity," commented a practitioner of Haute-Garonne in 1879.[62] Though one was free to bring charges against them, convictions were rare, for some enjoyed the protection of local officials or even that of legitimate practitioners, with whom they sometimes worked in concert. As Dr. Lesouef told the Senate in 1892: "The person who wants to practice medicine illegally often passes as a benefactor of humanity whom the physician seeks to keep from healing his patients, and the one who has law and justice on his side rarely has the last laugh."[63]

Nor should we forget the importance attached to the power of faith. There were the healing saints, who often changed specialties from one province to another.[64] Most of all, there were the clergy and the feminine orders, which, in theory, were limited to offering counsel on diet and hygiene or, in the case of a "simple indisposition," to providing balms, poultices, herbs, and "other harmless medications." That, at least, is how one bishop in the Vosges responded in 1890 to a letter from local practitioners, who had objected that country *curés* not only offered medical counsel to their parishioners but also made erroneous diagnoses, instituted treatment, and dispensed medicines: "In other villages, the sister, regardless of her order or duties, has taken the place of the doctor. She treats the whole commune, without discrimination, comforting and sometimes, by chance, healing but also in other cases placing the patient in danger."[65]

The medical press of the early Republic bristles with such complaints. A doctor in Morbihan insists that certain sisters are designated to engage in practice, that they have their own horses and buggies, and that their clients include aristocrats as well as peasants. Another in Haute-Garonne reports that almost all the congregations maintain a pharmacy, where they dispense free medical advice while charging dearly for their drugs. Another in Haute-Marne complains that a *curé* at Musseau treats twice as many patients as he does, that he dispenses tincture of digitalis and opium purchased illegally from a proclerical pharmacist, and that the sisters are so powerful that they have succeeded in ruining all his predecessors. Still another, this one in Loire-Inférieure, is compelled to admit a certain effectiveness on their part:

Right in the heart of a town of five hundred souls you can see sisters who I know have no diploma of any kind but who, from the incision of whitlows to the removal of tumors, perform more operations in a year than many of the surgeons in the town, and with good results, as I have seen myself. Just go a bit into the countryside and you'll meet up with sisters visiting, treating, and medicating their patients *usque ad mortem*. I've seen some making their rounds on horseback.[66]

Contemporaries could cite many examples in which clerical opposition had forced nonconforming doctors to abandon their practices. Those who survived were the ones who encouraged praying to the saints, conferred with the *curé* over the advisability of surgery for a parishioner, or consulted the mother superior before discharging a patient.[67] Others, usually the medical elites whose reputations lent them a certain immunity to retaliation, countered by attacking the sisters' motives and competence.

In Paris, for example, Bourneville's *Le Progrès médical* seldom appeared without new reports concerning the sisters' conduct. They were accused of changing prescriptions, administering chloroform on their own, and killing patients with overdoses of purgatives. They plastered the wards with portraits of the Virgin, wheeled the infirm to early morning mass in freezing chapels, and treated the insane as demonically possessed. They had last rites given to dying patients who had already declined them and, in general, behaved contemptuously toward the families of Jews, Protestants, and freethinkers. The sisters were especially fanatical regarding the baptism of newborns, Bourneville charged, to the point of pressing attending physicians to perform caesarean sections on women near death, even those in the third or fourth month of pregnancy.[68]

A widespread complaint centered on the sisters' treatment of other women, particularly prostitutes and victims of sexually transmitted diseases. In 1887, Bourneville himself visited a number of provincial hospitals in order to inspect their venereal wards. At the Hôtel-Dieu in Château-Thierry, he discovered that afflicted women were housed in the ward for the senile elderly; at Bar-le-duc, they lay in the attic; at Commercy, a garrison town, they were not admitted at all, and the mother superior was unable to tell him where they were treated. At Belfort, patients were confined to a small, isolated ward with barred windows, to which was attached a tiny room for examination by speculum. It was the same at the civilian and military hospital of Saint-Dié: "At the time of our visit, on September 12, it had only one patient, a poor working girl, who hid in shame and who certainly would not have caused any scandal if anyone had had the humanity to put her in the common halls."[69]

Léonard has pointed out that the sisters symbolized just one aspect of the pervasive medical power of women in the countryside. The profession, it is true, belonged to men. Although they were not excluded by law, it was only in the 1870s that women began earning degrees at the Paris faculty, and then only in small numbers. Yet, the fact could not be denied: In addition to the sisters, feminine forces counted the midwives and matrons, whose functions ranged from delivering babies to treating gynecological maladies. As a market, the latter remained inaccessible to faculty graduates, who were baffled by women's preference for folk healers of their own sex. Just as maddening was the boldness of the midwives. "Our midwives in Eure carry out natural childbirth, manipulations, application of forceps, and all obstetrical maneuvers," one doctor complained, adding that some advertised in the press as being specialist in the treatment of female disorders. He was not alone in bemoaning the loss of the obstetrical market or in assailing the midwives' skills. In the Senate, Dr. Lourties accused rural midwives of being the prime carriers of puerperal fever, smallpox, and diphtheria.[70]

Given these conditions, why would a doctor even bother making an effort to establish himself in the countryside? The answer is that many did not and tried their luck in the cities instead. As noted earlier, however, those in our group enjoyed several advantages, in particular their local origins and their status as property owners. All were convinced that their training had given them a superiority over other claimants to medical expertise, and all were eager to extend their own role. So vast was "this intervention of medicine in all acts of life," as Langlet of Reims put it, that it consisted of nothing less than overseeing the individual's growth from infancy to old age. That refrain was heard often among the physician-legislators. To Bouisson, the doctor was the representative of science to the peasantry and the pioneer of rural progress. To Gilbert Laurent, he was "a man of the elite" who had rescued the people from ignorance: "Always, night and day, you find the doctor at his post," he told the *conseil général* of Loire in 1908, "whether it is a matter of an infant in his cradle, an invalid in his bed of suffering, an old person on his litter. . . . He is a true lay priest who shuns not fatigue, poverty and misery, the danger of contagion."[71]

It was not enough for physicians to assert the universality of their role. There also had to be concrete efforts to change the attitudes of the peasants, starting with public education. This would stress the importance of hygiene, and it would help the people appreciate the value of doctors and the merit of such triumphs as smallpox vaccination, which the church consistently refused to endorse.[72] Thus, from the first days of their practices, great numbers of our doctors were involved in the crusade for rural enlightenment. They founded popular libraries and scientific societies, lectured in the public halls, served as members of departmental councils on education, and presided over the local branch of the Ligue d'enseignement. Dozens held such titles as officer of public instruction and officer of the academy, and several made public education their specialty in municipal and departmental assemblies. Others assumed direction of local literary societies or left a mark on the cultural life of their regions in other ways. For instance, Marius Loque of Vaucluse devoted himself to preserving the remains of the ancient theater at Orange, in the same way that Auguste Baudon tried to further the study of Roman sites in Oise. Louis Parisot, a member of the Society of Emulation of Montbéliard, surveyed geological formations around Belfort, and Jules Carret explored the caves and grottoes of Chambéry and was a member of the Savoyard Society of History and Archeology. At Riom, Dr. Girard, an ardent philhellenist, led a circle dedicated to the study of Greek history and culture.

Almost 58 percent of these doctors published books or articles beyond their medical thesis. Scientific and medical topics constituted the largest category; next came social, political, literary, and agricultural themes, in that order. The subjects on which they wrote exemplify the breadth of their interests, ranging from cooperative societies and penal laws to vagrancy and public assistance and representing a variety of physician-historians, poets, biographers, literary critics, and social theorists. Dr. Rey of Lot, for example, was passionately interested in the cathedrals of his department. Dr. Villard wrote on the history of surgeons and midwives in his hometown of Guéret, and Dr. Edmond Tiersot wrote on the post-1815 restoration in his native Ain. Several studied the events of the Revolution in their regions.

The record of our group provides other clues to the tactics that all doctors used in carving inroads into the medical wilderness. Besides magnifying the universality of their skills, they sought also to consolidate their moral authority, as by their leadership during outbreaks of cholera, which proved that self-sacrifice was characteristic of their profession – in the words of Bouisson, "one of the most noble and elevated forms of civil courage."[73] Testelin, who lived through several epidemics, once remarked: "I've gone to towns that had been abandoned by their foremost magistrates. There, where there existed a profound terror, where no one dared touch the sick . . . all that was needed was for one doctor to be present, to visit the sick, to give some consolations, in order to see the number of cases decline the following day."[74] The panic to which he alluded was real and could be seen during the summer of 1884, when Clemenceau and a delegation of deputies toured cholera-stricken coastal regions in the south.[75]

Numerous doctors in parliament boasted medals for their part in combating epidemics, and many of those who held the Legion of Honor (about a fourth of the total) had earned this distinction for the same reason. One finds instances of remarkable courage. The socialist Emile Dubois, who practiced in Paris, nearly died of diphtheria after treating stricken children during an epidemic of 1890. He was not the only victim, though he had worse luck than most, having been shot earlier by a deranged patient. Another was Maximilien Lesage, hospital physician at Beauvais in Oise, who caught typhus while combating a local outbreak the same year. He survived and went on to win election to the Chamber in 1895 but died of pneumonia two years later at the age of forty-three. Such fortitude endeared the doctor to the people, and it was not uncommon for voters to be reminded of it during political campaigns. The committee supporting Alfred Lombard at Dôle in 1885, for example, stressed the value of his services during an earlier cholera attack: "The city and its environs being decimated, the young physician knew how to do his duty valiantly, and the populations that never forgot his good conduct during these sad events soon rewarded his devotion by bestowing on him their confidence."[76]

War also provided opportunities for medical heroism. All together, 46 percent were involved in the war effort of 1870–1. In addition to 7 percent who fought in the ranks, 18 percent served as medical officers, assistants, and volunteers. Another 5 percent worked as ambulance directors and 3 percent as surgeons of the Paris National Guard. A few others served as prefects, subprefects, government administrators, and local mayors. The latter often had to organize makeshift hospitals in the rear, for along with the wounded came a flood of smallpox victims. Dr. Blatin, chief physician at the camp of Pont-du-Château on the banks of the Allier, witnessed the tragedy firsthand, as did Dr. Calès, director of army medical services at Toulouse.

Others did their part, including those still in medical school. Young Félix Ducoudray of Nièvre worked with ambulance units at the battle of Sedan and was later put in charge of the hospitals of Bourges. Liouville provided aid to the besieged inhabitants of Toul, and Félix Francoz of Savoie, an intern at Lyon, was with the surrounded garrison at Bitche that put up a fierce resistance to the Germans. A few others helped out during the siege of Paris, including Ferdinand Villard, an intern at Pitié, who served as a surgeon for the National Guard. Members of the faculty also pitched in, organizing ambulance brigades and giving hurried drills to army surgeons (at the School of Practice, Lannelongue had them extracting bullets fired into cadavers). Those too advanced in years to join up expressed their readiness: "I'm more than fifty years old and have never handled guns," Roussel wrote to the minister of interior:

I do not ask for a rifle, which can be put to better use in other hands, but I am a doctor, a former hospital intern, and an author of books that several times have been cited by the Academy of Sciences and for which I have received *la croix* under the Republic. I mention these titles so that they will serve to convince, without long examination, that I can usefully go to the help of the wounded on our battlefields.[77]

As with epidemics, a war record was of no small value in building a later career in politics. When Dr. Legludic ran for parliament in 1885, a local newspaper wrote, "Although in his capacity as a doctor he would have been able to attach himself to some village ambulance service, he wished to take his part in the common valor and dangers, and went to war with the troops of the canton of Sablé, which has not forgotten him."[78]

    Men of courage and sacrifice, our doctors especially cultivated an image of themselves as apostles of hygiene, which formed the basis of the authority they claimed in family life. We learn a good deal along these lines from those who wrote popular treaties on the subject, as in the case of Dr. Etienne Ancelon, deputy for Meurthe in 1871. His *L'Art de conserver la santé*, published almost twenty years earlier, is full of counsel as to how one can maximize the chances for physical well-being; his topics range from the proper care of babies to the advantages of bathing, a subject of no small concern to rural hygienists. Along the way, he remarks on the necessity for frequently trimming the hair and toenails, the inconveniences of wearing soiled underwear (vermin), the best cure for constipation (exercise and fresh air), the usefulness of wine for health (if taken in moderation), the best way to build a house (always facing southwest, with plenty of light and air), and the warmth of the classic cotton cap ("still the best headdress for the elderly at night"). One section of his guide provides a list of the most common household injuries and how to treat them.[79]

The attention to family hygiene led many physicians to consider the matter in a broader perspective, and as they gained experience they began to learn more about the maladies that afflicted the people of their own locality. The early writings of the physician-legislators attest to this tendency, particularly in the many books and pamphlets that they wrote on public health themes. Most had a local thrust and included numerous eyewitness accounts of epidemics – Ancelon on the cholera at Château-Voué (Meurthe) in 1850, Monteils on dysentery at Mende (Lozère) in 1857, and Empereur on typhoid at Peisey (Savoie) in 1883. Carret spent a lifetime studying goiters among his native Savoyards, whereas Morvan of Finistère went to such lengths studying a certain type of whitlow common in Brittany that the ailment eventually bore his name. Some wrote medical topographies of their homelands, like Guillemaut of Saône-et-Loire, who described the physical and hygienic conditions of his native Louhans.[80] Others concentrated on diseases of occupations in their districts: Henri Doizy of Ardennes, for example, worked on *schistose,* an ailment of coal miners and slate workers that was caused by inhaling silica.[81]

In short, medical men entered the realm of public hygiene, realizing, as Chautemps told the chamber in 1890, that "death and disease are not just individual accidents; they are social accidents."[82] The views of the surgeon and deputy Jean Peyrot on the relation of housing to tuberculosis were typical:

When one has visited the lodgings of the poor and seen a tuberculous father, a mother already beginning to cough a little and two children who are obviously already infected, one understands well that it is the slums, these ghastly, airless hovels preventing isolation of the mother and father, of the children from their parents, that are the origin of this evil.[83]

Others denounced the inadequacy of the diet of the poor, arguing that the war of 1870 had proved the physical inferiority of Frenchmen, as evidenced by the number of peasant conscripts rejected for duty. The solution was more and better food, a recurring theme in the writings and speeches of the physician–legislators.

Those belonging to *conseils généraux* played an especially active role as hygienists. Of sixty-one published reports that I have been able to find under their names, public health accounted for the largest percentage, of which most dealt with epidemics and water supplies, municipal sanitation, medical assistance, hospitals and asylums, and infant mortality. Most striking is the variety of problems on which the doctors established claims of expertise. For instance, in Seine-et-Oise, Amodru advised the *conseil général* on hospital construction. In Gard, Dr. Mallet helped make policies on education for the deaf. For Jean-Alfred Brugerolles of Cantal, it was the problem of foundlings. The same patterns were visible in the cities. Dr. Augagneur launched a vigorous hygienic campaign after becoming mayor of Lyon, just as Langlet had done at Reims, where he founded a municipal bureau of hygiene in 1881. In later years, his colleague Adrien Pozzi succeeded in creating a system of meat inspection, particularly for sausages, one of the vilest products of the industry.

Efforts after 1870 to extend claims of medical authority to society as a whole had their parallels within the family circle, where they began. The doctor no longer considered himself a mere healer or hygienic adviser; he was also a councillor and intermediary, a voice of reason and reassurance helping resolve the most private conflicts. Julien Noir argued in *Le Progrès médical* in 1907 that the growth of medical influence in the public arena rested on an expansion of the doctor's "old and noble role" within the family; mothers sought his advice on child development, fathers on choosing careers for their sons, young people on the desirability of certain individuals as marriage partners. That was not all: The physician had gradually replaced the *curé* in family life and had become "the high priest of the religion of science and health."[84]

There were several methods by which our doctors were able to erode traditional delineations of medical and priestly authority. One involved the confessional aspects of practice, which sprang from their ability to convince families that they were friends and confidants. Helping them achieve this goal was the legal obligation of confidentiality – *le secret médical* – which covered a vast and undefined terrain and thus multiplied opportunities for intervening in matters outside medicine. The ability to speak the *patois* was

an added advantage in this regard, as was the ability to manipulate
the peasants psychologically. That was not hard for doctors who
were themselves just a step or two removed from the soil. "As
for me," said Dr. Viger, "I was born among the peasants; I know
their faults well, but I profoundly admire their great qualities: their
love of work, their domestic virtues, their resignation in the face
of atmospheric accidents."[85]

The kind of charity described earlier formed another priestly
component of medical influence. In 1893, around eighteen million
citizens had no medical assistance of any sort, which meant that
in times of sickness, the poorest could rely only on the generosity
of the doctor. In this, the record of physicians was a source of
professional pride, as those in parliament liked to point out.
Bourneville portrayed medical men as the original socialists, who
had always made their skills available to the poor, without charge.
Cornil emphasized the rarity with which they billed families whom
they knew to be in financial straits, and he lauded their refusal to
make clients pay in advance, as lawyers did.[86] If practiced on a
grand scale, philanthropy might imply a variety of attitudes on
the part of the physician, including the sort of opportunism that
the Right considered it to be. A royalist deputy from Morbihan
complained in 1901, for instance, that for country doctors the
electoral period never ended and that even after the patient had
paid his bill he was still not free of the doctor: "He owes him a
little thanks, and this thanks is often translated into ballots."[87]
Even the syndicates railed against the tendency of wealthy, politically ambitious physicians treating patients free of charge, to the
detriment of poorer colleagues.[88]

It would be a mistake, however, to assume that the social conscience exhibited by many in our group sprang entirely from political ambition. In a "Letter to a Young Doctor" published by
L'Union médicale in 1872, a physician warned beginners that "each
day the practitioner sees touching dramas and cruel sufferings, and
although he is used to these sorts of scenes, it is impossible for
him not to become involved in the misfortunes he witnesses."
Clemenceau, whose defense of the workers during the 1880s surely
owed something to his early medical experiences, once recalled
the sadness he had felt while making his rounds in Montmartre,
whose malnourished inhabitants spent their lives going from infected lodgings to infected workshops: "I saw there, in the space

of a few years, all that one could see of infirmities and sufferings of life below."[89]

This description of the early medical careers of our doctors thus begins to uncover some of the broad sources of their growing authority. Their achievements in this domain necessarily involved ideological commitment; however genuine their wish to act as mediators, most had long abandoned any pretense to social neutrality and had come to accept the premise, as De Lanessan expressed it, the men of science were obligated to take sides in the "implacable combat" between past and future.[90] For the majority, the reality was less dramatic. As Hippolyte Jeanne noted in *Le Concours médical,* the doctor's routine dealings with municipal officials alone often made it impossible for him to resist involvement in politics – "sometimes for making sure our rights are respected (that's most often the case), at other times for pointing out the glaring shortcomings of an organization that's being sabotaged by incompetents."[91] We will turn now to the doctors' early political careers and to some of the specific ways in which their medical practices involved them in local affairs.

3

Early political careers

This chapter will examine the political activities of our doctors at the local level, before their entry into national life. After tracing their record in municipal and departmental offices, we will present some representative examples of their parliamentary campaigns, a sketch of their party labels, the relationship of these to their social and geographical origins, and the degree to which they reflected class values. Through an analysis of campaign platforms (the *professions de foi*), we will show the kinds of issues on which the doctors claimed special expertise when defending their qualifications. Our central goal is to discover those areas in which the doctor's professional concerns and his medical services to the community affected his political motivation and his prospects for success. It is thus important to determine whether his calling influenced his decision to enter public life and whether medical candidacies exhibited any distinguishing traits.

THE SOURCES OF POLITICAL MOTIVATION

Thus far, our analysis has stressed two sources for the doctors' political consciousness. The first is their class identity, the second their medical training and experiences. But none of this means that other motives, unrelated to medicine, had no part. Some doctors, for example, belonged to families that had a long tradition of officeholding. Jean Dêche, physician-mayor of Calonges, was careful to invoke his father's memory during the campaign of 1902, reminding voters that he was a "republican by tradition" and that the seat he held on the *conseil général* was the one that his father had occupied in 1848.[1] The importance of family political ties can be seen in the proportion having relatives in the Chamber or Senate (13 percent), which included several fathers and sons, such as the Allemands of Basses-Alpes and the Reymonds of Loire.

Nevertheless, there were those practictioners who believed that medical men should not become involved in politics. "It was not that I was uninterested in my country's affairs," one wrote later, "but I had neither the time nor the taste to get mixed up in party struggles."[2] The point was made frequently in letters to medical journals, many of them complaining about the competitive threat posed by physician-politicians. During the elections of 1910, a doctor in Roquefort lamented that he had searched in vain for a single contest that did not feature a medical man as "the first subject or impresario," and he voiced his contempt for *"les politiciens parasites"* of the profession, noting that in his department, thirteen of twenty-eight members of the *conseil général* were physicians and that in his immediate locale, seven of thirteen occupied an elective office. How did they get there? Through "bargain medicine," which worked according to the formula: "I treat you; vote for me."[3]

Others perceived an ethical conflict between politics and medicine. They advised their colleagues to maintain neutrality or, if they insisted on seeking office, to do so as private citizens – "under pain of passing at one and the same time as a bad practitioner and a bad politician."[4] In a speech to students at Reims in 1897, the pathologist Jean-Baptiste Duguet stressed that if the doctor did not resist – "if he does not remain profoundly and exclusively attached to the medical art, he's done for. Politics will absorb him and he will be devoured by it. As a doctor, he has only friends; when he becomes a politician, he will see his own friends turn against him." One of the worse fates was exposure to ridicule, as Duguet related in the case of a colleague: "Among us, when the question of his medical value came up, one always smiled but added: 'It appears that at the Chamber he's found his place.' On their side, the deputies, his other colleagues, laughed at his political naïveté but said among themselves: 'It seems that as a doctor he is not without value.'"[5]

The erosion of one's standing as a mediator in community life and, with it, the alienation of clientele were for many doctors sufficient reason to steer clear of partisan squabbles. As proof, one need only glance at the emotions unleashed during the campaigns of our group, among whom most had suffered the kinds of "passionate attacks and outrageous slanders" of which Dr. Empereur complained in Savoie. Clament of Dordogne, caught up in a bitter rivalry with a royalist *châtelain* at Bergerac in 1889, reminded the people that his father had practiced medicine for fifty years in the canton and that "the honor of my family puts me above the calumnies and lies that are being chalked up to my account by salaried agents and old offenders." Louis Amagat, forced into a runoff the same year in Cantal, assured citizens that his only goal in continuing the race was "to make of this arrondissement, troubled by a few egotists, one single family, while exhibiting to my adversaries a heart that is strong and generous enough to forget all the insults."[6] Some candidates even suffered injury, such as Dr. Vacher of Corrèze, who lost an eye at a political rally after being attacked with an umbrella. Clashes with sword or pistol were common, despite the ethical dilemma that dueling posed for medical men. In his youth, Dr. Chavoix of Dordogne actually killed an opponent.

Once in office, the doctor found himself drawn more deeply into the fray. If he held any hospital or public service posts, there was always the possibility that the loser would invoke the Organic Law of 10 August 1871. This measure barred from the *conseils généraux* all individuals who were "salaried or paid a subvention from government funds," such as departmental architects. Some administrators believed that this category also included any doctor who performed public services for pay, however small. Over the years, the Ministry of Interior tried to be flexible, applying the provision only to those receiving substantial salaries.[7] But there remained the even more heated issue of eligibility for the office of mayor. Before 1884, all "salaried agents of the commune" were excluded, a measure often invoked when it suited the political purposes of local authorities. Exempted were physicians and other professionals who performed part-time services for the commune or department, but medical men who held hospital posts faced a real conflict of interest, because the mayor served as president of the hospital administrative commission. That stopped few from trying, however, although in the process they risked losing their hospital positions.

Why were so many willing to assume the risks? Political scientists of the modern era have raised the question often in regard to all politicians. Their findings, derived from studies of legislators in France, Colombia, Brazil, and the Dominican Republic, provide insights into our own inquiry. An example is the work of Oliver H. Woshinsky on the modern French deputy, based on research and interviews carried out during the late 1960s.[8] Arguing that "a man's actions in politics are dependent on his reasons for being in politics," Woshinsky uses a method called *incentive analysis* in order to postulate four motivational sources in French politics. These four sources are *status* (the desire to increase one's personal prestige), *program* (the desire to work on public problems and to manipulate one's environment for the social good), *mission* (the desire to serve a quasi-religious cause transcending one's private interests), and *obligation* (the desire to expiate feelings of guilt by fulfilling the moral duties of citizenship). Overall, Woshinsky found less evidence to support traditional interpretations of the French deputy as being motivated by ideological goals than for the idea that his behavior was intensely personal and derived from "internal motivational forces."[9]

These findings help delineate broad patterns of behavior among the physician-legislators, in that they confirm the presence of two key forms of motivation – status and program – which for French practitioners of that era were closely linked. Accepting the view that what a politician does in office reflects his motives for being there, one is led to conclude that programmatic goals were of central importance in our doctors' motivation and that these goals were the logical corollary of their self-identity as social hygienists. Their zeal in this regard is reflected in their labors on behalf of health and welfare in local assemblies, and it becomes even more evident in their work as members of parliament. As we shall see later, the aggregate traits that they evinced there correspond closely to the identifying characteristics of the program participants as defined by Woshinsky: an interest in public policies, extensive involvement in committee activity, and immersion in the concrete details of problem solving.[10]

Nevertheless, it is hard to detach this programmatic theme from its ideological context, which for men of medicine involved more than abstract principles. I refer in particular to the nature of local politics under the Third Republic, which was marked by bitter quarrels among factions and which placed limits on the doctors' autonomy. How those in our group responded to these forces depended on their resources, professional as well as economic.

Few, however, could resist being pulled into the whirlpool that they created.

First, the hope of building a clientele often placed doctors of modest means in a position of dependency. For example, one physician estimated in 1901 that nine-tenths of his colleagues "rely entirely on a coterie, white or red, which calls them, patronizes them, supports them, maintains them by every mean." While one courted the clergy and the devout of the canton, he observed, another looked to the mayor, the municipal council, and the sub-prefect: "The doctor, as simply a doctor, without being a party man, is everywhere viewed poorly and held in suspicion by various coteries."[11] Dr. Edouard Duchemin, who practiced in a rural canton in the west, said much the same thing, describing the doctor's life as a constant struggle against "the secret but effective hostility of all the bigwigs who prevail like royalty over the spirit of the peasants and who can make or unmake a practice at will." To succeed,

you absolutely have to be part of a clan, either clerical or republican, and to be involved in politics, that is to say, to occupy yourself with elections, to drink by the bowlful in the favorite inn of the party, and to figure in all public meetings where the "bosses" appear.

Thanks to this, one will have on his side all the influence of the priests, and it remains great in this area. The other will benefit from all sorts of administrative favors and the support of government partisans.[12]

Occasionally, leaders of particular communities went so far as to seek out doctors who sympathized with local interests. *La Gazette des eaux* marveled in 1898 at the many advertisements in classified sections of medical journals seeking a "republican" or "conservative" physician. "The truth," it pointed out, "is that these requests disguise poorly the ridiculous pretensions of some country squire . . . or, worse still, the annoying need for a union of sectarian and ignorant mediocrities, ambitious and impatient to impose a forced regulation on the ideas of others."[13] Julien Noir warned beginners to be wary in accepting such invitations, especially when they came from the mayor, the pharmacist, of the *curé,* for they were often part of a scheme to undermine an established practitioner who had remained independent of their influence or who had crossed them in some way.[14]

Second, despite the centralization of French medical training, local governments had significant influence over the actual conditions of practice. The tendency of many officials to wink at illegal practice is one example, but even more important was their control over the administration of health and welfare. The mayor himself functioned as the country's chief hygienic officer by virtue of Article 471 of the Penal Code, which designated him as the individual responsible for carrying out the prefect's decrees involving the sanitary police.

As president of the administrative commission of hospitals, the mayor was also in a position to influence the awarding of hospital posts, which, as one doctor called them, were "the currency of the official candidature."[15] Under the Second Empire, and again during the *seize-mai* crisis of 1877, the victims of firings from medical posts were usually leftists; later, under the Republic, the targets shifted to Catholic practitioners.[16] Passage of the Medical Assistance Act of 1893 strengthened the mayor's powers in this respect, for, as Duchemin observed, it was often he who made up the lists of people who qualified for aid. This meant that he could punish his physician-opponents by refusing to send them patients. "One thing is certain," wrote Duchemin, "in order to benefit from assistance, it is essential to be a mayor, a municipal councillor, or at least an influential electoral agent."[17] Capturing the office of mayor, or just winning a seat on the municipal council, thus had distinct professional advantages. Among those in our group, 40 percent had served on municipal councils, and 47 percent had been local mayors.[18]

A municipal post was usually the first step on the road to national office. Next came the *conseil général,* where one proved himself worthy by his committee activities and speaking ability.[19] Just over 74 percent of our doctors had sat on *conseils généraux*; of these, over 15 percent served as presidents and 11 percent as vice-presidents. Throughout the period as a whole, the percentage of medical men in these assemblies ranged between 12 and 14 percent. Their strength can best be seen during the periodic elections that renewed half the membership, as in July 1895, when physicians accounted for almost 13 percent of all winning candidates. Their best showing came in the Massif Central (22% of the winners) and in the southwest (19%). In some departments, doctors represented nearly a third of all candidates, and in Corrèze the figure reached 40 percent.[20] If we assume the same patterns for the remaining half of the *conseils généraux*, which is suggested by the number of winning physicians in previous elections, the total would represent about 3 percent of all doctors.[21]

Those whose status as well-to-do landowners afforded them a certain immunity to local intrigues were susceptible on another front: the pressures put on them by political committees, which sought to capitalize on their popularity. A doctor's influence could hardly have passed unnoticed by local power brokers, who were quick to recognize the potential political value of his style and social identity. Our doctors, for example, featured an unusually large number of "characters," whose eccentricities probably enhanced their appeal. Some were not far removed from the images of popular literature, in which the doctor, in high hat and pince-nez, appears as a man brimming over with ideas and energy, as the local representative of culture who can quote Latin yet speak the language of the cultivator, who vaunts his disdain for the clergy while retaining the admiration of the pious, who could no doubt sense a heart of gold beneath the brusque facade.

One thinks of Jules Carret, who spent much of his life preaching science and atheism to his native Savoyards. Physician for a group of Savoyard irregulars in 1870, Carret won two elections to the Chamber and then lost interest in politics, retiring toward the end of his life to spend his time exploring caves. He willed his fortune to his hometown of Chambéry and stipulated that every three years it was to award a prize of ten thousand francs "to the young Savoyard girl who is best constituted from the physical and moral points of view."[22]

There were others, such as Philippe Grenier, a bachelor who practiced among the poor at Pontarliers in Doubs and later lived in Algeria, where he experienced a religious vision. Returning home and winning election to the Chamber in 1896, he appeared at the Palais-Bourbon dressed in the hooded white cloak of an Arab holy man, the first Muslim ever to serve in parliament.

And there was Alcide Treille, who so opposed the use of quinine for malaria that during the middle of a political campaign he went off to a German medical congress to denounce "the assassin drug." A bicycle fanatic and president of the Biking Club of Algeria, Treille once rode for a hundred kilometers and managed to deliver a speech immediately afterwards "without coughing, spitting, or drinking."

Oddest of all was the radical of Aube, Casimir-Laurent Michou, who could often be seen riding to the Palais-Bourbon on a velocipede, an early version of the bicycle. A miser who lived in a shabby Latin Quarter apartment, he often appeared in the marketplaces with a sack of vegetables slung over his shoulder. In parliament, he irritated his colleagues by stuffing his pockets with sandwiches from the Chamber canteen and eating them during sessions. Once, during a debate over providing fresh water for Paris, he denied that the Seine could cause typhoid and voiced his doubts that the average Parisian drank forty-eight liters of water a day, only to be reminded that some people used water for other purposes than drinking.[23]

So great was the local fame of certain of our doctors that they were able to make respectable showings just by allowing their names to be placed on the ballot. In 1902, Gustave Ravier, a small-town practitioner in Cher, received nearly 4,500 votes "without campaigning, without a committee, isolated." That was not enough to win, but as he boasted four years later, it proved his vote-getting ability as "a man of the countryside, who has always lived in the midst of you."[24] Running without a committee was unusual, however, as serious contenders had to rely on them for campaign organization and fund-raising. A typical membership was Dr. Clech's in Finistère during the elections of 1889, which included the vice-president of the *conseil général,* along with numerous mayors, *conseillers généraux,* municipal councillors, physicians, pharmacists, and other professional men. That of Sabaterie in Puy-de-Dôme in 1902 had a total of forty-one members, of whom thirty-six were local mayors; its officers included the president of the *conseil général,* and it had its own newspaper.

In some cases, committees were handpicked by the candidate, especially if he had money. In others, they were the product of regional congresses, which had extended to the candidate the invitation to run.[25] Such invitations, no doubt, were the fruit of lobbying on the part of some doctors, but on other occasions the initiative came from the committees themselves which, above all else, wanted a candidate who could beat the opposition.

Thus, Emile Guyot of the Rhône declared in his campaign manifesto of 1876: "If the central committee believes that my modest reputation, my feeble personality, can be useful to the cause, I am at its disposal, even if my medical position has to be sacrificed." Sabaterie spoke of "the insistence that true and sincere republicans of this arrondissement have strongly shown in wishing me to offer myself as a candidate." Pierre Bichon of Maine-et-Loire pointed to "the reiterated entreaties of a great number of old republicans." Aimé Evesque of Drôme alluded to the prompting of friends "who have spontaneously put my name forward while recalling the services that I have been able to render to the democratic cause and to the interests of our region."[26]

Local committees well understood the strategies for transforming the doctor's popularity into votes. Dr. Bavoux's backers in 1881 reminded citizens of Jura that "throughout his long career as a doctor, in the midst of the populations of our arrondissement, he has recognized neither rich nor poor, serving everyone with the same devotion."[27] The supporters of Dr. Girard at Riom in 1893 extolled his "forty years of public life as a doctor, a municipal councillor, a mayor, a *conseiller général,* years during which he has the conscience of having done his duty." And Dr. Sabaterie's campaigners in 1902 assured electors, "He is of the people by blood and by choice. You can be certain that he will never betray you."[28]

The efforts of committees to exploit the doctor's popularity, plus the doctor's own interest in defending his rights, thus help round out our explanation of why medical men in France were unable to resist the allure of public life. Those who succeeded freely admitted their debt to medicine. As Adolphe Pedebidou told the Civil Society of *Le Concours médical* in 1894, most doctors in parliament had "forced its gates thanks to sympathies acquired during the practice of our profession."[29] In all cases, however, the effort to win political office was carried out on an individual basis, which is to say that doctors did not run as representatives of their profession.

Some doctors thought it should be otherwise. One practitioner, writing in 1898, complained that "each time a doctor clears the gates of the Palais-Bourbon, his first concern is to forget his origins." He proposed that the profession sponsor "medical candidates" in each department who would subscribe to a professional agenda.[30] *Le Concours médical* admitted the difficulty of such an undertaking, because unlike workers, who tended to belong to the same political groupings, doctors ranged from republicans to monarchists. Still, it believed that common action was possible as long as it was based on mutual interests rather than ideology. Thus, in 1898, Cézilly and others at the Civil Society urged doctors to create local committees, which would spell out desired legislation and support candidates who promised their help. Subsequently, the Civil Society drew up an "electoral platform of doctors," which divided campaign issues into three areas: social questions, professional questions, and matters of public interest involving the medical corps. It singled out physician-candidates in particular, saying that pledges should be extracted from them to support this platform and to place themselves at the service of professional groups.[31]

In truth, such a strategy had little hope of success, for local politics under the Third Republic precluded anyone from winning office as the candidate of a particular profession. Dr. Doizy, deputy of Ardennes, reminded a medical gathering in 1912 that physicians were not the deputies of other physicians and that although they should try to be responsive to professional grievances, their electors had not given them a mandate to represent the medical profession.[32] If anything, once in office, many medical men had to disguise or even abandon their natural concerns in order to escape charges that they were promoting selfish professional interests. Emile Chautemps, deputy for Haute-Savoie, told the Syndicate of Physicians of the Seine in 1899 that because doctors who intervened on medical matters in parliament were considered suspect, he had deliberately sought out areas of activity that had little to do with medicine, such as the navy and colonies.[33]

PHYSICIAN-CANDIDACIES, CAMPAIGNS, AND POLITICAL LABELS

We will next consider how men of medicine conducted themselves as campaigners. In most contests in this period, the proportion of doctors among all candidates stood at 3 to 4 percent and occasionally ran higher. How do their rates of success compare with those of others? The French scholar Mattei Dogan has estimated that during the whole of the Third and Fourth Republics, close to forty thousand individuals ran for seats in the Chamber, some of them repeatedly, and that only six thousand, or 15 percent, managed to gain the prize.[34] By contrast (and insofar as one can

Table 3.1. *Physician-candidates for Chamber of Deputies, 1881–1914*

Election year	Number of candidates	Percentage of winners
1881	81	64.1
1885	113	42.4
1889	90	55.5
1893	92	73.9
1898	115	52.1
1902	121	47.1
1906	102	53.9
1910	128	46.0
1914	170	32.9

Source: Candidate lists by department in *Le Temps*

judge from the number who are identified as physicians on candidate lists in the press), doctors enjoyed fairly strong ratios of winners to losers. As can be seen in Table 3.1, their weakest performance came during the elections of 1885, when the system of single-member constituencies (the *scrutin d'arrondissement*), which favored doctors and others among the local elites, was temporarily abandoned in favor of departmental slates (the *scrutin de liste*).

No doubt, doctors enjoyed an advantage as campaigners because of their intimate knowledge of families. Addressing an elector by his first name or its diminutive, as Paul Vigné d'Octon later recalled, often sufficed in rural corners of the Midi to win over even the most hostile. But Vigné also remembered the hazards of campaign life – the endless rounds of toasts, the gaffes and unforeseen incidents, the insults, and especially the *coup de la dernière heure*. This last hazard developed into a veritable science under the Republic and represented a last-ditch effort to damage the opposition's chances, such as circulating rumors that its candidate had died or had been killed in a duel. Dr. Ferroul, socialist of Narbonne, was one of many to accuse his opponents of stuffing ballot boxes. For Paul Defontaine of the Nord, it was the mine owners' intimidation of his working-class supporters at polling places. In virtually all contests, republicans damned the interference of the priests, and on numerous occasions those in our group found themselves pitted against rich and powerful families who enjoyed the backing of the clergy, as happened in 1902 at Saint-Flour.

The incumbent, an obscure doctor named Pierre Hugon, faced Count Jean de Castellane, a stranger to Cantal, although his father had represented it during the 1870s. "Monsieur Jean" started early, dispensing largess throughout the communes in support of hospitals, fire halls, public fountains, and town clocks. His backers dealt harshly with Dr. Hugon, describing him as the offspring of rapacious peasants who had schemed and saved in order to advance themselves, selling their barley sugar for a *sou* while adding to their houses and lands. The doctor, they said, had an annual income of 20,000 francs, yet took his meals in the Chamber canteen to save money and had made the arrondissement of Saint-Flour "a laughingstock among the deputies and ministers." Hugon's supporters, including most of the mayors and members of the *conseil général*, in turn attacked "this haughtily rich noble" as the spokesman for reactionary Catholics in Saint-Flour, even accusing him of having taken money from Prussia. The doctor himself said little, seemingly befuddled at being made the symbol of the Republic and the means by which to keep the rich from making the town their fief. He lost, but he need not have worried, as republicans in the new legislature annulled Castellane's election on the grounds that he had tried to buy his way into parliament. The count offered a rational defense, pointing out that Hugon himself had boasted of having dispensed at home 62,000 francs in public monies during his previous tenure as deputy. As for donating a clock to the town hall of Malbo, "It chimes for my adversaries as it does for my friends."[35]

Invalidation was a favorite tactic of the majority in Paris, often extricating the party faithful from a sticky situation at home. Almost any protest was sufficient to prompt an investigation. The right-wing doctor Eugène Livois, mayor of Boulogne, was among the lucky few. He had roundly whipped his republican adversary by almost four thousand votes in 1877, only to find his admission to the Chamber threatened by a committee report that attributed his victory to clerical interference. Livois spoke in his own defense during the hearings, quoting the violent attacks that had appeared in his opponent's journal and crediting his victory to his own popularity as a medical practitioner of twenty-five years standing.[36]

Similarly, a Bonapartist physician of Gironde named Alcée Froin, who in 1889 beat a local republican mayor, faced a protest accusing him of having enjoyed the support of wealthy vineyard owners who had pressured their servants and workers into voting for him. The protest also accused his backers on the *conseil général* of buying an additional five hundred votes by promising relief funds to farmers whose pigs had been killed by swine fever. During the parliamentary inquiry, Froin attributed the charges to the conniving of a local pharmacist and a justice of the peace, ascribing his success to the fact that he had practiced medicine free of charge for thirty-seven years and had never refused aid to a sick person, whatever the patient's political opinions. Froin lost his case but got revenge the next month by defeating his opponent.[37] In contrast with the unfavorable ruling in his case, complaints from conservatives about the tactics of republican doctors usually fell on deaf ears.[38]

In several instances, doctors were the chief actors in long-standing family rivalries, as occurred at Mende in Lozère. On one side was the monarchist Amédée Monteils, who had practiced since 1849 and who enjoyed great influence as municipal councillor and president of the Society of Agricultural Arts and Sciences of Lozère. On the other was the Bourrillon family, fiercely republican and long prominent in the region's economic life. Monteils won a seat in the Chamber during the *seize-mai* crisis of 1877 on a platform of "Religion and Liberty," beating a member of the Bourrillon family. The latter took revenge in 1881, but the doctor triumphed again four years later. Parliament nullified the results, however, and although Monteils ran once more in 1889, he received few votes and then retired from politics for good. By then, a younger member of the Bourrillon family, Maurice, later to become a deputy, was already creating a thriving practice and enjoying growing influence on the municipal council.

If the sight of physicians ripping at opponents troubled many in the profession, worse still was to see two doctors in combat. One example, in Allier, involved Cornil and a young protégé named Jules Gacon, who, in 1878, had opened a practice in Donjon and had quickly gained a reputation as a militant radical. After capturing the office of mayor, he went on to win a seat on the *conseil général,* where he attracted the notice of its president, Senator Cornil. With his backing, Gacon entered the Chamber in 1889 and began making a name for himself on committees, at the same time continuing to build his base in Allier. By 1898, he was strong enough to wrest the presidency of the *conseil général* from his mentor. The final blow came five years later, when he successfully challenged Cornil for his Senate seat. Cornil accepted his eclipse with his usual grace, but that was not the case for the aging Dr. Theulier of Dordogne who, in a bitter contest in 1906, was beaten by his former friend and protégé, Dr. Sireyjol, after trying to stage a comeback. During the campaign, the latter's posters had portrayed Theulier as the puppet of a reactionary coterie guided solely "by their personal interests, their malice, and their tenacious hate."[39]

Such examples illustrate the realities of office seeking and the extent to which personal rancor often defined campaigns. Once embarked on the campaign trail, it was impossible for medical men to assume that their calling would afford them any immunity. This was especially the case insofar as the Right was concerned, for many Catholics saw doctors as materialists and radicals. Most dangerous of all was the *médecin de campagne,* who was in daily contact with the masses. Witness the alarm sounded by one conservative newspaper in 1876:

Medicine is the absolute applied to the treatment of disease, just as radicalism is the absolute applied to the organization of society. You can thus say that radicalism and medicine have a reciprocal attraction and that there exists between them a natural affinity. Medicine subjects the human body to experiments; radicalism does the same thing to society. In both cases, those doing the experimenting care little for the subject, and the subject's final state matters little to them. The doctor always has an advantage in that if the experiment goes badly, the subject disappears without complaining. . . .

This explains why medicine constitutes such an excellent preparation for radicalism. A doctor who kills his patient without flinching is ready for radical politics. He'll vote for the most enormous propositions: the income tax, the suppression of all religion, and the abolition of private property.

The author then sketched a picture of the country doctor, which is typical of that drawn by conservative spokesman in parliament well into the twentieth century:

Doctors, especially in the provinces, are the most active agents of radicalism. . . . There are many villages, lost in the fields or woods, where politics would never have penetrated without the doctor.

When you see him in the countryside coming toward you in his one-

Table 3.2. *Political ideology of doctors and type of membership in parliament, 1876–1914*

Political ideology	Percentage of deputies only (N = 233)	Percentage of senators serving first in Chamber (N = 71)	Percentage of senators only (N = 52)
Right	1.6	0.0	5.7
Conservative republican	9.5	9.6	11.5
Moderate republican	38.0	50.0	71.0
Radical	45.0	40.4	10.1
Socialist	5.7	0.0	1.4

horse gig, you can say to yourself: "Here comes the apostle of radicalism." Somewhere, there in his carriage pouch, next to his black bag and medicines, he has a stack of radical pamphlets. He has over the inhabitants of the countryside the ascendancy of a man whom everyone believes to be very learned, whom one sees only in very grave circumstances, like birth or death, and whom in both cases people are used to viewing as a sort of god. With all that going for him – and if he doesn't charge his patients too much or pressure them to pay before the end of the year – he can congratulate himself on holding his clients in the palm of his hand insofar as politics is concerned.[40]

On what is this legendary image based? If we consider the percentages for all 358 physician-legislators, including the more conservative elements who sat only in the Senate, we discover in the following list that moderate republicanism was their most dominant ideological characteristic:

Right (monarchist, Bonapartist)	2.8%
Conservative republican	11.3
Moderate (opportunist) republican	48.2
Radical, radical-socialist	34.4
Socialist	3.1

The degree of radicalism increases, however, if we focus on those doctors who served only in the Chamber. The latter owed their seats to universal manhood suffrage, and they accounted for the great majority. Table 3.2 illustrates this pattern, showing that half of those who served only in the lower house identified themselves as radicals, radical-socialists, or socialists. The popular view of doctors as radicals was thus not without foundation.

The explanation for this leftist orientation has many facets, several of which were touched on in Chapter 1. For the moment, let us probe the matter in light of Dogan's argument that a deputy's social origins, as defined by his father's occupation, constituted a more important determinant of ideology than did his profession. Dogan contends that before 1914 the social composition of the Chamber showed a marked decline of the nobility, whose representatives had accounted for one out of three deputies during the early 1870s. By 1893, nobles made up 23 percent of all deputies, but by 1919 just 10 percent. A slower decline occurred within the ranks of the *haute* bourgeoisie (36% in 1871 down to 30% in 1919). Judged by the backgrounds of cabinet ministers, this class, aided by the *moyenne* bourgeoisie and the nobility, ruled the country during the pre–1899 "Republic of Dukes," afterwards sharing power with the *moyenne* and starting the search for support within the *petite*. It was the two latter classes that showed the most consistent gains after 1871, and it was from them that over two-thirds of all radicals in parliament came.[41]

In regard to our doctors, Dogan's thesis can be confirmed by analyzing any of the legislatures of the period. That of 1893 provides a good example. According to Dogan, 30 percent of the deputies who belonged to it came from the *moyenne* bourgeoisie and 10 percent from the *petite*. The respective figures for physician-deputies were 52 and 41 percent, and even these figures include within the *moyenne* all those whose fathers were professional men or rural *propriétaires,* many of whom certainly ranked among the *petite*. Not one physician-deputy came from the nobility, and only 1.6 percent came from the *haute* bourgeoisie.

Explanations of ideology that are derived solely from social class, however, tend to ignore the degree to which work and other forms of experience affect one's view of the world. These include not only the theoretical values of particular professions but also a range of attitudes that grow up during one's interaction with clients. Gaudemet has suggested this idea in alluding to the tendency of lawyers of that era to view human problems within a conservative and juridical frame of reference.[42] As we shall see later, that tendency contrasted with the more pronounced prag-

matism of the physician-deputies, who were somewhat more open
to legislative innovation in areas in which social and hygienic
reforms departed from precedent or from traditional assumptions
regarding individual liberty and contractual rights. The lay ethos
that characterized the great majority of such doctors was most
certainly related to their professional lives.

There remains the matter of geographical origins, whose influence overlapped with that of class and profession. A fourth of our
doctors, for example, won election in those departments where
republican and radical ideas had deep roots.[43] Along with Paris,
these included parts of the southeast and the Mediterranean Midi,
plus several departments of the Center. The latter rallied to republicanism later than the Midi did, but it could boast a fairly
consistent leftist tradition from the 1870s on. The Left was also
at home in the Pyrénées and Massif Central, although, as François
Goguel notes, several departments of the latter long retained their
prochurch sentiments. Rightist tendencies were most pronounced
in the west; in our group, the west had the weakest proportion
of radicals and contributed the largest share of monarchists and
conservative republicans. The southwest, a region of unstable
opinion, can be characterized as conservative in outlook at the
birth of the Republic, although leftist ideas were strong in Dordogne and Haute-Garonne and, after 1900, in Landes and
Gers.[44]

Because 80 percent of the doctors represented the department
where they were born, their regional distributions in parliament
resembled those for their regional origins. Overall, the departments that had the most physician-deputies were (in percentages)
the Seine (5.0), Dordogne (3.3), and Haute-Vienne (2.2), followed
by the Nord, Rhône, and Saône-et-Loire (1.9 each), and Allier,
Basses-Alpes, Corrèze, and Puy-de-Dôme (1.6 each). After Paris
and the Massif Central, the leading provinces were Aquitaine,
Bourgogne, the center plains, Jura, and Languedoc. Focusing exclusively on those who sat in the Chamber yields the distributions
in Table 3.3.

Table 3.4 shows a cross tabulation of the physician-deputies'
region of representation by political orientation. We see that the
most leftist (radicals, radical-socialists, and socialists) constituted
over half their respective proportions in Paris, the Center, the

Table 3.3. *Region of physician-deputies' representation, 1876–1914*

Region	%
North	7.1
East	10.4
Paris region and the Center	16.1
West	12.9
Southwest	11.5
Massif Central	14.0
Lyon region, Savoy, and Dauphiné	12.9
Mediterranean region	10.0
Overseas colonies	4.6

Table 3.4. *Cross tabulation of region represented by physician-deputies' political ideology, 1876–1914*

Region	Right (%)	Conservative republican (%)	Moderate republican (%)	Radical (%)	Socialist (%)
North	5.5	5.5	44.4	33.3	11.1
East	0.0	7.6	50.0	34.6	7.6
Paris region and Center[a]	0.0	6.8	31.8	50.0	11.3
West	3.1	12.5	46.8	37.5	0.0
Southwest	6.4	19.3	38.7	32.2	3.2
Massif Central	0.0	8.8	32.3	55.8	2.9
Lyon, Savoy, and Dauphiné	0.0	13.7	31.0	51.7	3.4
Mediterranean region	0.0	0.0	38.4	53.8	7.6

[a]Of the eighteen doctors elected in Paris, eleven were radicals and four were socialists.

Massif Central, the southeast, and the Mediterranean Midi. The minority conservatives typically won election in departments in the north, west, and southwest.

Although there are no dramatic correlations between medical specialties and ideology, one can discern a few tendencies (see Table 3.5). Nonpractitioners had the highest proportions of rad-

Table 3.5. *Cross tabulation of type of practitioner by political ideology*

Practitioner	Right (%)	Conservative republican (%)	Moderate republican (%)	Radical (%)	Socialist (%)
Country doctors	3.0	6.7	46.7	41.5	1.5
Town doctors	2.6	15.4	53.8	24.4	3.0
Big-city doctors	0.0	4.9	41.5	43.9	9.7
Professors	0.0	22.6	41.9	32.3	3.2
Agriculturalists	0.0	16.6	58.3	25.0	0.0
Former army	18.1	27.3	45.5	9.1	0.0
Former navy	0.0	10.0	70.0	20.0	0.0
Administrators	8.3	8.3	41.6	41.6	0.0
Nonpractitioners	0.0	11.1	22.2	44.4	22.2

icals and socialists, followed by those who practiced in big cities, except for professors, of whom more than two-thirds embraced a moderate-to-conservative republicanism. Close to 42 percent of the country doctors ran under radical banners. The most conservative were former army and navy doctors, along with the *médecins-agriculteurs*.

In the next chapter, I will examine more closely what these labels actually implied in parliamentary life, how they compared with those describing lawyers, and how their meanings changed over time. For now, our concern is with their general implications, for although the issues that the doctors raised during their campaigns were diverse, certain values remained constant among moderates and radicals alike.

POLITICAL IDEAS AND CAMPAIGN THEMES

Among the sentiments expressed most frequently in the campaign literature of the physician-legislators was that of *laïcité*, a term that appears in almost three-fourths of their platforms. In tracing the doctors' vision of a society purged of clerical influence, it is impossible to measure religious attitudes with any precision, for anticlericalism did not, in itself, imply the absence of belief. For instance, Bernard Lavergne, long an opponent of the clergy in Tarn, considered reason alone to be incapable of satisfying human needs and argued that most people still believed in God and an afterlife.[45] Still, there are a number of clues. Of the eighty cases for which good information is available, 13 percent were devout Catholics, 36 percent conformist Catholics, 5 percent nominal Protestants, and 44 percent freethinker, which included an assortment of deists, agnostics, and militant atheists. Devout Jews made up only 1 percent; a handful of others with Jewish backgrounds considered themselves freethinkers.

The truly pious thus represented only a small minority in our samples, and most of these were distributed among the ranks of monarchists, Bonapartists, or right-wing republicans. Topping the list was the Vendean Paul Bourgeois, legitimist and Catholic to the core, followed by Urbain Clédou, mayor of Navarrenx in Basses-Pyrénées, who called himself a "resolute conservative" and declared his program to be the defense of "religion, property, and the family." Adrien Michel, mayor of Yssingeaux in Haute-Loire, ran under the banner of "God and Country" in 1902, denouncing freemasons and promising to work toward abrogating the laws on the congregations and reestablishing the Falloux law. The anti-Semitic and anti-Freemason physician of Mayenne, Charles Daniel, was the brother of a priest and ran for parliament with the support of local clerical authorities.[46]

The religious conformists tended to keep silent on matters of dogma, occasionally condemning the excesses of clericals and anticlericals alike. Though favoring the separation of church and state, Félix Martin of Saône-et-Loire rejected the notion that "religious nihilism is a civic duty" and condemned those who mocked families that attended mass.[47] Most in this group tried to maintain neutrality in religious quarrels, but sometimes the campaign brochures of even these contain a thinly veiled hostility toward the church. In Puy-de-Dôme, Léon Chambige proclaimed himself "tolerant in religion, respectful of all beliefs, but firmly resolved to require of the clergy the same respect for our institutions." In Côtes-du-Nord, Charles Baudet employed a simple formula: "The mayor at his office, the priest at the church, the teacher at the school." In Dordogne, Dr. Clament dismissed as "the same old hypocritical nonsense" the accusation that he was an enemy of religion, arguing that his record had proved his support for liberty of conscience: "Where are the demolished churches? For my part, I see a number of new ones being built or repaired thanks to the subventions that I have been able to obtain; you will agree that favoring the building of churches is a new way of being the enemy of religion."[48]

The most vociferous priest-baiters were generally found among the scientific elites. Materialist and positivist, their ranks included many of the best-known figures in medicine and politics of the Third Republic, such as Augagneur, Bert, Blatin, Bourneville, Cornil, Debierre, Langlet, Naquet, and De Lanessan. De Lanessan, proclaiming that "observation kills faith," contended that France lagged behind Germany in the sciences because its educational system was "manacled" by religion, and his bitterness on this score was fanned anew by the founding of a Catholic medical faculty at Lille in 1878.[49] Equally outraged was the positivist Debierre, who taught at Lille, and who for years afterwards continued to denounce "the complicity of a hospital administration composed of clericals."[50] Such types were found in all the faculties and schools. The exception was the faculty of Montpellier, as Dr. Amagat, who once taught natural history there, could confirm. An outspoken materialist, he had gotten into trouble in 1880 for talking in class about his beliefs. His suspension provoked demonstrations and the closing of the faculty, in the midst of which he announced that he would continue to teach his courses off campus. This led to a hearing before university authorities, who fired him for insubordination.[51]

Although many rural practitioners tried to steer clear of religious controversies, one does find exceptions. Dr. Carret's *Démonstration de l'inexistence de Dieu,* published in 1912, was a pointed, often funny, assault on belief. Among other things, he denounced the priests for always having sided with the rich against the poor, and he ridiculed the church's teachings on purgatory, which, he said, had exercised a greater influence over history than had gunpowder or printing. He also attacked the church fathers, disputing their view that the perfection of the human body signified a divine creator. To wit: Human eyesight was poor, much inferior to that of owls and hawks, and teeth did not replace themselves. Moreover, the proximity of the tubes in the throat for taking in food and air showed careless design, as was true also for the dual function of the male sexual organs for both reproduction and the elimination of wastes. Most of all, the author could not understand how a perfect God could condemn to hell all humanity in order to expiate the sin of Adam and then, changing his mind, send his

Son to die in order to appease his own sense of justice and, after all this, admit to heaven only a tiny number of those who were born after Christ and who had been baptized.[52]

Though rarely so blatant, other provincial doctors left little doubt where they stood, even in Catholic strongholds. Pierre Le Monnier, vice-president of the *conseil général* of Sarthe, stated in 1881: "I am today what I was yesterday and will be tomorrow – a devout servant of the Republic, an ardent and convinced defender of lay society which, under the clerical and jesuitical banner, is being assaulted by all the partisans of fallen regimes." René Cazauvieilh of the Gironde promised in 1889 to support authorization only for those religious congregations "whose members know how to stay out of our political struggles." In Finistère, Dr. Dubuisson openly referred to himself as an adversary of clericalism, arguing that "the role of religious powers is to occupy themselves with affairs of religion and not with the affairs of government."[53]

Almost a fourth (24.5%) of the physician-legislators were Freemasons.[54] Although not all radicals and freethinkers belonged to Masonic lodges, the movement's tendency after 1870 to abandon the deistic premises of an earlier age and, in place of the "Grand Architect of the Universe," to substitute a positivist and materialist philosophy, made it attractive to medical men, who praised Masonic doctrines as being "founded on reason, the conquests of science, and social progress."[55] The doctors in our group were active in dozens of the more than three hundred lodges existing by 1880, but they were most visible in the work of the Grand Orient of Paris, which was the central authority of the societies. Augagneur, Baudon, Blatin, Fernand Dubief, and Meslier all had sat on its Council of the Order, and Debierre had served as its president. These were only a few of the more prominent Masons; others were Bamberger, Bert, Cazeneuve, Chautemps, Chevandier, Combes, De Lanessan, Dufour, Frébault, Marmottan, and Georges Martin, the last of whom founded the lodge Droit humain in 1894, which stressed the antireligious mission of Freemasonry and was the first lodge to admit women.[56]

Another way of measuring the doctors' religious attitudes is to consider the kinds of funeral ceremonies they specified. The choice of a lay service, for example, served as a final statement to the world, if not a parting gesture of defiance, for we find numerous cases like that of Testelin, who declared that his services were to be civil, that there were to be no orations, and that his body was to be burned.[57] A church burial, by contrast, might imply true piety, or it might mean simply that the deceased had wished to spare his family any pain or embarrassment. In our group, one finds few if any last-minute conversions, as some said had happened to Claude Bernard.[58] On the other hand, several known unbelievers received religious burials because their families ignored their last wishes. At the death of Dr. Laussedat at Moulins in July 1878, for instance, a local magistrate barred his widow from giving him the civil burial he had desired, after other family members intervened on behalf of church services.[59] In Ain, Charles Robin received a religious burial, despite the fact that his will had specified a civil funeral to be followed by an autopsy.[60]

Of the known and probable cases, 35 percent received religious burials and 65 percent civil burials.[61] About 15 percent of the latter were cremated. Cremation was both a hygienic and an ideological cause, particularly because Catholics, concerned about the resurrection of the body, viewed the practice as one of the most extreme statements of medical materialism. Cremation advocates such as Bert or Blatin took pleasure in invoking the names of saints who had been burned at the stake, suggesting that if God had created the body he could also put it back together again. Bourneville went further: In November 1880, he and a group of Parisian doctors, lawyers, and engineers founded the Society for the Propagation of Cremation, which aimed to make this form of burial a matter of private choice in the eyes of the law. Bourneville served as the society's vice-president and later president; other members were Cornil, Georges Martin, Henri Chassaing, and Brousse. At Lyon, Dr. Augagneur, then a member of the municipal council, pushed for funds to build a crematory and founded a society similar to that of Bourneville's.[62]

Along with their belief in *laïcité,* one finds in the doctors' writings and speeches certain recurring political themes. For most, the Revolution of 1789 stood as the watershed of the modern epoch, and ownership and inheritance of property were among the most sacred of the rights that it had bequeathed to society. These were indissolubly linked with the institutions of marriage and the family, in which property regulated private relations and in which even the mother's milk, as Félix Martin pointed out, belonged, by right, to the infant.[63] As one might expect, the duties of women figured more prominently than did their rights in this way of thinking, a view heavily influenced by physiological dogma. In typical fashion, Dr. Lavergne professed to believe in equal pay for equal work but insisted that women were too weak to perform many kinds of labor. Their claim to equal education, moreover, conflicted with feminine "nature" and with "the goal that this nature assigns her in society." Were women to be admitted to the professions, it would damage the family and the sacred ideal of domesticity.[64]

Most of the doctors recognized that the lower classes had not yet shared in the benefits of the Revolution and believed the resolution of this social question to be of the utmost urgency if bourgeois civilization were to survive. Specific solutions varied, but underlying them was a moderate rationalism that saw liberty and science as the keys to resolving human inequities. For the most part, the cures these doctors offered differed little from those of other moderate republicans and were based on prevailing notions of social solidarity. "I desire a society in which, far from showing one's teeth and fist, a person extends his hand," proclaimed Adrien Pozzi at Reims, "We must work not to exasperate but to conciliate the differences of employers and employees."[65] The 1902 platform of Paul Pourteyron in Dordogne embodied the standard rhetoric: "Realization of works of mutuality, of insurance, of assistance by the union of capital and labor, by harmony and solidarity."[66] Others urged state subventions to mutual-aid societies that could provide capital for old-age pensions, or they voiced support for more direct forms of medical aid to the old, particularly during the two elections preceding passage of the 1893 law concerning rural medical assistance. Candidates in industrial departments, such as Gustave Dron of the Nord, emphasized factory hygiene and safety, housing, protection of pregnant women in industry, and indemnification for victims of labor accidents. In the same department, Defontaine vowed to promote extension to industrial diseases of the 1898 law pertaining to labor accidents.[67]

Above all, the doctors affirmed their commitment to private property, which Delpierre of Oise called "the extension of personality and the essential condition for liberty, initiative, and human activity." It is not surprising that few doctors figured in the ranks of the Guesdists or other collectivist factions. Such doctrines, argued Dr. Ricard of Côte-d'Or, threatened to "suppress liberty, competition, and personal autonomy." Gabriel Chevalier of Saône-et-Loire condemned them as "destructive of individuality, initiative, liberty, the family, and public wealth." For Sabaterie of Puy-de-Dôme, their proponents were "the sort of demented visionaries who, in defiance of the natural laws of evolution, dream of the brutal and instantaneous transformation of society by spoliation."[68]

Added to these traits was an agrarian mentality bordering on physiocracy. Campaign tracts brimmed over with admonitions regarding the importance of the land and the need to maintain the agrarian spirit. Lannelongue proclaimed agricultural prosperity to be "indissolubly linked" with the grandeur of *la patrie,* and Vacherie saw the land as "the source of all wealth, the mother industry of all industries." Dr. Mandeville, a graduate of the Toulouse faculty who worked his own farm at Fronton, pictured agriculture as the key to restoring France's commercial and industrial greatness. The first step, he said, was to abolish the free-trade agreements left over from the empire, followed by nationalization of the Canal du Midi, lower railroad tariffs, agrarian credit, and retirement funds for agricultural workers: "As a property owner, I will defend the protection of all our agricultural products weighed down by foreign competition. . . . I am, and will remain above all else, an agrarian candidate."[69]

The appeal for protective tariffs was especially strong in the platforms of 1889 and 1893, that era having been one of crisis for agriculture as a result of a general depression and the phylloxera vine epidemic. Running a close second was the call for agrarian banks offering low rates of interest. In the opinion of Dr. Rey, president of the Agrarian and Industrial Society of Lot, the absence of such institutions was the chief barrier to France's entry into scientific farming.[70] Dr. La Cote of Creuse held the same view, believing that agrarian banks could accomplish for agriculture what the Bank of France had done for commerce and industry. Like Rey, he urged the founding of schools for teaching scientific agriculture, reminding voters of the one he had created in his own locality.[71]

For many doctors, a healthy agriculture produced more than social harmony and national strength; it was also the precondition for physical and emotional well-being. This attitude was central to the agrarian cosmology, which, however much it decried rural poverty and disease, regarded city life as worse. Roussel, for one, argued that the rural exodus had been the cause of terrible anguish and that many of those who flocked to the cities ended up as alcoholics or wards of insane asylums.[72] Other doctors, remembering the lessons of 1848, warned of the social dangers. In urging the creation of agrarian banks in 1889, Marius Isoard called on the government to help halt the rural flight, which was "ruining our country inhabitants and which, by the influence of unemployed workers, crowded into the big cities, constitutes a veritable menace."[73] So concerned was one member of our group, Legal Lasalle of Côtes-du-Nord, that he penned a novel in tribute to rural bliss. Entitled *L'Héritage de Jacques Farruel,* the book focuses on a farm owner in the commune of La Roche, who starts from nothing and has only one ambition – "to live long enough to transmit to his children, free of all debts, the beautiful farm he had created." In the end, after many twists and turns of plot, the children manage to withstand the temptations of the city and, after their father's death, remain on the soil, where they became more and more attached to agrarian life, "happy in work, well-being, and duty, under the watchful eye of God."[74]

Sectional rivalries loomed large in the political campaigns of medical men, and most of these rivalries involved conflicts between north and south over sugar, alcohol, and wine production. In Hérault, Vigné d'Octon assailed "the league of deputies from the north whose interests are so divergent and who have only one goal: to crush the Midi economically." In Loire, Gilbert Laurent denounced the "incessant encroachments on the wines of the Midi" by northern sugar manufacturers.[75] Northerners responded in kind. Defontaine warned of a "coalition of interests" that was threatening sugar production, while Dron assailed "the efforts of winegrowers in the Midi to impose on the alcohols of the north higher tariffs than those placed on their products." In Pas-de-Calais, Victor Morel promised that if elected, he would not only defend the interests of his region against the south but would also strengthen his efforts "to establish equality before universal suffrage, so that the Midi, with an equal number of electors, will not have 30 to 40 percent more deputies and senators."[76]

The *professions de foi* talked much about alcohol production but never broached the subject of alcoholism. On the contrary, most professed sentiments similar to those of Pascal Bourcy of

Charente-Inférieure, who called vineyards "the wealth and glory of France." Indeed, the doctors took pains to portray themselves as friends of alcohol-producing interests in their region. Vigné d'Octon promised, "If you accord me your votes, I will not forget that a great part of the arrondissement of Lodève is a region of vineyards." Lannelongue, who elsewhere spoke eloquently about the threat of alcoholism to future generations, told the voters of Gers: "I will defend energetically the right of a property owner to make brandies outside all control and to dispose of them according to his pleasure so long as they do not enter into public circulation." At Narbonne, the socialist Ferroul, whose own party often lamented the damage wrought by alcohol among workers, promised that he would work to protect winegrowers by means of tariffs on foreign grapes and on any substances used in manufacturing artificial wines.[77]

Far from denouncing the rights of the *bouilleurs de cru,* or home brewers, which many hygienists regarded as a leading cause of alcoholism, physicians often singled out these rights as worthy of special protection. Auguste Cachet, a former army doctor who practiced at Domfront in Orne, demanded in 1902 "the absolute liberty of home brewer's rights, a very strong reduction of taxes on natural brandies and on the license fee for dealers." Four years later, Edmond Chapuis, mayor of Lons-le-Saunier in Jura, set as his priorities the passage of laws against the manufacture of artificial wines, restrictions on the use of sugar in wine making, and an end to all regulation of the rights of home brewers. At Toul the same year, Gustave Chapuis (no relation to Edmond) reminded voters that he was president of a group of deputies who had organized themselves in order to protect home brewers.[78]

Few doctors, in fact, waged their campaigns around public health topics, narrowly defined. Exceptions can be found among a handful of urban candidates, such as Emile Dubois of Paris, who made factory hygiene a central focus of his 1902 campaign, or among a sprinkling of radicals in impoverished rural districts, such as François Dellestable of Corrèze, whose plea for cantonal hospitals and medical assistance in 1885 prompted charges that he was promoting state tyranny "over the child at school, over the poor at the hospice."[79] In most instances, discussions of health and hygiene took place only in very general terms, the 1892 platform of Bernard Thonion in Haute-Savoie, for example, promising "to give a great place to private and public hygiene, to medical assistance in the countryside, to unhealthy lodging, to rural industries."[80]

The elections of 1902, for which there exists a fairly complete collection of *professions de foi,* illustrate the kinds of issues that medical men addressed. Although many platforms include specific mention of medical and hygienic topics – typically, pure drinking water, hospitals, school hygiene, and medical assistance – their main concerns are those of the voters to whom they are addressed. Thus, they appear to differ little from the platforms of other candidates. Most prominent are discussions of local affairs, which usually center on roads and railroads, school construction, communal loans, disaster aid, court costs, and hunting and fishing rights. Problems of the land also loom large, including agrarian banks and credit, insurance, tariffs, agricultural associations, and mutual-aid societies. There are frequent calls to lower municipal taxes and to reduce the time spent in military service.[81]

Because many physician-candidates already enjoyed reputations as hygienists by the time they ran for parliament, their lack of attention to health matters in the *professions de foi* does not mean that they deemed them unimportant. As we have seen, most thought of hygiene in the broadest sense, envisioning the building of schools and roads as essential first steps toward rural amelioration. In Seine-et-Oise, Dr. Amodru stressed his lifelong desire to better the overall material conditions of the people, "a task that is dear to me and to which I have especially applied myself, notably in taking the initiative for creation of hospital services, of mutuality, of maternity that functions today in our department to the satisfaction of everyone." In Lot, Rey proclaimed help for the sick to be the duty of society: "It is not right that the agricultural worker, having given a long life of toil to the task of feeding and clothing his family, should be allowed, when age and sickness have reduced him to nothing, to die of hunger and misery." In Dordogne, Denoix promised that "the organization of public assistance in the countryside will occupy my total attention. The workers of the fields, like those of the cities, must be able to have for themselves and their families, aid and protection against sickness and poverty."[82]

The emphasis on rural misery blended with another trait; that is, the doctor's special appeal to the voter, based on his long medical services. The words of Dr. Clament in Dordogne during the 1902 campaign touch on almost all the relevant ideas:

Reared in the country, having practiced medicine in the canton of Laforce after the example of my father who, for fifty years, treated the rich and the poor with the same devotion, I know your needs. A property owner and viticulturist, your interests are mine. My house is unreservedly open to all those who want to do me the pleasure of coming to see me, and it is not a deputy puffed up with his situation that you'll meet, it's a neighbor, a friend, a child of the people like you who has only one desire: to be kind to you and to prove his gratitude in placing at your disposition his influence with the administration and the public powers.[83]

These themes may be summarized in order of their frequency. First, the doctor was a man of the people. Merlou of Yonne described himself as a farmer's son who had always lived in the midst of workers and peasants; "I have learned to know them; I have loved them. In the various offices that have been awarded to me, I have defended the cause of the weak and the disinherited." Bichon of Angers presented himself as the offspring of a family of workers: "I found my clientele among the people, and my interests have always been tied to those of workers." Michel of Haute-Loire stressed the nature of his work and the fact of his local origins:

For more than thirty years... I have been established in the *chef-lieu* of the district where, in a rather extended range, my profession has placed me in daily contact with the rich and the poor, with the inhabitants of the towns and the fields.... In addition, I was born in the canton of Montfaucon of a family that for several generations lived a simple, honorable, and laborious life there as farmers of our region, like you.[84]

Second, the doctor was witness to the physical and material anguish of the people. At Nancy, Dr. Henri Henrion told voters in 1893 that his profession had given him firsthand knowledge of their suffering and promised to spare no effort toward improving the material conditions in which they lived. To the citizens of Riom, Dr. Girard proclaimed, "Not only have I had, throughout my already long life, a great sympathy for the suffering poor... but I would go so far as to say that this has been perhaps the result of a personal conception on the origins of human miseries." Hippolyte Rouby, mayor of Laplaeu in Corrèze, portrayed his life as having been passed entirely in the midst of the downtrodden, which had "initiated me into their sufferings and needs and furnished the occasion to know their aspirations."[85]

Third, the doctor knew what was needed in order to cure the economic and social ills of the people. In Corrèze, Dellestable urged citizens to vote for men like himself "who, having lived in the midst of the working populations of the countryside, draw their inspiration constantly from their needs and desires." A similar appeal came from Bourrillon in Lozère: "Having practiced medicine for close to fifteen years in the midst of your working populations, I have been able to know their needs and to impress these needs upon myself, which I will defend with zeal and devotion." Pascal Bourcy of Charente-Inférieure stressed the knowledge he had gained in thirty-eight years of medical practice: "President of the *comice agricole,* living in the midst of farmers, a witness of their incessant labors and often of their disappointments, I will know to be guided by their needs." Baudet of Côtes-du-Nord also emphasized his sympathy for the peasants, noting that he himself had often walked behind the plow and that he would work to better the lot of small property owners and farmers. In Puy-de-Dôme, Sabaterie reminded voters of the twenty years he had given to alleviating human woes, as a result of which he had come to know the desires of "workers, farmers, small businessmen, small industrialists, and petty functionaries, who toil and struggle in a labor that is often disproportionate to their forces and means."[86]

Such appeals were effective. Still, the passions of the campaign did not disappear once the winner took his seat, and for doctors the inevitable clash between the world of politics and that of reasoned professional judgment was to compromise further their self-proclaimed image as social arbiters. This will become clear as we examine their record at the national level.

PART II

In parliament

4

Patterns of medicopolitical careers in parliament

What distinctive traits marked a physician once he entered parliament? In order to answer this question, it is necessary to compare the doctors with members of other occupational groups and, once again, to determine whether their behavior expressed any unique marks of professional identification. To do so requires us to focus on their primary characteristics as legislators – from age and length of service to voting patterns and committee work – and on the ways in which their concerns as doctors affected their performances as deputies or senators. The goal of this chapter is thus to provide an overview of their parliamentary careers, which will serve as a basis for the more detailed analyses of specific areas of activity in later chapters.

GENERAL CHARACTERISTICS

Mattei Dogan, whose study of deputies under the Third Republic provides a convenient starting point for our own inquiry, has stressed the degree to which intellectuals dominated parliament.[1] Whether lawyers or doctors, journalists or teachers, engineers or architects, almost two-thirds of all deputies between 1871 and 1914 may be broadly classified as intellectuals. This was a matter of concern to many contemporaries, who decried the theorists' hold on the country's political life and believed that the weakness in parliament of its "natural representatives" from commerce, industry, and agriculture stood as a prime cause of national weakness.[2]

For most of the professional men who served, election to parliament normally spelled a suspension, often permanent, of their private careers. As André Tardieu observed later in *La Profession parlementaire*, political office during the Republic was not perceived as a mandate of limited duration but as a *métier* in itself.[3] Here and there were a few who managed to maintain a semblance of professional life; the *avocat*-deputy pleading cases in court was not an unusual sight, and several in our group, such as Cornil and Bourneville, continued to hold teaching and hospital posts during their time in office. Those whose home departments were near Paris had an advantage in this respect. For example, Anatole Guindey, hospital physician at Evreux in Eure, had a rich clientele that he refused to abandon after his election in 1891; instead, he spent his mornings with patients, then boarded the Paris train to attend afternoon sessions of parliament, and returned home the same night. A few of the poorest tried to generate modest clienteles in Paris on the side.

The possibility of resuming private practice in case of defeat was not at all a certainty, or was less so for doctors than for lawyers. Of the known cases, barely a fourth returned to medicine after a stint in parliament; another fourth, usually from among the eldest, retired from all activities. Six percent won appointments to government posts, which were often awarded as consolation prizes to losing candidates who had been loyal to the government. Local assessors and tax collectors included numerous physicians whose calling cards bore the title *ancien député,* but the best positions bore some relationship to one's profession. On his defeat in 1881, Dr. Bamberger was appointed assistant librarian of the Museum of Natural History. Joseph Grisez of Haut-Rhin, beaten in 1893, was named director of the insane asylum of Sarthe au Mans. Chavanne of Rhône won the prize of Senate physician. These were the lucky ones. Vigné d'Octon has recalled the sad scenes in the Salle des pas perdus at the opening of each legislature, where former deputies, unable to live off their modest pensions, mingled among journalists and favor seekers in search of their just compensation.

A little over 44 percent of all physician-legislators died while in office, which, in part, reflected their advanced ages on first entering parliament (an average of 48.2 years for deputies and 55.8 years for senators). This, in turn, was a product of their long years of medical training (an average of 7) and practice (an average of 23). During the whole of the Third Republic, around a third of all deputies were under 40 when first elected; another third were between 40 and 50; and a final third were 50 or over. Among

Table 4.1. *Comparative ages of physicians in the Chamber of 1898*

Age	All deputies (%)	Doctors (%)
25–29	2.9	0.0
30–39	20.5	12.6
40–49	34.3	38.0
50–59	29.4	34.9
60 and over	12.9	14.2

physicians, only 19 percent were under 40 when first elected; 40 percent ranged between 40 and 50; and 41 percent were 50 or over. Table 4.1 compares the ages of medical men in a single legislature – that of 1898 – with the ages of the other deputies.[4] As a group, the doctors in the Chamber were older than the lawyers, owing to their longer periods of study. In the Chamber of 1898, about 65 percent of all jurists were under fifty years old, and for doctors, the figure was 50 percent.

If the professional risks of becoming a deputy at middle age were great, so were the dangers to one's peace of mind. Parliament remained in session between eight and twelve months a year, and though absenteeism was high, a deputy had to spend four or five days a week in Paris in order to carry out his duties. Committee work was only a small part of it, for much of one's time was spent drafting handwritten replies to inquiries and complaints from voters (it helped to have a secretary who could duplicate one's handwriting). Even more burdensome were the endless rounds of visits to ministers on behalf of favor seekers. Tardieu described this function as that of the *ambassadeur-courtier* and called it "the substance of the parliamentary profession." Vigné d'Octon later described the special need to cultivate ties with low-ranking staff members in cabinet offices, to inquire about the health of their wives and children, and – an advantage for doctors – to give free medical advice and, on occasions, even physical examinations.[5]

In addition, anxiety over reelection spelled constant efforts to control the political situation at home – to keep in touch with committees and subprefects, to monitor the activities of the opposition, and, especially important, to appear whenever possible at local fairs and fêtes. It helped if, in addition to occupying a seat

Table 4.2. *Length of physician-deputies' parliamentary careers,*
1876–1914

	Number of times elected as deputy						
	1	2	3	4	5	6	7 or more
Physician-deputies (N)	116	59	45	25	15	6	3
Percentage of distribution	42.9	22.2	16.6	9.2	5.5	2.2	1.1
Term (years)	4	8	12	16	20	24	28–35
Actual years of service	387	353	467	372	261	130	89
Percentage of distribution	18.7	17.1	22.6	18.0	12.6	6.3	4.3

in parliament, one held a political office at home, which most did,
even though the jealously guarded tradition of *cumul* served as a
distraction from more urgent tasks in parliament.

Dogan found that of the 4,892 deputies who represented con-
tinental France during the whole of the Third Republic, 46 percent
won election for one term (usually 4 years), 21 percent for two
terms, and 33 percent for three or more. The figures illustrate the
insecurity of one's tenure there. Over two-thirds had relatively
short careers – around 8 years at a maximum. This was true also
for the 269 doctors who held seats in the Chamber: 43 percent sat
for one term, 22 percent for two, and 35 percent for three or more.
The average number of years served (9.5) was slightly higher, the
maximum being 35. The vast majority of those who won two or
more terms served them in sequence; only 8 percent (7% for all
deputies) had discontinuous terms. An additional 6 percent interrupted their careers in the process of going from the Chamber to
the Senate.

Table 4.2, which is modeled on Dogan's table for all deputies,
shows these patterns in detail. The figures provided here are only
the years served during the pre-1914 period; in all, just over 16
percent had careers in parliament extending beyond that date.

These calculations confirm for the doctors what Dogan showed
for all deputies. First, although continual changes in parliament's
composition resembled, in his words, "the movement of sand
dunes," there existed a core of "cemented sand" that was not so
easily moved by the wind. Put another way, 852 of the 2,059 years
served by doctors in the Chamber derived from 49 individuals

with four terms or more. The 24 who served five terms or more had a greater proportion of the total years (23%) than did the 116 who were elected just once. Second, there was a direct link between a doctor's duration of service and his political significance, a fact that becomes readily apparent when one understands the influence exercised by a small elite whose accomplishments far overshadowed those of the others.

Most visible were the cabinet ministers, who represented 3.6 percent of the physician-legislators and who accounted for 8.6 percent of the total years served by doctors. As a rule, individuals who achieved ministerial rank in the early Republic came from the wealthiest ranks of society and, as Estèbe discovered, often held high positions in the worlds of industry, banking, railroads, and mining. It was only during the post-Dreyfusard era that this pattern began to change, as illustrated by the advent of Combes, and later Clemenceau, to the office of prime minister. Together, their tenure lasted six years; otherwise, the premiership was monopolized by lawyers, who headed up two-thirds of the cabinets that were formed between 1873 and 1920. Around three-fourths of those who presided at interior were lawyers, which was only slightly higher than the proportions for commerce and industry or for public education. Justice was almost their exclusive preserve. By contrast, doctors had few cabinet-level opportunities to exercise their professional skills, as would have been the case had a ministry of health existed. In 1906, Clemenceau did succeed in creating a post for labor and social welfare, but that also became monopolized by lawyers.[6]

Doctors who won ministerial appointments exhibited a number of common traits, aside from their generally modest social origins. Well over half served for four terms or more, and most had served on one or more of the big standing committees, such as labor, foreign affairs, agriculture, colonies, or the budget. The intensity of their committee work and their success at the polling place denoted a certain ambition and capacity for survival on their part, both of which were essential to gaining high office. Yet, neither in itself was sufficient. Well-to-do country doctors, like many of their colleagues on the medical faculties, often lacked the talent, or taste, for the intrigues that accompanied the forging of new ministerial combinations – hence, the absence of men of known ability, such as Rey, Ricard, Cornil, Roussel, or Liouville. Doubtlessly, there were those who found stimulating the all-consuming struggles for position. Judging from his journal, Dr. Lavergne of the Tarn was one of them, his account of political life during the 1880s abounding in the endless small detail of factional infighting, in which he himself was often caught up.[7] Lavergne, however, was a veritable professional whose tenure in parliament went back to 1849, and Ferry loyalist though he was, not even he managed to secure a place in government. Of Dr. Lannelongue, it was said that achieving a cabinet post represented the last, great ambition of his long and distinguished career, but he, too, failed to win the prize.

The ones who did so displayed an extraordinary versatility. Bert and Combes made their marks at the Ministry of Education, an office that touched on numerous interests of the medical corps and that called forth an expertise common to many of its members. The same was true for the Ministry of Agriculture, where Gadaud, De Mahy, and Viger held posts, or for the Ministry of Commerce and Industry, where Dubief and Lourties served. Curiously, the largest single group was in two related ministries – the navy and colonies – where De Mahy, Chautemps, De Lanessan, Armand Gauthier, and Augagneur won appointments. The latter two also held ministerial rank at public works, posts and telegraphs. With the exception of Bert, Combes, and Clemenceau, however, few were able to leave behind any substantial record of accomplishment, and only rarely were they able to focus explicitly on tasks that reflected medical concerns, such as De Lanessan's efforts to lower alcohol consumption in the navy, or those of Viger and Gadaud to safeguard the purity of the nation's meat supplies.

The problem was the frequency of cabinet turnovers. Bert lasted only a year as minister of public education and religion under Gambetta. Gadaud and François De Mahy at agriculture and Lourties at commerce and industry also stayed for just one year. Merlou survived for only a year at finance, having served with success as undersecretary of state for the preceding four years. Chautemps had a ten-month term as minister of the colonies but managed only five days as minister of the navy in 1914. De Mahy put in a year at the latter post, which was bettered only by De Lanessan, who had three. Viger served four years as minister of agriculture during the 1890s, but under three different cabinets. Following Combes, prime minister during the era of the *bloc des gauches*,

Table 4.3. *Physician-orators in parliament*

Number of speeches	Number of doctors
0	138
1	94
2	44
3	21
4	14
5	9
6	7
7 or more	31

Dubief put in fourteen months at commerce and industry and then interior, his post being assumed in 1906 by Clemenceau, who ruled the country for the next three years.

It was within the committee structure of parliament that the doctors exerted their greatest influence. Twenty-three served as presidents of major committees of the Chamber, of whom almost half had four or more terms in parliament. They accounted for 13 percent of the total years served by doctors, and if we add eighty-five others who were reporters for major bills, the figure rises to nearly 50 percent.

Within these two groups lay an even smaller contingent – around forty individuals all together – whose years in parliament may be described as "very active" or "extremely active." In addition to their role as committee presidents, reporters, and authors of bills, they ranked higher than average in the number of speeches that they gave at the tribune, as can be seen in Table 4.3.

Making speeches was of prime importance to one's visibility and influence, but it had its risks. Vigné d'Octon related the case of a prominent physician who, though a brilliant speaker at local rallies and in committees, was terrified at the thought of appearing at the tribune. He claimed his fear grew out of an unusually high regard for the sanctity of parliament. More likely, Vigné pointed out, it was a natural reluctance, common to many deputies with thin skins, to expose himself to the barbs and sarcasms hurled from the floor.[8] The most impassioned debates usually occurred when a member of parliament attacked a specific action of the government and called for a vote of confidence. This was the

Table 4.4. *Physician-radicals in the Chamber of Deputies,*
1881–1910

Legislature	Radicals (%)
1881	30.8
1885	47.3
1889	48.3
1893	50.7
1898	66.7
1902	62.5
1906	68.3
1910	61.5

famous *interpellation,* of which a total of forty-six physician-deputies were authors.

Among professional types, the professors and the well-to-do country doctors served the longest in parliament. Just under a fourth of the total in each category had four terms or more. A glance at the names of those who were "very" or "extremely" active in parliamentary affairs confirms that as a rule, the most influential physician-legislators came from this blend of professional and rural elites. Among them one finds big-city surgeons and members of prestigious medical societies, alongside property-owning *médecins de campagne.* As we noted earlier, the feature that both types usually shared was their status as rural property owners. What they also shared, and what allowed them to leave their mark in politics, was their staying power at the polls. For the lower house, one could cite the names of Augagneur, Bert, Gustave Chapuis, Chautemps, Chevandier, Devins, Dron, Dubief, Empereur, De Lanessan, Levraud, Rey, and Viger. Examples in the Senate include Combes, Cornil, Dellestable, Guyot, Labbé, Lannelongue, Lourties, Félix-Martin, Roussel, and Testelin.

I mentioned the proportions of medical men in the Chamber who associated themselves with advanced political opinions. I should add here that the percentages in each legislature who identified themselves as radicals and radical-socialists increased steadily over time, as is illustrated in Table 4.4.

How did doctors compare with lawyers in the political groupings of this period? Figures 4.1 and 4.2 focus on the Chambers of

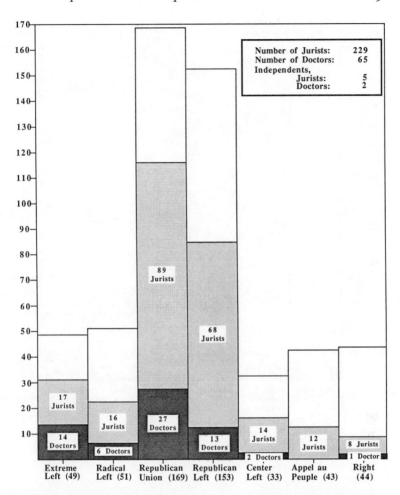

Figure 4.1. Political affiliations of doctors and jurists in the Chamber of 1881. (Proportions for jurists are from Gaudemet, *Les Juristes et la vie politique de la IIIe république*, p. 95.)

1881 and 1906. In both, we see that the proportion of doctors tends to increase as we move to the left along the spectrum, a pattern that was not nearly so pronounced among men of law. In 1881, for example, around 22 percent of the doctors (as opposed to 7.2% for the jurists) belonged to the extreme Left. If we combine the two most advanced groups (dual registration was common), the proportion for doctors rises to 32.3 percent and for jurists to only 14.4 percent. Figures for Gambetta's Union répub-

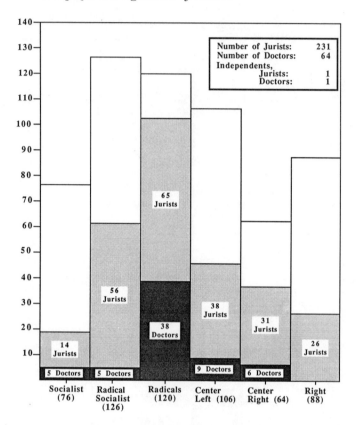

Figure 4.2. Political affiliations of doctors and jurists in the Chamber of 1906. (Proportions for jurists are from Gaudemet, *Les Juristes et la vie politique de la IIIe république*, p. 96.)

licaine were closer (41.5% and 38.8%), but unlike jurists, doctors were almost entirely absent from right-wing groups.

The proportion of physician-radicals in the Chamber of 1906 was even larger, although as we shall see later, their overall posture suggests a drift toward the center. By then, around 23 percent ranked themselves among conservative groups of the center Left and center Right. Only a handful sat on the extreme Left, a position now occupied by the socialists. Around 59 percent, it is true, still called themselves radicals, but the political implications of this label had changed over time. Whatever his profession, the radical of 1906 usually displayed more moderate and conservative traits than did his predecessor of the 1870s, when the battle to secure the Republic and to achieve social reform still lay ahead.[9]

We will now explore the meaning of these affiliations as they related to the doctors' everyday political behavior in parliament. A good way to do this is to look at their voting records, to compare them with those of the lawyers, and to discover ways in which they changed over the years.

VOTING RECORDS

Voting records provide useful clues to understanding the doctors' political tendencies, but one must be cautious. Poor attendance at sessions meant that many routine ballots were cast by proxy, a task performed on behalf of each parliamentary group by deputies known as *boîtiers*. The process was baffling to many, to say the least. Dr. Michou of Aube, who never understood the workings of *vote par procuration,* expressed repeated bewilderment at how a person could cast a ballot without being present at the session. At other times, parliamentary groups showed little cohesion, each member making his decision on the basis of practical considerations that bore no relationship to ideology.[10] Even when the hall was packed during moments of high drama – from passage of a key bill to the fall of a ministry – the outcome often reflected the dominance of group tactics over principles.

We thus look to votes on those bills and amendments in which the attitudes of doctors revealed themselves with greatest consistency over an extended period, beginning in 1871. Again, it is essential to grasp the relative nature of political labels, for, in the royalist-dominated legislature of that era, even conservative republicans were viewed as men of the Left. Nevertheless, physicians stood out in the vanguard of democracy. The proportion on the Left (33%) was higher than that for men of law (13%). Whereas, 38 percent of the jurists associated themselves with the monarchist or Bonapartist Right, only 9 percent of the doctors did so.

These patterns are reflected in Table 4.5, which is based on the votes used by Jacques Gouault in *Comment la France est devenue républicaine.* They show clearly that on issues that stood as hallmarks of radicalism in 1871, starting with opposition to the treaty with Prussia, doctors exhibited stronger leftist leanings than did parliament in general or lawyers in particular.

Table 4.5. *Comparative voting records of physicians and* avocats *in the National Assembly, 1871–6*

Vote	Percentage of physicians			Percentage of *avocats*		
	For	Against[a]	Abt.[b]	For	Against[a]	Abt.[b]
Peace treaty with Prussia (March 1871). Approved, 547–107	47.0	**41.1**	11.7	85.3	**12.8**	1.8
Repeal of laws on exile of Bourbons (June 1871). Approved, 472–97	30.7	**61.5**	7.6	73.5	**21.6**	4.7
Constituent power of National Assembly (August 1871). Approved, 434–225	18.1	**81.8**	0.0	49.2	**46.8**	3.9
Ban on civil burial during daylight hours (June 1873). Approved, 413–251	13.6	**86.3**	0.0	46.0	**51.7**	2.1
Wallon amendment establishing republic with president having 7-year term (January 1875). Approved, 353–352	**87.5**	12.5	0.0	**65.1**	32.2	2.6
Constituional laws creating machinery for a republic (February 1875). Approved 425–254	**87.5**	8.3	4.1	**72.1**	24.4	3.4

[a] Bold type indicates a leftist vote.
[b] Deputies appearing under this heading either abstained or were absent, a matter unspecified in the *Journal officiel.*

Because the majority of 1875 envisioned a republic as an interim measure until the monarchy could be restored, the Left managed to paper over its differences, making preservation of the new regime its first order of business. Forty-three doctors (including 18 who had served in the National Assembly) were victorious in elections to the new Chamber in February 1876, more than two-thirds of them being veterans of political battles against the Second Empire. Their devotion to the Republic was evident during the *seize-mai* crisis of 1877, when President Patrice MacMahon dissolved the assembly and called for new elections. All but two associated themselves with the 363 deputies who denounced the government's actions, and all but three of those who did so re-captured their seats during the ensuing campaign.

It was only with the triumph of the Republic in the late 1870s that the fundamental divisions on the Left came to the fore. Mod-erate or "opportunist" republicans who formed the majority in parliament were determined to move slowly on political and social reform, to the dismay of the radicals. The role of doctors in this regard cannot be determined solely by group affiliation; of those elected in 1877, for example, 77 percent had their primary asso-ciation with groups of the moderate Left, primarily Gambetta's Union républicaine, and only 18 percent with the more advanced radical faction led by Clemenceau and Louis Blanc. Yet, the doc-tors' voting records show higher levels of radicalism than these affiliations suggest, because there existed among Gambetta's fol-lowers a core of soft support for proposals sponsored by the ex-treme Left.

A good way to measure the doctors' attitudes is to see how they fared in Clemenceau's *La Justice,* one of the most influential mouth-pieces of radicalism. Before each election, *La Justice* published the voting records of outgoing deputies on issues it deemed of special significance, many symbolizing key tenets of early radical ortho-doxy. Table 4.6 compares the votes of doctors and lawyers on a number of these issues for the legislature that was elected in 1877, following the *seize-mai* crisis. On average, about 47 percent of the doctors cast their ballots in accordance with radical orthodoxy. This proportion was almost identical to their record on sample votes used by *La Justice* to evaluate the subsequent legislature of 1881–5.

Doctors thus showed comparatively strong levels of support for advanced measures, but as the figures indicate, the degree of ap-proval varied according to the issue and, as with all deputies, rose or fell in response to changing circumstances. In 1881, for example, only 28 percent of the doctors favored revising the constitution, although by then the extreme Left had made reform or abolition of the Senate one of its chief goals. As this drive gained momen-tum, however, the proportion of doctors supporting it increased. In three separate votes between June and December 1884, 47 per-cent declared themselves in favor of unlimited constitutional re-form, 49 percent in favor of popular election of senators, and 65 percent in favor of curbing the upper house's financial rights. Even

Table 4.6. *Comparative voting records of physicians and* avocats *in the Chamber of 1877–81 on issues selected by* La Justice

Vote	Percentage of physicians			Percentage of *avocats*		
	For[a]	Against	Abt.	For[a]	Against	Abt.
Prosecution of Broglie–Fourtou cabinet over *seize-mai* affair (11 March 1879). Defeated, 317–159	58.6	39.1	2.1	35.7	58.7	5.5
Popular election of judges (19 November 1880). Defeated, 241–199	71.4	20.4	8.1	29.0	47.3	23.6
Revision of constitution (31 May 1881). Defeated, 245–184	28.0	54.0	18.0	20.7	71.5	7.6
List voting (*scrutin de liste*) for election of deputies (19 May 1881). Approved, 267–102	50.0	38.0	12.0	53.4	35.8	10.6
Freedom of assembly and legality of political clubs (29 January 1880). Defeated, 257–180	31.2	56.2	12.5	20.4	68.5	11.0
Full amnesty for communards (Blanc motion of 11 February 1880). Defeated, 350–99	41.3	41.3	17.3	24.0	68.4	7.5
Legalizing divorce (initial Naquet motion of 9 February 1881). Defeated, 247–216	68.7	25.0	6.2	44.6	43.0	12.3
Banning of religious instruction in public schools (Barodet amendment of 24 December 1880). Defeated, 277–137	54.1	31.2	14.5	37.2	48.0	14.7
Lowering salaries of cardinals, archbishops, and bishops (Duvaux amendment of 30 July 1879). Defeated, 242–186	63.2	24.4	12.4	46.0	39.6	14.2
Elimination of post of French ambassador to the Vatican (30 July 1879). Defeated, 319–112	37.2	39.2	23.5	38.0	46.2	15.6

Table 4.6 (*continued*)

Vote	Percentage of physicians			Percentage of *avocats*		
	For[a]	Against	Abt.	For[a]	Against	Abt.
Separation of church and state (23 June 1881). Defeated, 348–83	**48.0**	25.0	26.9	**18.1**	65.9	15.9
Protection of railroad workers from arbitrary firings and loss of pensions (3 March 1881). Defeated, 310–228	**52.9**	25.4	21.5	**52.9**	30.5	16.4
Ten-hour day in industry (Villain amendment of 29 March 1881). Defeated, 309–133	**30.7**	50.0	19.2	**26.8**	55.2	17.9
Trade union rights (Cantagrel amendment to abolish penalties for unions not registering with government, 17 May 1881). Defeated, 251–168	**24.0**	54.0	22.0	**11.6**	69.4	19.4

[a] Bold type indicates a radical vote.
Source: Voting samples selected from *La Justice*, 1 to 16 August 1881.

as late as February 1889, after the movement had peaked, 65 percent voted against a motion to postpone further discussion of constitutional revision.[11]

Related to this issue was the drive to abolish single-member constituencies. Here was a favorite leftist theme, many radicals believing that the *scrutin d'arrondissement* favored local, conservative elites and that voting for lists of candidates on a department-wide basis would spark the growth of disciplined republican parties. Although half the doctors supported the idea in 1881, it never generated much enthusiasm, simply because most owed their seats to their influence within the arrondissement. For example, Gambetta's inclusion of the scheme in his plans for modest constitutional reform drew a lukewarm response, a fact of no small importance when the fate of his ministry was decided in early 1882. His downfall came on a committee motion that exceeded his own ideas on the subject, and only 40 percent of the doctors supported him, despite his popularity within the medical community. The *scrutin de liste* was finally tried in 1885, but first-ballot successes among monarchists led parliament to restore the old system four years later, which gained approval from 63 percent of the doctors.

The theme on which the physician–deputies exhibited the greatest consistency was anticlericalism. Around half (48 % in 1881 and 52% in 1885) voted to support radical proposals for separation of church and state. Even those who wished to maintain the Concordat in 1801 as a means of control were often prepared to endorse assaults on clerical privilege coming from the extreme Left. An amendment by Dr. Justin Labuze in May 1881 to abolish draft exemptions for members of the clergy won the support of 55 percent of the physicians who voted. The proportion in favor of severing diplomatic ties with the Vatican rose from 37 percent in 1879 to 51 percent in 1883, and nearly 62 percent supported a motion by Bert in February 1885 to reclaim from the church, on behalf of the public schools, all property that the state had ceded to it in the past.

The depth of these sentiments is illustrated by votes on Jules Ferry's anticlerical legislation. Doctors gave overwhelming support to the crusade for free and obligatory primary education; the same was true for virtually all antichurch laws that were passed during the Ferry era, from the banning of teaching among unauthorized congregations to the laicizing of cemeteries, hospitals, and charitable institutions. Table 4.7 compares the percentage of doctors who supported the Ferry laws with that of parliament as a whole.

Most doctors in parliament remained skeptical of the church's later grudging recognition of the Republic. Gacon of Allier echoed the sentiments of many others in 1893: "We must guard against the leaders of the old opposition parties which, after having spent their last forces in a campaign of insults and calumnies, wish to perform an outflanking movement." Bizarelli of Drôme called the *ralliés* "masked enemies," and Denoix of Dordogne warned that application of their program would be "the death of the Repub-

Table 4.7. *Voting records of doctors on the Ferry laws, 1879–82*

Vote	Percentage of doctors in favor	Percentage of Chamber in favor
Training schools for lay teachers (Bert proposal, 20 March 1879)	90.0	71.5
Banning of teaching activities among members of unauthorized congregations (Article 7, Ferry bill on higher education, 9 July 1879)	88.6	67.0
Exclusion of clergy from academic councils and Superior Council of Public Instruction (19 July 1879)	93.0	73.3
Free primary education (29 November 1880)	91.8	74.7
Compulsory primary education (24 December 1880)	91.1	71.0
Abolition of denominational cemeteries (7 March 1881)	91.6	73.7
Secularizing administration of hospitals and charitable institutions (30 July 1879)	95.0	76.7
Divorce law (19 June 1882)	85.3	70.5

Source: JOCD, 21 March, 10 July, 20 July 1879, pp. 2297–8, 6432–3, 7071–2, respectively; 30 November and 25 December 1880, pp. 11729–30 and 12879–80, respectively; 8 March 1881, pp. 443–4; 31 July 1879, pp. 7832–3; 20 June 1882, pp. 966–7.

lic."[12] Only four physician-legislators associated themselves with the Catholic *ralliés*. The rest were quick to abandon any prime minister who tried to introduce a spirit of tolerance into religious affairs, as was the case for Jean Casimir-Périer, who had 60 percent of the doctors ranged against him (as opposed to 52% for the whole assembly) when his cabinet was toppled in May 1894. Over 64 percent voted against his successor, Charles Dupuy, for similar reasons.

A final example can be found during the post-1901 parliamentary coalition known as the *bloc des gauches*. Numerous votes could be used to illustrate the doctors' growing commitment to separation of church and state, as can be seen in Table 4.8. These samples show that the proportion of doctors favoring anticlerical laws, though slightly lower than it had been during the Ferry era,

Table 4.8. *Voting records of doctors on church-related issues during* bloc des gauches, *1901–5*

Vote	Percentage of doctors in favor	Percentage of chamber in favor
Law on associations (religious communities could not be formed without legislative authority, and unauthorized communities could not teach; 28 June 1901)	85.0	57.5
Confidence in Combes ministry (12 June 1902)	92.3	72.5
Prohibition of all teaching by religious orders (28 March 1904)	82.0	55.9
Separation of church and state (3 July 1905)	73.0	59.4

Source: JOCD, 29 June, 1901, p. 1673; 13 June, 1902, 1841–2; 29 March 1904, pp. 1002–3; 4 July 1905, pp. 2701–7.

was still significantly higher than that of the Chamber as a whole. The final break with the church, coming in 1905, found almost three-fourths of them in favor.

If doctors were consistent in promoting the goal of a secular society, the same cannot be said concerning their attitudes toward the workers. These traversed several stages, each conditioned by changing tactics within the labor movement and by the doctors' own belief in social order and private property. At first were the memories of bloodshed during the Paris uprising of 1871, which for many bourgeois politicians symbolized the reality of the threat from below. However deep their revulsion at these events, the medical men who sat in the assembly at Versailles exhibited a spirit of conciliation toward the city, and all but three of them voted a few months later in favor of a losing motion to move parliament back to Paris.

More crucial was the fate of thousands who had been arrested, imprisoned, or deported, but it was not until after the new Chamber had convened in May 1876 that a bill appeared providing for amnesty. Its author was François-Vincent Raspail, and it received only fifty votes, ten of them cast by doctors. On a separate proposal, also heavily defeated, 51 percent voted in favor of a limited plan to free those arrested for political or press crimes. A motion in November to halt further indictments (except for murder, arson, or theft) was backed by 93 percent of the doctors. Thereafter, the proportion favoring radical motions for total amnesty constantly increased and was always higher than that for the Chamber as a whole. A bill by Louis Blanc to this end in February 1879 won support from 38 percent, and another in February 1880, from 53 percent. The final amnesty bill, passed on 22 June 1880, found 88 percent of the doctors voting in favor.

Physicians responded with guarded optimism to renewed working-class activity during the late 1870s. Despite the growth of collectivist ideas on the Left, they were confident that the Republic would be able to meet the challenge and, like Gambetta, who hoped to associate the interests of artisans and wage earners with those of small farmers and businessmen, believed that improvements for workers could be achieved in a spirit of social solidarity. The doctors in parliament thus formed an important part of what one historian has described as a reform-minded, university-trained elite, most of whom had modest bourgeois origins and who were committed to promote worker self-help under the regime to which they owed their rise.[13]

Such attitudes prompted a majority of medical men to support the legalization of trade unions in 1884, though with typical caution, only 24 percent were willing to abolish penalties for unions refusing to register with the government. Great numbers could be found among the early proponents of measures to end public ignorance of labor conditions: Two-thirds voted in favor of a controversial proposal by Clemenceau in 1884 for a parliamentary investigation of social and economic conditions in France, and many were enthusiastic supporters of Camille Raspail's efforts to create a ministry of labor, whose function would include gathering facts about working-class life. In parliamentary debates, doctors often cast themselves as spokesmen for small producers.[14] Bills to encourage cooperative and mutual-aid societies invariably won their praise, as did early attempts to create pension programs for industrial workers, miners, and the elderly. Among the first private bills for workers' pensions are several in which physicians acted as sponsors or cosponsors: De Lanessan in 1880, Chavanne in 1882, Edouard Isambard in 1891, Chautemps in 1893, and Chassaing in 1894.

In addition, many physicians in parliament condemned the tax structure for its unfairness and its impositions on the poor, and they were consistent backers of some form of income tax. In votes on income tax bills on 12 July 1894, 10 July 1896, and 9 March 1909, the proportion of doctors voting in favor was 63 percent, 73 percent, and 89 percent, respectively. Suspicion of the "financial feudality" was evident among them on numerous occasions – in 1881, for example, when 53 percent approved a radical motion blaming the railroad companies for the arbitrary firings of workers, or in 1883, when the same percentage refused to approve a new state contract with the Compagnie du Midi. Attacks by Alexandre Millerand on the railroad companies for violating union rights during the 1890s found over half the physician-deputies on his side.[15]

Although the doctors often showed sensitivity to the plight of the workers, it was difficult for most to overcome an innate distrust of state intervention in economic life. This was illustrated by their reactions to efforts aimed at reducing the twelve-hour working day. During the early years of the Republic, a majority of them had been willing to change the law as it applied to women and children – to limit the working day of women to eleven hours and of children to ten, for example, and to establish a minimum working age of thirteen. Seventy percent had voted in favor of the latter in January 1889; the previous year, 68 percent had voted to ban night work for women (16 June 1888). In a vote on 2 February 1891, however, only 27 percent approved an amendment that would have limited the working day of women and children to eight hours, and during the same session, only 38 percent were willing to apply it to children under fourteen.

Less than 31 percent voted in favor of an amendment in March 1879 that would have applied the ten-hour day to all industrial workers, and only 23 percent favored an amendment by the socialist Jules Guesde in June 1896 to establish an eight-hour day and a six-day week. Over time, the doctors did come to accept the necessity for a shorter workday, but this was true for most members of parliament. Nearly 77 percent of physician–deputies, for example, approved an eight-hour day for miners in February 1902, which the Chamber passed by 322 to 201. In a vote on 4 July 1912, 80 percent finally expressed their willingness to adopt a ten-hour day for all workers. A successful amendment by Dr. Delpierre of Oise, however, to exempt industries having fewer than twenty employees, gained the support of 52 percent of the doctors, about the same as for the whole Chamber.

The doctors' votes almost always displayed a conservative bias when it came to socialist proposals, whatever their merit. A proposal by Jean Jaurès on 23 June 1897, for instance, to establish a bank for agricultural credit got approval from only 30 percent, and another requiring the Bank of France to extend credit to labor unions got only 35 percent. A purely symbolic resolution from Vaillant on 20 June 1901 to affirm the right of all citizens to social guarantees "against handicaps, injury, old age, sickness, and accidents" was supported by less than a third, although many who voted against it had on other occasions expressed identical sentiments.

For doctors, as for many others, the growing incidence of labor violence during the 1880s provoked a backlash. A majority (51%, with 24% abstaining) approved the government's decision in early 1884 to send in troops to break a strike at the coal mine of Anzin. Similar events at the Decazeville mines two years later found 74 percent approving the government's conduct.[16] The same attitudes prevailed in all subsequent episodes of labor unrest. In a committee response to a private bill of 1897 that would have granted amnesty to arrested strikers, the radical Dubief wrote that such an action "would have no other result than to undermine the workings of justice, to the great damage of respect for laws."[17] A motion by the socialist Alexandre Zévaès in June 1900 to create a parliamentary commission to investigate strike violence at Chalon-sur Saône received the backing of only 22 percent of the physician-deputies.

The most dramatic illustration of the physician-deputies' attitudes came during the wave of labor violence that hit the country during the first Clemenceau ministry. To each socialist challenge of the government's use of force to crush the strikers, the physicians in the Chamber responded with overwhelming votes of confidence, and the proportion that did so was even higher than it had been at the time of the Anzin and Decazeville strikes of the 1880s. Plainly, the conservative response to strike violence had only intensified over the years, as Table 4.9 shows.

A final point should be made in regard to those doctors who sat in the Senate. As one would expect, they exhibited more conservative voting traits, though here, too, they usually showed a

Table 4.9. *Voting records of doctors on strikes during the first Clemenceau ministry, 1906–9*

	For (%)	Against (%)	Abt. (%)
Confidence in cabinet (Jaurès *interpellation* of government policy toward strikers; 21 June 1906). Passes, 400–88	86.5	7.6	5.7
Motion for amnesty for fired postal workers of Paris who had gone on strike, 11 July 1906. Fails, 335–140	29.7	51.0	19.1
Confidence in cabinet (socialist *interpellations* of workers' affairs; 14 May 1907). Passes, 323–205	82.6	15.2	2.1
Confidence in cabinet (socialist *interpellations* of government actions toward striking vineyard workers in the Midi; 18 June 1907). Passes, 389–153	79.1	16.6	4.1

Source: JOCD, 22 June and 12 July 1906, pp. 2042–3 and 2256–7, respectively; 15 May and 19 June 1907, pp. 1021–2 and 1415, respectively.

more pronounced leftist orientation than did their fellow senators. Like their *confrères* in the lower house, physician-senators tended to be comparatively radical concerning motions aimed against the church. Well over two-thirds supported Ferry's anticlerical laws, and in 1905 nearly 89 percent voted in favor of separation of church and state. Most other measures aimed at achieving a secular society found them in support; the divorce law, for example, voted by the Senate on 24 June 1884, received the backing of 89 percent.

Social issues were another matter. Although physician-senators were unanimous in approving the trade union bill of 1884, seven years later only 17 percent stood ready to endorse penal sanctions against employers found guilty of violating trade union rights. On a proposal defeated on 4 February 1897, 57 percent voted against creating an annual commission to investigate labor and welfare conditions in France.

What conclusions can be drawn from this survey of voting records? Despite the political pressures that often rendered a deputy's autonomy an illusion, it is clear that doctors showed more leftist tendencies than was true for the assemblies in which they sat and, more specifically, for the lawyers who dominated them. Except for anticlericalism, on which the doctors maintained a remarkable consistency, their radicalism appears to have been most pronounced on voting samples taken from the pre-1893 era. The chronology no doubt reflects the demise of the generation that had cut its political teeth under the Second Empire, but such crises as boulangism and the Panama scandal also played a part in toning down radical idealism, just as did labor's growing hostility toward the bourgeois Republic.

Ironically, physicians who sat in post-1893 assemblies had a higher proportion of radicals and radical-socialists than did those who belonged to earlier legislatures (54% as compared with 32%). Yet, as noted before, the meaning of these labels had changed. With the exception of the clerical issues revived by the Dreyfus affair, the votes of medical men after 1893 tend to suggest a more conservative social and political posture than had been the case during the regime's formative years.

THE FORMS OF PROFESSIONAL IDENTIFICATION IN PARLIAMENT

Although doctors in parliament did not consider themselves to be the political arm of the medical corps, it would be wrong to conclude that their work as legislators bore no relation to their professional identity. Certainly, critics who complained of their presence in French political life thought of them as something more than ordinary politicians who just happened to hold degrees in medicine. In committee deliberations, as in open debate, doctors had to proceed cautiously, knowing that their actions would be interpreted by some as an effort to promote professional interests. "Our legislators share some of the prejudices of the population," Testelin told a medical society in the Nord in 1877, "Because, by their studies, the doctors have touched on a multitude of questions and thus play an effective role in many committees, everyone regards them as intruders. 'These doctors,' they say, 'are everywhere!' "[18]

Of all occupations represented in parliament, physicians seemed the most susceptible to caricature, and other deputies and senators were quick to indulge in jesting at their expense or to invoke the sarcasms of Molière. A debate between Cazeneuve and Vaillant in 1904 over the dangers of apéritifs, for example, prompted one minister to remark that it was always easy to find one practitioner to confound the other: "In the old days it was Hippocrates and Galen; today, it's Dr. Vaillant and Dr. Cazeneuve."[19] A sure source of hilarity was to quote Beaumarchais's adage that doctors were the most fortunate of all people because "the earth covers their mistakes." Nor was there any reluctance to remind them of the less-glorious chapters of their professional past. Thus, the rightist senator Hervé de Saisy said in 1892 that although he was only "one of the uninitiated" amidst so many doctors, his study of their record had convinced him that "behind this claim to a monopoly in medical science there exists nothing but a chimera."

Can we not recall some of our great doctors, like Bocquillon, who applied axioms of the following kind to his patients? One day, upon entering the wards of the Hôtel-Dieu, he said to the students who were following him, "Well, what shall we do today?" And answering himself, he said, "Today we are going to purge all those on the left and bleed all those on the right."[20]

Medical men could be especially annoying in their habit of indulging in medical and scientific technicalities. Naquet's efforts in 1873 to lecture the National Assembly on the physiological causes of alcoholism provoked protests that parliament was not the Academy of Medicine. The debate on Liouville's proposal for obligatory vaccination in 1881 drew the same response, as did Bert's attempt three years later to instruct the Chamber on the causes of cholera. A lecture by Cornil on microbes, fermentations, and the chemical composition of sewer wastes, illustrated with flasks of contaminated and purified water, led an exasperated minister of public works to complain that "methods that are legitimate in the biological sciences are not . . . applicable to the same degree when it is a question of social facts."[21]

As legislators, doctors exhibited two forms of professional identification that distinguished them from other deputies and senators. The first may be termed *private-occupational* and was grounded in their own individual interests as medical men. The second is *public-corporate* and describes a more formal, collective attitude toward professional groups outside parliament, in particular the AGMF and the medical syndicates. We will begin with the first, which was the more dominant of the two.

It is not surprising that the areas in which doctors tended to specialize as legislators were usually related to their professional aptitudes, despite the number who made themselves experts in fields outside medicine. Examples of the latter include Bert and Combes in education; Viger, Rey, and Ricard in agriculture; Dron, Cosmao-Dumenez, and Camille Raspail in labor questions; Merlou in finance; Lourties in cooperative societies; Marmottan, Edouard Lachaud, and Labbé in army matters; and De Lanessan and Chautemps in the navy and colonies. Even for these individuals, however, the cultivation of nonmedical specialties did not preclude interests in fields more closely tied to their concerns as medical men, as the most active were normally involved in a variety of legislative endeavors.

All, without exception, devoted a substantial part of their efforts to purely local affairs. Those from rural departments, which is to say the majority, also followed matters of agricultural policy, at least insofar as these affected their own districts. Beyond that, certain multiterm deputies tended to develop one or more specialties, as reflected by their committee memberships and reports, their authorship of bills and amendments, and their speeches. Judging from these criteria, one finds high levels of activity among doctors in all areas touching on public health and social welfare, whether as a primary or a secondary field of specialization. Again, however, it is important to remember that many specialties overlapped with broader hygienic concerns. Labor problems, for example, often demanded expertise on a host of medical questions, from the need for obligatory rest for pregnant women working in factories to the physiological consequences of the twelve-hour day.

The interest of medical men in health and welfare is best seen in their committee activities. Before the emergence of standing committees at the end of the century, the business of the Chamber was conducted by ad hoc, or select, committees, each formed to consider proposals emanating from the government (the *projet de loi*) or from private members (the *proposition de loi*). The latter, less prestigious than the former, first had to pass a committee of initiative, but in both instances, proposals underwent brief discussion within the eleven *bureaux* of parliament. These, chosen each month by lot and including all deputies, in turn designated one and sometimes two of their members for service on new select committees, which then chose their own presidents and reporters.[22]

The large number of doctors in each legislature ensured that

Table 4.10. *Physicians on Chamber select committees dealing with health and welfare, 1876–1900*

Subject[a]	Percentage of doctors on committees	Number of presidents	Number of reporters
Reform of medical profession (4)	83.3	2	4
Reform of pharmacy profession (7)	37.6	1	3
Reform of veterinary profession (3)	18.1	0	0
Health administration, vaccination, housing, factory hygiene (7)	37.5	1	2
Rural medical assistance (1)	45.4	1	1
Rural hygiene, sanitary police (1)	63.6	1	1
Army and navy hygiene, medicine (3)	9.0	1	2
Water supplies, sewer systems (4)	18.1	0	2
Food processing, wine fraud (6)	21.8	0	3
Insanity laws (5)	40.3	1	5
Cemeteries, burials (6)	19.6	0	5
Protection of infants (4)	29.5	1	0
Old-age pensions, industrial conditions, women in industry, child labor, mendicity (7)	12.4	0	2

[a]Numbers in parentheses indicate number of committees considering bills on topics listed.

most of the *bureaux* had access to the services of several medical men. That the latter were consistently named to almost all the select committees dealing with hygiene and social welfare indicated more than a simple regard for their formal qualifications. As we shall see, physicians often brought their interests and specialties to the attention of parliament, by either offering amendments during debate or preparing their own bills. Like others, they frequently served on the very committees that were formed to consider their own bills.

Table 4.10 pinpoints medical membership on those select committees that examined health and welfare proposals in the Chamber between 1876 and 1900. It shows the proportion of doctors in the total membership for each category and the number of physician-presidents and physician-reporters. The figures in parentheses denote the actual number of committees that considered bills related to the topic in question; these were sometimes carried over from previous legislatures but in each case necessitated the creation of new committees. The table does not reflect the work of doctors on the Labor Committee or on the Social Insurance and Welfare Committee, which became permanent institutions in the 1890s.

After 1900, physicians could be found on all new standing committees, including those for agriculture, customs, railroads, public works, the army, and the navy. They normally comprised about 12 percent of the Labor Committee and 10 percent of the Budget Committee, which, unlike the others, dated from the early years of the regime. Doctors were more evident on the Committee on Social Insurance and Welfare (18%), but their greatest visibility lay on the Committee of Public Hygiene (43%). Created as a standing committee in 1898, it invariably had a medical man as president, and most of its reporters were doctors. Several belonged to it over the course of two or more legislatures, among them a core of committee activists who were prominent on the Left, including Vaillant, Levraud, Delbet, Chopinet, Eugène Villejean, Hugon, and Vacherie. An additional number of pharmacists (three to four per legislature) also sat on the committee.

Physician-senators exhibited similar interests to those of their colleagues in the Chamber, although the paucity of social measures originating in the Senate meant that their work was usually done in response to bills passed by the lower house. The proportions of doctors on both select and standing committees were also akin to those of the Chamber and, as in the lower house, usually ran high when the legislative task pertained to areas of their professional competence. During the 1890s, for example, doctors made up 60 percent of those committees considering measures to reform the medical, pharmacy, and veterinary professions. In public health, the percentage usually stood at around 25 percent, though this varied. It was lower on those dealing with controversial bills arousing entrenched economic interests, as in the areas of factory hygiene, labor accidents, and pure food and drink. It was higher (often close to 50%) in the domain of rural medical assistance, public health administration, and reform of insanity laws.[23] That the Senate was not a center or concern for public health should not cause us to underestimate the role of its doctors. On the contrary, the difficulty of getting health measures approved there served to enhance their importance, and frequently it was owing only to the persistence of doctors like Roussel, Cornil, Denoix, Cazeneuve, Lourties, or Labbé that certain bills could be salvaged.

Among all physician-deputies and senators, 8.6 percent served as committee presidents and 35.7 percent as reporters during the period as a whole. It was the *rapporteur* who performed the most difficult tasks, as he (or his aides) not only wrote up the committee's findings but also introduced and defended its final proposals on the floor. Many of these reports – replete with tables, graphs, and breakdowns by department – provide a wealth of information on the physical condition of French citizens, despite numerous flaws in the government statistics on which they often relied. Some earned for their authors a certain reputation in parliament, as was true for Bourneville, whose report of 1886 on a bill to purify the waters of the Seine was for years afterwards cited in parliament as a model of clarity and research.

Counting all major reports by doctors in the National Assembly, Senate, and Chamber between 1871 and 1914, we find a total of fifty that concerned public health, over two-thirds of them dating from the post–1890 period. Ten others dealt with reform of the medical and allied health professions, and an additional eight applied to social legislation whose articles touched on health and hygiene. The importance of this work is attested to by the number of bills that were eventually enacted into law – a total of twenty-six – on which doctors had at some stage worked as reporters. As we shall see later, these laws represent a significant share of the social legislation passed during the pre-1914 era. Well over half dealt with hygienic issues, from the law of 1881 on the sanitary police to that of 1902 on the protection of public health. A fourth centered on issues of social welfare, such as that of 1874 on regulation of wet nursing, of 1893 on rural medical assistance, and of 1905 on assistance to the old, infirm, and incurable.

In addition to committee work, physicians were active as authors and coauthors of numerous private bills. Although many of these concerned strictly local affairs, others were national in scope and often became the seed for future laws, despite the years that elapsed between their introduction and promulgation. There are numerous examples: Roussel on wet nursing and (with Dr. August

Morvan) on rural medical assistance; Chevandier on the liberty of funerals (1887) and on the reform of the medical profession (1892); Liouville on obligatory vaccination and on the protection of public health; Raspail on the Office of Labor (1891); Rey on assistance to the old, infirm, and incurable (1901); Chavoix on the regulation of slaughterhouses (1908); and Labbé on antityphoid vaccination in the army (1914). In addition, the doctors' private bills often were part of a group of related bills that ultimately resulted in laws. Examples include those by Marmottan on the military health service, which contributed to passage of legislation on this subject in 1889; by Roussel and Couturier on protection of mistreated and abandoned children (law of 1889); by Dron and Peyroux on the job rights of working mothers (law of 1913); and by Chautemps, Defontaine, Isambard, Goujon, and Chassaing on workers' pensions (law of 1895).

I have been able to identify all together eighty substantive bills by doctors (see Table 4.11). These demonstrate the strength of their programmatic interests while serving in parliament, as defined by Woshinsky for all legislators.

None of this is meant to suggest that physicians were the only members of parliament to show an interest in the nation's health. One could cite the names of numerous others who specialized in social issues, such as Jules Siegfried, Richard Waddington, Martin Nadaud, Jules-Louis Breton, and Paul Strauss. Yet, doctors could rightfully claim to have played a part in almost all health-related issues that came before parliament, and even those bills that ended up on the back burners, becoming void at the expiration of each legislature, served as periodic reminders of national problems. One thus should not judge the doctors' work simply by the number of overnight successes but, rather, by the degree to which it contributed to a political momentum that often took years to bring them near their goal.

The second form of professional identification was what I described as a public-corporate consciousness, which, though weaker than the first, could be seen as early as 1871. The election of thirty-three medical men to parliament that year raised hopes in the profession that these individuals would become its natural defenders. In August, Amédée Latour, secretary general of the AGMF, urged Roussel to rally his *confrères* against legislation threatening the medical press. He repeated such appeals on several occasions, citing an "avalanche" of social measures before parlia-

Table 4.11. *Private bills of doctors concerning health and welfare, 1871–1914*

Subject[a]	%
Medical and health professions	10.0
Public health	67.5
Administration, contagious diseases, vaccination (10.0)	
Rural medical assistance (6.2)	
Sanitary police (1.2)	
Army and navy hygiene (5.0)	
Pure water supplies (5.0)	
Food and wine purity (8.7)	
Insanity laws (5.0)	
Health protection for children, elderly (12.5)	
Worker health and hygiene (10)	
Population (3.7)	
Social welfare	22.5
Regulation of workshops, mines, railroads (11.2)	
Women and children in industry (2.5)	
Old-age and accident pensions (6.2)	
Indigent children (1.2)	
Reform of penal code (1.2)	

[a]Numbers in parentheses are percentages.

ment that would ultimately rest on medical practitioners and re-duce the profession to chaos. Ambroise Tardieu, president of the AGMF, had already written to local societies encouraging them to lobby on behalf of an amendment by Chevandier and Bouisson to place physicians on all administrative commissions of local hospitals and hospices. He also called attention to the bill to create new medical faculties and asked that each society make its views known to the deputies of its department.[24]

As the next chapter will show in more detail, these early efforts, which were poorly coordinated and dependent on just a handful of physician-legislators, proved to be symptomatic of the problems that later leaders of the profession would face in this respect. Chevandier and Bouisson did try to persuade the assembly to approve the seating of doctors on hospital administrative commissions, but their amendments were defeated on the grounds that local medical rivalries would disrupt the work of these commissions.[25] At the same time, and with hardly a glance at the AGMF, parliament proceeded to create new medical faculties, despite the reservations of Latour, who complained that Bert's report on the subject had exaggerated medical shortages and had ignored the problem of illegal practice.[26] In speeches to the annual meeting of the AGMF in April 1873, both he and Tardieu warned that their colleagues in parliament were powerless to help them, as evidenced by their failure to win approval for amendments to strengthen bills against public drunkenness and for the protection of children in industry.[27]

The election of forty-three doctors to parliament in early 1876 temporarily dispelled the gloom. At the AGMF's annual meeting in May, Paul Brouardel, vice-secretary, pointed out that twenty-three of these doctors were members of the AGMF, including three local presidents and four vice-presidents. Most important, one of them, Joseph Soye of Aisne, had taken the initiative in organizing a *groupe médical parlementaire,* which had already met with the minister of public education to discuss a bill revising laws on medical practice. Brouardel was euphoric: "I don't think I'm deluding myself in saying that right now we have the goodwill of the legislative powers and probably that of the executive."[28] Such optimism was still in evidence at the next year's meeting, when Cornil, Liouville, and Laussedat, the leaders of the new group in parliament, appeared at AGMF sessions and banquets bearing pledges of solidarity. Henri Roger, the new AGMF president, voiced his hopes that the parliamentary doctors would be able to win passage of new laws against charlatanism, despite the suspicion with which the political establishment had thus far greeted all proposals from them.[29]

Meanwhile, the *groupe médical parlementaire* had been holding weekly meetings, having chosen its officers during the summer. Laussedet was named president, Soye, vice-president, and Liouville, treasurer. Thirty-four physicians in the Chamber and Senate joined, and although regular attendance seldom approached half that number, the initial enthusiasm appeared to run high. At the outset, the group defined its purposes as being threefold. First, it would serve as a clearinghouse for ideas and information, which would enable the doctors to forge common strategies. Second, it would exert pressure on individual cabinet ministers, both to enlist support for specific measures of interest to the medical profession and to insist on more rigorous enforcement of present laws. Third, it would serve as a liaison between parliament and medical societies throughout the country, soliciting advice and receiving letters, reports, and petitions.

Over the next few months, the *groupe médical parlementaire* enjoyed a fairly active life, owing mostly to Laussedat, Soye, Liouville, Roussel, Chevandier, and Cornil. It appointed committees to examine two bills before parliament (on mineral waters and on rural medical assistance) and to report their recommendations to the full body. In addition, members of the group tried to arrive at a common agreement on bills dealing with army hospitals, welfare councils, and medical practice by foreigners. It also began considering loopholes in the law regulating wet nursing and in January 1877 sent a delegation to the minister of interior to complain that many departments were not obeying its provisions. Finally, it began to make itself known to the profession, sending out notices to local AGMF societies and urging them to submit ideas for possible legislative action.[30]

The realities of parliamentary life soon disappointed these initial hopes. For one thing, the *seize-mai* crisis of 1877 resulted in the dissolution of the Chamber, which sent deputies scurrying to regain their seats. For another, it was by no means certain that the leaders of the medical corps completely trusted a small group of politicians, even fellow doctors, on the matter that was uppermost in their minds, namely, the reform of medical practice. Latour, for instance, criticized a proposal by Cornil to this effect in 1877 as being unrepresentative of the ideas held by most doctors.[31] As will be seen in the next chapter, the AGMF leaders were by then already soliciting support from the government and within a year had formed their own commission to study the issue.

Most important, the demands on a deputy's time and the diversity of interests he represented made it impossible for him to perform the tasks envisioned by the founders of the *groupe médical parlementaire*. The group did reconstitute itself after the new Chamber convened in 1877, but fewer than half the doctors joined, and only a dozen or so bothered to appear at meetings, now scheduled on a monthly basis. "They're preoccupied on the committees to which they belong and by the political questions that most concern them," Chevandier explained in 1880, noting that most of their remaining time was spent attending to requests from constituents.[32]

Throughout most of the following decade, the *groupe médical parlementaire* remained inactive. Théophile David, deputy for Alpes-Maritimes, attempted to revive it after the elections of 1889, urging his colleagues to create a new and more vigorous union that would focus on reform of medical practice, rural assistance, and public hygiene. His efforts produced few results, and it was only in 1894 that the group finally began to renew its activities. This time the initiative came from *Le Concours médical* and a dozen or so deputies who belonged to its Civil Society. The journal stressed that its support was part of a larger strategy to enhance the profession's parliamentary influence, which was being undermined by frequent changes in cabinets and in the committees considering medical legislation. Thirty-seven of the seventy-one physicians in parliament now associated themselves with the new group, choosing Berthelot as honorary president, Labbé as president, and Cornil and Lannelongue as vice-presidents. A circular drawn up by the board of directors of *Le Concours médical* and sent out to all doctors in parliament specified six areas of concern: the first year of instruction in the faculties, military service of medical students, public health laws, organization of medical assistance to the poor, application of the 1874 law on wet nursing, and reform of laws dealing with the practice of pharmacy.[33]

As in 1877, however, the initial fanfare quickly died away, and by the end of the legislature those who had hoped to create an effective professional coalition in parliament had nothing to show for their efforts. Only three meetings, all in 1894, were ever held, and the only specific action taken by the group was a visit to the minister of public education to plead for scholarship aid for children of doctors serving in the *lycées*. In later years, the *groupe médical parlementaire* did manage to maintain an existence as an organized caucus. But the broad social vision that underlay its original creation had largely vanished, and it survived to 1914 as only one of many "extraparliamentary" groups formed to defend special interests.[34] Its infrequent meetings were dominated by a handful of doctors having ties with the syndicates and *Le Concours médical*,[35] and even these meetings were usually called only in response to pressure from groups outside parliament – in 1899, for instance, when the Union of Medical Syndicates tried to encourage the group to defend the rights of medical syndicates, or in 1907, when students in Paris sought to enlist its support in the fight to reform medical studies.

Eventually, most physicians outside parliament gave up hope of ever seeing the *groupe médical parlementaire* become the political voice of the profession. "I regret to say that many of them have forgotten that it was through medicine that they came to politics," Dr. Jeanne wrote in 1898, reflecting a sentiment heard with increasing frequency in the medical corps.[36] In reality, few of the critics seemed to grasp the problems that a physician-deputy faced in trying to help his profession. In all, only 52 percent adhered to the *groupe médical parlementaire* at any point in its existence. The number taking any part in the affairs of the group was much smaller, consistent with the modest proportion that had been active in the medical syndicates before entering parliament.

Several features of the doctors' overall record have been firmly established at this point. We have seen that on entering parliament they tended to be older than most other deputies and that, for the majority, this step marked an effective end to private practice. We have seen also that their ranks included a small but important elite, drawn mainly from professors and well-to-do country doctors, which enjoyed a relatively long tenure in parliament and was thus able to play a dominant role in its committee activities, particularly in the realm of health and welfare. Our preliminary survey of actual laws in whose making doctors had a part leaves little doubt about their influence, just as our analysis of their voting record has established without question a political and ideological outlook more radical than that of lawyers. These patterns will become even clearer as we examine in more detail their actual legislative accomplishments on professional, hygienic, and social issues.

5

Reform of the medical profession

What influence did our doctors have in strengthening the French medical profession before 1914? We will begin our examination of their legislative record by focusing on their individual and collective contributions to professional reform, starting with the campaign to abolish the institution of health officer (the *officiat*) during the 1870s. Afterwards, we will trace their deteriorating relations with the medical syndicates and the AGMF following passage of the Medical Reform Act of 1892, and we will conclude with a look at their activities in corollary efforts to reform pharmacy and nursing. Our aim is to show that the physician–legislators did play an important part in the post-1870 reorganization of the medical profession but that their ability to serve as defenders of its political and economic goals was greatly limited by the practical demands of a career in parliament and by the pressures each faced as a spokesman for rural interests.

THE DEFENSE OF PROFESSIONAL INTERESTS

As we saw earlier, the appearance of physicians among the national political elites during the 1870s was a cause of great rejoicing among leaders of the AGMF. Their optimism in regard to the future of the medical corps in general under the new Republic found numerous parallels among the professional classes, and it extended even to the workers, who saw the consolidation of the regime in 1877 as the prelude to political and economic emancipation.[1] For medical men, the promise ahead arose not only from their expectations for increased political participation but also from their belief that a natural link existed between their desires as doctors and the social goals of the Republic, ranging from primary schooling to urban sanitation, smallpox vaccination, and medical assistance in the countryside. Providing a powerful underpinning to this link was the historic record of doctors as champions of republicanism, a matter often alluded to by those in parliament, whose ranks included several who had been arrested under the Second Empire. For instance, during his campaign for the Chamber of Deputies, Dr. Bavoux of Jura reminded voters of his own fate during the coup of 1851, when gendarmes had bound him in chains and marched him to the sea. Dr. Le Monnier, who had practiced medicine as "a veritable priesthood" in Sarthe, had likewise suffered, having been fired from his hospital post, jailed at Nantes for eighteen months, and then deported to North Africa. It was this sort of country practitioner, Dr. Turgis reminded the Senate in 1891, that had been "the pioneer of the republican ideal."[2]

The question facing leaders of the profession in 1871 was whether this prestige could be translated into practical gains. At that point, the fundamental law governing medical education and practice in France was still that of 10 March 1803, which had created the system of faculties and preparatory schools and divided practitioners into two orders. Efforts to change the system had started as early as the Restoration and had peaked with the Paris Medical Congress of 1845, which had voted to unite the two orders. A bill to this effect, though backed by Paul de Salvandy, minister of public education, had aroused intense opposition in parliament, however, and the revolution of 1848 had ended further debate. The only significant reform had come six years later, when the government abolished the method of apprenticeship for future health officers and began requiring them to undergo formal training in a school or faculty. That change had marked the beginning of a decline in the number of graduating health officers.[3]

The birth of the Third Republic revived the question in earnest, owing mainly to the efforts of doctors in the National Assembly. The first to raise it was Alfred Naquet, radical of Vaucluse, who, as a freethinker and Jew, was hardly one to inspire enthusiasm in the conservative assembly. True to form, he proposed not only to abolish the *officiat* but also to do away with all provincial medical schools and faculties in order to concentrate resources in Paris. Naquet acted without consulting leaders of the profession, and his ideas took a drubbing in the medical press.[4] Still, some of his ideas touched a sensitive nerve, especially those concerning France's loss of medical and scientific preeminence to Germany. Thus, in February 1872, two other physician-deputies – Chevandier of Drôme and the monarchist Bourgeois of the Vendée – joined him in proposing the creation of a special commission to study the whole of medical reform. A committee of review, which included eight doctors, endorsed the idea,[5] but the Consultative Committee of Public Hygiene, which advised the government, was less enthusiastic. In a report dated August 1872, it conceded that reform was needed but warned against abolishing the second order, saying the resultant gap in practitioners would not be filled by an increase in the number of doctors.[6]

Meanwhile, leaders of the AGMF had issued a call to all affiliate societies urging them to express their own views. The results, published by Brouardel in 1873, showed near unanimity for abolishing the *officiat*.[7] By then, however, the National Assembly had put an end to hopes for immediate reform. In March 1873, after defeating a move by Chevandier and Bouisson to place doctors on all hospital administrative commissions, it vetoed the idea of a special commission to study medical reform. Later, it went on to reject Naquet's original bill.

Thereafter, only one topic proved capable of generating interest in this area in the assembly. That was the drive to create new medical faculties, which had been prompted by monarchist efforts to end the state monopoly over higher education. For republicans, the prospect of new Catholic faculties provided a powerful incentive to improve state institutions. The first bill pertaining to medicine thus came from a republican attorney of Lyon named Philippe Le Royer, who in the fall of 1871 proposed to transform the preparatory school of his city into a medical faculty. His was followed by similar bills on behalf of Bordeaux, Toulouse, Nantes, Lille, and Marseille. In June 1873, the assembly named a committee of fifteen to consider these, which counted six medical men (Bert, De Mahy, Naquet, Roussel, Thomas, and Bouisson). Almost all agreed on the need to decentralize medical education and to improve the number and quality of provincial schools; the exceptions were Naquet, who argued that creating new faculties without reforming teaching would perpetuate old abuses, and Bouisson, who feared that a faculty at Lyon would damage that of Montpellier, where he was dean.[8]

The reporter, Paul Bert, had his hands full in keeping the group's attention focused on the country's health needs, rather than on the municipal rivalries that had arisen among those cities wanting new faculties.[9] His final report, the product of an immense effort, pointed to a decline in the number of all types of practitioners since mid-century, which had been caused by a decrease in the number of health officers and by the tendency for the number of doctors to remain at the same level. Overall, Bert noted, the ratio of both to population had risen from 1 per 1,895 in 1847 to 1 per 2,341 in 1872. Yet, none of this reflected reality, for only a tiny minority of rural communes had a doctor. The cause was the reluctance of both doctors and health officers to practice in poor districts.

The report went on to argue that medically impoverished departments were generally those located great distances from medical faculties. Creating new ones, close to the student's home and less costly to his parents, would thus help alleviate the problem. Because most doctors practiced in the department of birth, it would have the added advantage of creating new medical families in isolated regions. The report recommended creating two new mixed faculties (of medicine and pharmacy) – one at Lyon and the other at Bordeaux – both of which offered excellent hospital resources for teaching. In addition, the preparatory schools of Marseille, Nantes, Toulouse, and Lille would eventually be allowed to become *écoles de plein exercise,* which would offer a four-year doctoral program without granting degrees.[10]

Doctors voted overwhelmingly in favor of Bert's proposal, which survived the required three readings in June and December 1874.[11] On the whole, reaction within the profession was favorable, although some journals insisted that no real shortage of doctors existed but that the real problem – unequal distribution of personnel – arose from the prevalence of illegal practitioners, which Bert had not addressed. AGMF spokesman Amédée Latour, for one, was quick to challenge Bert's statistics, contending that no one knew the precise number or distribution of practitioners in France.[12]

The failure of the physician-legislators to achieve further medical reform was a source of much frustration among leaders of the profession, which was only partially eased by organization of the *groupe médical parlementaire* in 1876. Even then, two years passed before officers of the AGMF took the first steps toward changing the law of 1803. That was the naming of a special study commission, which included Roger and Latour and had an important link with parliament in Dr. Dufay, deputy for Loir-et-Cher and former president of his local chapter. The sluggish pace of this group, however, convinced the newly organized Civil Society of *Le Concours médical* to take matters into its own hands. In August 1881, therefore, it appointed its own study group, this one led by Cézilly and counting among its members the physician-deputies Chevandier and Soye, both of whom belonged to the Civil Society.

The Civil Society's report, which was addressed to the doctors in parliament as "the natural intermediaries between the medical corps and the legislative power," gave a bleak account of circumstances in the medical corps. It argued that the condition most essential to improving them was the abolition of the *officiat,* followed by the enactment of stiffer punishments for those who practiced illegally. Such people included the religious orders, village matrons, itinerant charlatans, and all others who "take part in the treatment of medical or surgical maladies and afflictions, as well as in the practice of childbirth, either by habitual counsels and directions or by operations, application of dressings, or delivery of medications." Foreign doctors living in France were also singled out as illegal competitors.[13]

As Cézilly cranked up public support, Chevandier began drafting a bill that incorporated the report's main provisions. In the fall of 1883, he presented a draft of it before the study commission of *Le Concours médical,* where it won unanimous support and its author was praised for having provided "a good and salutary example to his *confrères* in parliament."[14] Although it used many of the same arguments contained in the report, Chevandier's bill placed greater emphasis on the extent to which the training of health officers now approached that of doctors. Existing health officers were thus to be allowed to continue as before or, if they had the requisite secondary degrees and six years of practice, to acquire their doctorates after passing two additional examinations and writing a thesis. Otherwise, only those with doctorates that had been earned at a state faculty and registered in the department of residence would be permitted to practice. In addition, foreign physicians would have to meet all requirements for the degree. The bill employed the commission's definition of illegal practice and adopted the same penalties it had prescribed. To the dismay of some, it also rejected any limitations on the right of women to enter the profession, pointing out that they already dominated obstetrics. Women, Chevandier observed, had never been explicitly barred from the practice of medicine, simply because "the legislator of 1803 never thought them capable of doing so."[5]

In the Chamber, Chevandier's bill was sent on to a committee chaired by Dr. Léon Joubert, deputy for Indre-et-Loire. In all, nine of the eleven members were medical men, including Chevandier, who was elected reporter. Then in his early sixties, Chevandier possessed a keen intellect and years of parliamentary experience, and he prided himself on having a firsthand knowledge of the problems of doctors, based on own earlier practice in the Drôme. With others on the committee, he tried to hammer out a bill that would meet the profession's legitimate demands and still stand a chance of passage. From their first meetings, the members were inundated with letters and petitions from the syndicates, AGMF affiliates, and individual doctors. They also had before them another report – this one the product of the almost-forgotten AGMF commission created in 1878. Focusing exclusively on issues of medical practice rather than teaching, the AGMF document likewise called for abolition of the *officiat,* while acknowledging that the idea was now opposed by a fourth of all affiliates, mainly those in departments with preparatory schools. On other matters, it proposed to make it more difficult for health officers to earn a doctorate, and it contained an additional article to create a degree in dentistry.

Chevandier's final bill, presented in June 1885, tried to incorporate a number of these and other ideas that had been brought before his committee by assorted professional groups. One provision, for example, stipulated that health officers who were still in practice after abolition of the *officiat* would no longer be restricted to a single department, even if they chose not to obtain a doctorate. In addition, a state diploma would be required of all future dentists, although this would take effect only after degree-granting programs had been in place for two years. Foreign doctors who had practiced for at least four years in their native countries could do so in France, but only if they passed a prescribed course of examinations. A final section obliged local prosecutors to bring illegal practitioners to court; fines and jail terms were spelled out in detail and made to increase in severity with each conviction.[16]

Chevandier resubmitted his bill shortly after the elections, adding an article that banned the dual practice of medicine and pharmacy. By February 1886, a new committee had been chosen, which counted ten doctors and again named Chevandier as reporter. The political situation he faced was not an easy one; for one thing, the elections had increased the number of radicals in the lower house, some of whom believed that the healing arts should be unregulated, as they were in America.[17] Another problem was whether the committee should introduce an article ensuring the legality of the medical syndicates, a matter of special urgency in light of a recent court ruling that stated that the trade union law of 1884 did not apply to doctors. The ensuing storm had already spilled over into parliament: In March 1885, leaders of the Union of Medical Syndicates had met with several physician-legislators to voice their complaints, and in February 1886, Dr. Destin Dupuy, deputy for Aisne and president of the union, had brought to the Chamber an amendment allowing doctors to form unions. He and Liouville had also presented a petition to this effect, which bore the names of 1,373 doctors.

The most formidable challenge came from the government itself, which had asked the Consultative Commission of Public Hygiene to prepare a bill based loosely on that of Chevandier, but taking care to "safeguard all the interests at stake." The subcommittee that performed this task counted only one doctor in parliament (Liouville); the rest typified the medical elites, and their report, written by Brouardel, departed from Chevandier's views in several ways. That is, it recommended that matters pertaining to teaching not be inscribed in the law, as these changed quickly in accordance with new directions in science. It also preferred a stricter regulation of dentistry and the limiting of its practice to those having the degree of health officer or doctor. Although it agreed with Chevandier in banning the dual practice of medicine and pharmacy, it refused to apply the restriction to those who already held both degrees. Nor did it spell out penalties for illegal practice, preferring to let the local courts decide. Most important, it urged retention of the *officiat,* arguing that otherwise the total number of practitioners might decline by a fourth. This was so, Brouardel said, because poor families, who now provided the bulk of recruits to the *officiat,* would be unable to afford the costs of the doctorate.[18]

Encouraged by Cézilly, Chevandier unleashed a stinging attack on Brouardel's report, refuting each of the arguments he had made in defense of the *officiat,* from its alleged services to rural France to its part in providing careers for the poor. Only one thing mattered: the right of citizens to receive from the state a guarantee of competence on the part of those to whom it awarded diplomas. In regard to possible shortages, Chevandier contended that if such a threat existed, the solution would be to make medical study more easily available, to eradicate illegal practice, and to continue building a national system of roads and railroads that would bring health care to all the people.[19]

These points were part of the revised bill that Chevandier submitted in early 1888, which also included a provision giving doctors the right to form unions. On the primary issue – abolition of the *officiat* – it got unexpected help from the military law of 15 July 1889, which required three years of service for those intending to become health officers. Students for the doctorate, on the other hand, were permitted to fulfill their obligation if they served one year before starting their medical education and if they received their degree by age twenty-six. The new law thus crippled defenders of the health officers, as Brouardel himself admitted, because poor parents could not afford to support a son whose studies might be prolonged to age twenty-eight.

Although Chevandier had succeeded in keeping alive the issue of medical reform, parliament's distractions over the boulangist controversy and other matters again kept his bill from reaching the floor. With the help of the physician–deputies Dellestable, Michou, De Mahy, and Marmottan, Chevandier renewed his efforts after the elections of 1889. The government followed suit, though without the provision for maintaining the *officiat.* The bills were sent on to yet a new committee, for which Chevandier retained the post of reporter.[20] Significantly, seven of its eleven doctors belonged to the Civil Society of *Le Concours médical,* and throughout the deliberations Cézilly kept up a steady lobbying effort, urging all doctors in the Chamber to join the newly revived *groupe médical parlementaire.* Professional reform also served as the theme of the annual banquets sponsored by the Civil Society and the Union of Medical Syndicates, at which Cézilly ensured that a select group of parliamentary doctors, including several committee members, was always on hand. Chevandier was the most active, but numerous others took part as well.[21]

By the spring of 1891, the committee had finished its work. Its members were unanimous on both maintaining state regulation of the profession and abolishing the *officiat*. They also recommended legalizing medical unions; on the other hand, they compromised with the government in accepting the need for strict regulation of dentistry and in abandoning efforts to reform medical studies. In March, the proposal finally reached the floor. In his opening remarks, Chevandier insisted that the issues at stake were those of humanity, not of the medical profession: "There is, in fact, only one category of sick people; there should be only one category of doctors. The equality of the sick before science is a democratic right that the Republic cannot ignore."

Because the government had dropped its objections and because it was able to convince deputies from departments with preparatory schools that these would be protected, the article to abolish the *officiat* passed with surprising ease. But this was not the case for the proposal to confine dental practice to doctors, health officers, and holders of a special state certificate. Edouard Isambard, physician–deputy of Eure, for example, balked at requiring dentists to have a doctor present when administering anesthesia, saying this would increase costs and thus "make the suppression of pain the privilege of those favored by wealth." Chevandier agreed, but Brouardel, the government's expert in the debate, delivered such dire warnings on the dangers of chloroform and cocaine that the Chamber approved the article. It also supported an amendment by the monarchist René Le Cerf to eliminate the bill's wording on illegal practice, specifically its ban on providing "habitual counsel" to the sick, which Le Cerf argued could never be enforced among families living great distances from a doctor. In addition, the majority endorsed an amendment compelling doctors to perform forensic services when asked to do so by local courts.

Numerous other articles that benefited the medical profession passed with scarcely a murmur of dissent. Among them were the right to unionize and the right to take up to five years in bringing nonpaying clients to court. Foreign doctors were to be subject to strict regulation, and the dual practice of medicine and pharmacy was to be outlawed, except to doctors residing in areas without a pharmacy or whose patients lived more than four kilometers from one. In any case, all would be permitted to carry certain drugs from an approved list.[22]

All eyes now turned toward the Senate, where the bill was submitted in May 1891. Here the key figure was Cornil, who headed a nine-member committee that counted seven doctors. These soon came under pressure from representatives of the preparatory schools, who portrayed the *officiat* as essential to provincial teaching. At the start of its deliberations, the committee was divided; Cornil thus proposed that the *conseils généraux* be polled on whether their populations would suffer if the *officiat* were ended. The results, presented to the committee in October, showed fifty-nine departments answering no and twenty-one yes. An additional seven expressed a willingness to see the *officiat* abolished as long as measures were taken to protect the preparatory schools. As a result, all but one of the doctors on the committee voted in favor of abolition. The majority also supported the right of doctors to form unions but chipped away at numerous other items. Although it retained the ban on dual practice of medicine and pharmacy, for example, it allowed those currently in practice to continue. It also reduced from five to two years the length of time a doctor could take to bring court action against patients.[23]

The Senate debate occupied two readings in March and April 1892.[24] Cornil dominated much of it, after first fending off an amendment to maintain the *officiat*. This motion lost by 146 to 92, and all but a handful of doctors voted with the majority. The Senate went on to accept state regulation of dentistry but decided to eliminate a provision requiring the presence of a doctor during the administration of general anesthesia. Dr. Lesouef, citing the needs of rural practitioners, also tried to defeat the article banning the dual practice of medicine and pharmacy. Cornil answered that the problems posed by dual practice seldom arose in the countryside but, rather, in the cities, where doctors gave "free" consultations and then charged extra for the drugs they prescribed. The ban passed by 107 to 57, with only two doctors voting with the minority.

The most heated debate came on the matter of medical unions. Supporters of the provision were apprehensive on this score, having learned on 19 March that the cabinet had voted to oppose it on the grounds that doctors were employed by state and local governments and so should not be allowed to strike against the public interest. Cézilly had immediately fired off a letter of protest to Prime Minister Emile Loubet, and Chevandier had paid the prime minister a visit in order to assure him that his fears were groundless.[25] Loubet stuck to his guns during the debates, but the most telling blows were delivered by Henri Tolain, a specialist in labor issues who had served as reporter for the trade union law of 1884. Gently mocking Cornil's attempt to compare doctors with industrial workers, Tolain remarked that he could accept the article in question only "if it were possible for the sick to organize themselves into professional unions in order to resist the doctors." The provision was defeated by a single vote. Physicians were overwhelmingly in its favor.[26]

Chevandier and Cézilly had one last chance to reverse this defeat, and that was in the second reading, scheduled for April. *Le Concours médical* called on each of its members to write to those who had opposed the article, and Cornil and his entire committee met with Loubet and Henri Monod, director of public assistance. Finally, a solution was reached: Doctors were to be allowed to unionize to defend their interests, but with the stipulation that they could not do so against the state, the departments, or the communes. Shortly afterwards, Cézilly called a meeting of the directors of *Le Concours médical* and the governing board of the Union of Syndicates, both of which accepted the compromise and began writing to each senator justifying the need for doctors to unionize.[27]

These efforts paid off during the second round of debate. Cornil argued that the country had nothing to fear from unionized physicians, even those holding public service jobs, and that the chief goal of the profession had been only to protect itself against illegal practitioners. Loubet expressed satisfaction with the new version, and the Senate approved it by voice vote. It went on to pass the rest of the bill, despite repeated attacks from the Right, which portrayed the measure as endorsing an official state medicine designed to protect the rights of doctors.

Indeed, the Chevandier law represented an important victory for the medical corps. As Martha L. Hildreth has shown, it advanced private practitioners in France closer to a true monopoly over the practice of their craft and, in so doing, helped them become "powerful arbitrators of the medical care system."[28] At the same time, the new law stimulated the political expectations of the medical corps, encouraging doctors to step up their pressure for new reforms. Léonard has placed special emphasis on the latter phenomenon, noting the host of special studies and congresses that were held after 1892 and whose focus was "the medical condition" and the need to narrow the gap between medical prestige and medical incomes.[29]

For the doctors in parliament, the victory marked a high point in their collaboration with the medical corps, one in which they had proved to be of great help in winning state support for the attack on sources of competition. Politically, the task had not been easy; yet, the physician-legislators had been able to draw on an old and powerful political theme, which was defending professional goals by referring to social needs and egalitarian ideals. A case in point was Chevandier's attack on the *officiat* as a denial of equality in health care. As we shall see later, the force of this idealism diminished as the medical corps began to articulate its goals in terms of a more narrowly defined self-interest.

None of this was yet apparent in the aftermath of the 1892 victory. That November, delegates attending the annual meeting of the Union of Medical Syndicates chose Chevandier and Cornil as honorary chairmen, in recognition of the part that each had played in guiding the bill through parliament. Cornil, offering a toast to professional solidarity, pledged his continued support, and Chevandier eulogized the law as an important step toward reaching the goals first laid out by the medical congress of Paris in 1845.[30]

Chevandier's death in early 1893 cast a temporary pall over this euphoria, but the gap he left was soon being filled from among the great numbers of doctors who entered the Chamber that year. There would be a total of seventy-one during this legislature: Joined with the thirty-six doctors already holding Senate seats, this represented their numerical high point for the period as a whole. Among the new deputies were several who had long been active in professional affairs, including Bourrillon, Chantelauze, Gueneau, and Pedebidou, the latter a practitioner from Hautes-Pyrénées who soon began assuming the mantle of Chevandier. These, plus seventeen others belonging to the Civil Society, exhibited a strong interest in professional life and took an active part in the meetings and banquets of the syndicates and other medical groups outside parliament. At Cézilly's urging, they reorganized the *groupe médical parlementaire,* which chose Labbé as president. At a banquet held in June 1894, a total of thirty-six physician-deputies and senators pledged anew to work together on issues affecting the profession.[31]

Following earlier patterns, however, the *groupe médical parlementaire* soon ceased to meet, and only Pedebidou and a few others could be counted on to take a consistent interest. *Le Concours médical* tried to revive it again in 1898, complaining on 18 June that "the physician-deputies have almost completely forgotten their origins" and that since passage of the Medical Reform Act few had spoken up to defend their profession. Such was also the opinion of the Syndicate of Doctors of the Seine, which in March 1899 hosted a banquet for the physician-legislators in an effort to persuade them to become the "natural representatives" of the profession. Several of the twenty-one physician-deputies and senators in attendance joined Pedebidou in promising cooperation, and shortly afterwards the *groupe médical parlementaire* was revived under Cornil's presidency. Only two meetings were held during the remainder of this legislature, however.[32]

The group's only sustained period of activity came after the elections of 1906, when it was led by Pedebidou and Dubuisson. The latter, deputy for Finistère, had by then become one of the profession's most outspoken defenders in parliament. Both he and Lannelongue served as the group's two vice-presidents, under Labbé, and by 1914 the group had increased to fifty-nine physician-deputies and thirty-seven physician-senators. Following a suggestion made by Cézilly, it had even divided itself into three sections, focusing on medical studies, professional interests, and public health. Yet, despite the best efforts, the group never managed to become a cohesive and influential parliamentary caucus.

Eventually, professional militants learned to look less to the doctors as a group than to certain individuals who were willing to draft amendments or to defend particular points of view in committee. It is easy to identify these physician-legislators, as *Le Concours médical* often singled them out for praise. Their numbers seldom rose above twenty, and most belonged to the group (about 15 percent of all physician-legislators after 1906) that was associated with the Civil Society or that had been active in local syndicates.[33] In addition, it was this minority, joined occasionally by sympathizers from among the elites, that exhibited the greatest ardor in championing the medical corps in its battles with the bureaucracy and the courts. Roussel, president of the Society for the Protection of Victims of Medical Duty, sponsored bills that would have treated as war widows the wives of doctors who died fighting epidemics, thereby entitling them to pensions.[34] Cornil condemned the inequities of forensic practice, especially after doctors at Rodez were fined for refusing to cooperate with judicial authorities in determining whether a murder victim had been raped.[35] He and Pedebidou were also active in winning a presidential pardon for a practitioner named Lafitte, who, despite his protests of innocence, had been sentenced in 1894 to three years in prison for performing an abortion on a patient he had been treating for a uterine disorder.[36]

On other issues troubling the medical corps after 1892 – in particular illegal practice and professional overcrowding – the physician-legislators could offer little help. In regard to the latter, for example, few were willing to address the root causes, which included easy access to the faculties. That point had arisen during a meeting of the parliamentary doctors with the medical syndicates in May 1899, where Cornil and others had rejected the idea of limiting the number of students by means of an initial *concours*.[37]

Capturing far more attention was the sporadic rioting of medical students at the Paris faculty. Though usually touched off by complaints against particular professors, its deeper causes lay in the structure of medical education and in the fact that most students, not interested in scientific careers, found themselves excluded from any sustained hospital experience. A requirement for a year of study in the science faculties, implemented in 1893, had rekindled old passions on this score that refused to subside with the passage of time. Students complained that the sciences absorbed more than half their time and that the system seemed bent on turning out scientists and scholars rather than practitioners. The resulting turmoil had implications extending beyond the faculty. As George Weisz has noted, this merged into a larger revolt of French practitioners against the dominance of the scientific elites, which the Right sought to exploit as part of an attack on the whole structure of republican educational institutions.[38]

Doctors in parliament repeatedly expressed their sympathy for the medical students' problems. Almost all backed the efforts of Labbé and Lannelongue in 1894, for example, to extend the draft deferment age for medical students from twenty-six to twenty-seven.[39] The same year, 68 percent supported a motion by Dr. Gadaud attacking a plan to transfer the teaching of physics, chemistry, and natural history from the medical to the science faculties.[40] Once again, however, their ability to offer solutions was limited. In 1904, after new protests had prompted the government to close the Paris faculty, a delegation from the Corporative Association of Medical Students of Paris met with leaders of the *groupe médical parlementaire* to ask for their help. The latter promised to intercede on behalf of those who were threatened with immediate military induction and to protest in parliament the closing of the faculty, but their intervention had little effect.[41]

Subsequently, members of the *groupe médical parlementaire* did help persuade the government to name an extraparliamentary commission on medical studies. Created in March 1907, the commission included nine prominent physician-legislators (of sixty-seven members), plus ten other members suggested by *Le Concours médical*.[42] Over the next year and a half, the group succeeded in putting together a series of recommendations that formed the basis for a decree reorganizing medical studies. But this decree fell far short of making the hospital the center of training, and in any case, it made no provisions for financing the proposed changes.

Continued turmoil at the Paris faculty, plus a vigorous press campaign by the syndicates, finally prompted the government to issue a new decree in 1911. Though essentially a repeat of the earlier one, it at least provided for the creation of the Superior Committee of Medical Instruction to oversee matters of application. Its seventy-five members counted nine prominent physician-deputies and senators, but the majority still consisted of the Paris elites. In the end, the causes of student frustration remained untouched, despite growing criticism of the Paris faculty from doctors in parliament.[43] On balance, and notwithstanding the repeated interventions of a small group, the physician-legislators proved to be a diminishing force for professional advancement of the kind envisioned by militant leaders in the afterglow of the 1892 victory.

THE ATTEMPTED REFORM OF THE ALLIED HEALTH PROFESSIONS

If the post-1892 efforts of the physician-legislators to defend the interests of the medical profession were limited, the reform of pharmacy and nursing, in which only a minority was involved, was even less vigorously pursued. Although the work of this minority was not without significance for the future of the two professions, our main interest in it is to demonstrate the degree to which parliamentary attitudes toward the health professions were defined by professional rivalries and electoral pressures.

As with medicine, the laws regulating pharmacy dated from 1803 and were equally defective from the standpoint of training and practice. Two orders existed: Students of the first had to have a diploma in letters or science and to spend three years in a faculty, a superior school of pharmacy, or an *école de plein exercice*. Students of the second needed only a certificate of studies and could fulfill all their requirements in a preparatory school. Although the second-class degree limited one's practice to a single department, it had a strong appeal for young men from poor backgrounds and in sheer numbers had always overshadowed the first. Testifying before a Senate committee in 1894, Brouardel pointed out that of approximately eight thousand pharmacists in France, 66 percent held the second-class degree. Like health officers, they tended to reside in the cities, where they constituted over two-thirds of the total.[44] The pattern had been noted by Bert in his report to the National Assembly of 1874; he had also warned of a deterioration in the profession's scientific standing, contending that the advent of patent medicines was reducing its members "to the role of simple warehouse retailers."[45]

Naquet and Chevandier had wished to include pharmacy as part of their proposed study of medical reform during the 1870s. Although parliament rejected the plan, the minister of commerce later asked the Council of State to prepare a bill revising those parts of the law dealing with practice. Completed in 1880, this report recommended keeping the second order while liberalizing the sale of patent medicines. In the meantime, the General Association of Pharmacists had been at work on another proposal, which was debated at a meeting in 1882. Delegates agreed on the desirability of abolishing the second order but were split over a proposal to allow the state to regulate sales of patent medicines and secret remedies. This hesitation caused the government to delay submitting a bill, prompting Hippolyte Faure, a pharmacist and deputy of the Marne, to offer one of his own. His bill proposed keeping the second-class practitioners, on condition that they be banned from cities of over ten thousand people. It also outlawed the dual practice of medicine and pharmacy, except when the patient lived at least six kilometers from a pharmacy. Those pharmacies located in hospitals or religious orders were to be forbidden altogether to engage in public sales.[46]

Faure's proposal went to a select committee of the Chamber, which now had before it bills from both the government and the General Association of Pharmacists. The committee, which chose Naquet as its reporter, favored abolition of the second-class degree while acknowledging the threat that this posed to future recruitment. To enhance the profession's appeal, therefore, it proposed that veterinarians no longer be permitted to dispense their own drugs and that strict laws be enacted against all forms of illegal practice. The committee also concurred with the ban on dual practice but adopted a more liberal attitude toward the sale of patent medicines, requiring only that their formulas be inscribed in the *codex*. Finally, it endorsed the idea of forbidding pharmacies in hospitals or religious orders from selling to the public.[47]

Naquet's bill survived only a committee of initiative before the term of parliament ended; it was left to the pharmacist-deputy César Duval to resubmit it after the elections of 1885 and, when it failed to reach the floor, to do so again after the elections of 1889. The committee that finally considered it, which was chaired by Duval, also had before it a revised government proposal to maintain the two orders, while preserving the right of veterinarians to practice animal pharmacy. Duval agreed with the latter but rejected keeping the second-class degree. At the same time, he and his colleagues faced such stiff resistance from the pharmacy profession regarding the ban on dual practice that they eliminated the article entirely, giving in to those who argued that this constituted an assault on property rights.[48] On the other hand, the committee kept a proposed ban on the sale of all French or foreign medicines whose names and formulas were not registered with the Academy of Medicine, despite a protest from over three thousand pharmacists.[49]

Leaders of the medical profession were equally upset with the report, insisting that dual practice most often injured the economic interests of doctors. Worse still in their eyes was the plan to allow pharmacists to sell freely all nontoxic drugs, while limiting the right of country practitioners to dispense medicines to their own patients. As if these issues were not enough, by the second reading of the bill in the summer of 1893 a new dispute had arisen, this one over a proposed ban on the right of hospital pharmacies to sell drugs. It was this that concerned most deputies, who stressed the importance of this source of income for the work of the hospitals in their own districts. Although a majority was willing to approve the bill, it reaffirmed the rights of hospitals in this regard.[50] The matter now went to a Senate committee, chaired by Cornil.

To this point, the physician–legislators had played only a limited part in the debates. By 1893, however, the medical syndicates had started to worry that an expansion of the rights of pharmacists would come at their expense and had begun appealing for help from the doctors in parliament. In November, delegates of the syndicates came before Cornil's committee to request that the ban on dual practice be reinserted. They also urged limits on the types of drugs that pharmacists could sell without prescription, and they asked the senators to reaffirm the Chamber's decision to abolish the second-class degree, whose holders were pictured as the ones most often involved in illegal medical practice. Members of the General Association of Pharmacists also appeared before Cornil, focusing their attacks on that part of the bill allowing hospital pharmacies to sell to the public, which they denounced as a boon to the religious orders that would lead "fatally to the ruin of several thousand pharmacists."[51]

In the midst of this controversy, Cornil tried to steer a middle course. In the fall of 1894, he presented an amended bill on the floor of the Senate. This version accepted abolition of the second-class degree, and although it agreed that hospitals should not be allowed to operate public pharmacies, it proposed a ten-year grace period before such a prohibition would take effect. The bill also stipulated that individuals who were now engaged in dual practice could continue but that this would be banned in the future. In addition, pharmacists were to be allowed to sell across the counter any simple medication that appeared on an approved list. On the question of how far away a pharmacy had to be located in order for a doctor to furnish drugs to his patients, the proposal recommended six kilometers, as a compromise between the four asked by doctors and the eight asked by pharmacists. Cornil did express sympathy for rural practitioners on this score and promised that in any case, they would always be allowed to carry with them certain essential drugs, from ether to quinine.

On the main point – suppression of the second-class degree in pharmacy – the Senate agreed by a vote of 170 to 68, with only 1 doctor joining the minority. An amendment to allow doctors in rural areas to continue practicing pharmacy passed by a single vote. To the anger of many in the medical profession, only 23 percent of the physician-senators voted in favor of the amendment, and an additional 30 percent abstained.[52]

This bill might have become law had the Chamber been willing to accept it without changes. The medical syndicates denounced it, however, demanding that pharmacists be allowed to sell without prescription only those medicines that were included on an official list.[53] *Le Concours médical* especially criticized Cornil and other physicians in parliament for trying to accommodate pharmacists, though it was pleased to learn in early 1896 that two of its own members – Pedebidou and Bourrillon – had been named to the new Chamber committee that would review the amended bill.[54] In fact, Bourrillon and his colleagues (there were five other doctors on the committee) not only altered the Senate text but even changed a number of articles that the Chamber had already approved. Complicating matters further was their attempt to clarify the legal status of patent medicines, which only intensified the debate among pharmacists themselves. Faced with the difficulty of getting the whole bill passed, the committee reported out only the single article calling for abolition of the second-class degree. As reporter, Dr. Bourrillon argued that to have accepted a government plan to solve the problem by restricting second-class pharmacists to rural areas, where it was hard to earn a living, would have been an inducement for them to practice medicine, thus driving out the doctors. In March 1898, the Chamber approved the partial measure.[55] Otherwise, the reform movement in pharmacy achieved few of its goals, despite several attempts after the turn of the century to regenerate the momentum.[56]

In regard to the other health professions, medical reformers in parliament worried less over professional rivalries of this kind than over the political realities in their own districts, particularly among voters who continued to prefer lay practitioners to graduates of the schools. A case in point was veterinary medicine, a matter of no small importance to the nation's health. In a report to parliament in 1895, Dr. Gadaud suggested that up to two million head of cattle were afflicted with bovine tuberculosis alone. A few years later, Dr. Villejean, deputy of Yonne, observed that the disease was of "extreme frequency" in certain regions, infecting up to 50 percent of the herds. France, Cornil warned the Senate, was losing a fifth of its cattle wealth to contagious diseases.[57]

Only three training centers for veterinarians existed – at Alfort, Toulouse, and Lyon – all founded early in the century to meet the needs of the cavalry. These, however, produced very small numbers of graduates: In 1894, the total number of state-trained veterinarians was estimated at 3,400, many of them located in cities.[58] Who, then, treated animal diseases? The answer can be found in the multitude of unschooled practitioners who flooded the countryside. Although some were useful, having specialized as farriers or gelders, others posed a danger, such as those empirics whom the minister of agriculture described in 1886 as "using all the means that their greed can suggest for gaining the confidence of their credulous victims."[59] The competition that they posed made it hard to recruit young men to the profession. Still, as Dr. Guillemaut reminded the Chamber, many rendered invaluable services to agriculture and could not be replaced.[60]

Other physicians in parliament recognized this reality, even though they gave lip service to the idea of strengthening the rights of state-educated personnel. Physician-deputies who helped forge the law of 1881 concerning the local sanitary police, for example, agreed that only licensed veterinarians should oversee the quarantining or destruction of animals suffering from certain contagious maladies, such as foot-and-mouth disease, glanders, farcy, scabies, anthrax, and rabies. Even so, the committee reporter, Dr. Félix Mougeot, warned that twenty-five of the seventy *conseils généraux* in favor of the bill had expressed concern over the lack of enough state veterinarians to carry out the law.[61]

During their stay at the Ministry of Agriculture, both Viger and Gadaud found themselves indeed handicapped by the shortage of state veterinarians, especially in the battle against bovine tuberculosis. Gadaud, for example, presented a bill in 1895 stipulating that all cattle exhibiting the standard clinical signs of the disease be slaughtered. Suspect animals were to be injected with a tuberculin devised by Robert Koch and, if positive, were also to be destroyed; cattle that seemed healthy but that had been exposed and tested positive could be sold for slaughter, providing this was done within a year so as to ensure that the disease had remained localized.[62] Such efforts were a step in the right direction, but they could succeed only with the help of qualified veterinarians, who were needed to organize local epizootic services and to introduce newly discovered methods, such as vaccinations for anthrax, glanders, swine fever, and rabies.

By the turn of the century, only thirty departments had services of this kind, at a time when animal losses to disease were costing owners fifty million francs a year. Doctors in parliament were among the strongest backers of a private bill of 1906 to place epizootic services in the hands of veterinarians chosen by competitive examination.[63] This bill became law three years later, but many parts of the nation remained untouched. As the Committee of Agriculture concluded in 1914, the continuing problem of epizootic diseases in France mirrored a breakdown in animal sanitary regulation, at the heart of which was the absence of qualified veterinarians.[64]

As difficult as this issue was, nursing presented an even greater challenge to those physician–legislators who hoped to introduce scientific reforms to patient care. For nursing was the turf of the sisters, whose influence had been on the rise since the Second Empire. In 1881, their membership stood at over eleven thousand, and it was they, not the doctors, who dominated the life of the wards. Few physician–legislators could ignore the risks involved in attacking the very popular sisters, and few had any ideas as to who would replace them. Even assuming that state schools could be built, there remained the question of who would pay the higher fees that the lay graduates demanded.

For these reasons, the campaign against the orders originated in an even smaller minority of our group, most of them radical ideologues who typified neither the elites nor the rank-and-file practitioner. The majority came from the cities, where they had served as mayors or municipal councillors before entering the Chamber and where, unlike other physician–legislators, they enjoyed a certain immunity to retaliation. Even then, things could be difficult. At Lyon, Augagneur's efforts to introduce lay nurses into the hospitals earned him the undying enmity of the local monarchists, as did those of Langlet at Reims. Paul Laurens, physician-mayor of Nyons in Drôme, even received death threats. But the person who most inflamed feelings was Bourneville of Paris.

Robust and barrel chested, his head tilted back as if in defiance, Bourneville was unyielding in his assault on the orders, arguing that their expulsion was an indispensable complement to school reform and to the social program of the Republic.[65] In his thinking, the sisters would never be able to meet the demands of modern medicine and surgery, for along with the technical knowledge these required was the need for new ways of thinking, which had already proved their worth in the lay services of Germany and England. Of no less importance was the issue of power, for non-clerical personnel would be more malleable than the sisters were – in his words, the former would be "capable and obedient auxiliaries to the doctor."[66]

Paris was the logical starting place, for its three thousand lay hospital personnel already outnumbered members of the orders by six to one. Thus, in 1877 Bourneville persuaded the municipal council, to which he had been elected, to send him and several others to London to study English nursing as laid out by Florence Nightingale, whom he admired. The next year, he created two new training centers – at Salpêtrière and Bicêtre – with a third being added at La Pitié in 1880. Together, their enrollments soon reached around four hundred women a year. Along with modest sums voted by the municipal council were funds from Bourneville's own pocket. Besides running the schools, he also wrote much of their instructional materials, including the well-known *Manuel pratique de la garde-malade et de l'infirmière*. In addition, he persuaded a number of friends, among them Charcot and Liouville, to donate time and money.[67]

In the meantime, Bourneville and other radicals on the municipal council were pressing the city to move against the clerical hospital personnel. First to go were the resident hospital chaplains; then, in December 1880, came the first of several efforts to replace the sisters themselves. This provoked an outcry, not all of it from the Right, for among the elites holding hospital posts in the capital were several republicans who condemned the campaign as disruptive and who included from our group Cornil, Lannelongue, Labbé, and Pozzi.[68] The most violent protests, however, emanated from the eccentric surgeon of Charité, Armand Després, who soon emerged as one of the warmest defenders of the orders, despite his Protestant origins and his reputation as a freethinker. Showing a combative zest matching Bourneville's, Després denounced the latter as "the worst enemy of our hospitals," at one point accusing him of protecting a lay nurse who had been caught stealing, at another questioning the honesty of his expenditures at Bicêtre. In the press and in the municipal council, to which he was elected in 1884, Després kept up these attacks, which Bourneville answered in kind.[69] The duel continued in parliament after Després was elected deputy for Paris in 1889 on a platform of keeping the sisters in the hospitals.

There were doubtless many physicians in parliament who sympathized with Bourneville's efforts, but there was also truth in Després's charge that those who did so ignored the nursing orders in their own departments, knowing that they could not be replaced. The issue came before the Senate in May 1881, when Lambert de Sainte-Croix pressed the government on whether it associated itself with the actions of the Paris municipal council. He argued that the sisters had long ago proved their worth and that what had prompted the attacks was not a matter of incompetence but of religion, and only because republican doctors were "much more worried over this sort of contagion than over smallpox or diphtheria." Ernest Constans, minister of interior, defended Paris, adding that the government did not wish to set the precedent of interfering in local hospital management. By a vote of 135 to 120, nevertheless, the Senate approved a resolution favorable to the sisters. None of the doctors voted with the majority.[70] In the lower house, it was Bourneville who most often introduced the issue. He contended that the state should laicize the staffs of all institutions under its control, from navy hospitals to insane asylums, and he was especially eager to rid Charenton of its resident chaplains.[71]

Després's moment came in December 1890, when he attacked the government as having abdicated its authority over the Paris hospitals. He described the lay nurses who had replaced the sisters as being incompetent, claiming that there had been six deaths in the wards due entirely to their negligence. By contrast, one could always count on the sisters. True, there were those who prayed with patients and occasionally tried to convert them, but this he regarded as harmless and, for terminal cases, even useful. Whereas the lay nurse went home at the end of her shift, the sister remained at the bed of the dying, who was usually alone in the world and for whom the sister represented the only family:

A woman who has neither family nor pecuniary interest, who doesn't even have a name and is called simply "Sister," who lives the life of a prisoner, sleeps in a dormitory, eats in a dining hall the same food that the sick eat, and who, 365 days a year, from four in the morning until ten at night, cares for the sick with clockwork regularity, have you replaced that? No! and you will never replace it.[72]

Despite Després's failure to win over the Chamber, the campaign in Paris was already starting to falter. During the municipal elections of 1890, supporters of the sisters formed a committee and began circulating a petition that within three years had accumulated 600,000 signatures.[73] Bourneville kept up the fight, despite losing his Chamber seat. In 1895, he created a fourth program at Lariboisière and was soon boasting that the number of graduates from the four schools had reached 3,070.[74] Meanwhile, the sisters were holding their own at the Hôtel-Dieu and the Hôpital Saint-Louis, and in the provinces their numbers had actually increased. Bourneville assailed the Paris municipal council for its failure to expel them, and he charged departmental legislatures with having sacrificed the welfare of the sick because of selfish concerns over the cost of replacements.[75] By 1903, he was pleased with the decision of Dr. Combes, then prime minister, to laicize Charenton. While admitting that France still had far to go, Bourneville pointed with pride to nursing programs that now existed in twenty towns and cities.[76]

That same year, Combes signaled the start of a new push against the orders with a circular to prefects urging the creation of nursing schools in all cities where a medical faculty or preparatory school existed.[77] Although nothing came of this, he did approve plans to remove the orders from the navy hospitals of Cherbourg, Brest, Lorient, Port-Louis, Rochefort, and Toulon. By that point, however, many practitioners were beginning to conclude that modern nursing would never take root in France so long as ideology dominated the question. Dr. Jeanne, for one, argued that many physicians were allowing their political prejudices to blind them to the fact that in certain regions, like the west, both patients and practitioners would be without nurses if the orders disappeared. As it had done with primary education, Jeanne pointed out, the state must provide alternatives, and he appealed to the *groupe médical parlementaire* to begin preparing these by sponsoring laws regulating nursing education.[78]

Few medical men in parliament were willing to take up the cause, however, even though the doubtful legal status of the nursing orders following the Combes era created uncertainties for both practitioners and local governments. In 1911, Jeanne observed that many physicians who were mayors and presidents of hospital commissions or who ran their own clinics would have liked to hire members of the orders but had hesitated to do so in light of government threats to move against the orders. The problem was most delicate regarding unauthorized congregations, whose applications often went unanswered. Jeanne appealed to the *groupe médical parlementaire* for help in facilitating these requests.[79]

Only in 1912, after rumors began circulating that all nursing orders would be banned, did the physician-legislators attempt to take a stand, and then only because of protests from *Le Concours médical* and other journals assailing government intrusions into the affairs of private clinics.[80] On behalf of the *groupe médical parlementaire,* the physician-deputy Amédée Peyroux wrote to the minister of interior in July condemning any plans to ban the sisters from these clinics. Prodded by the AGMF and the Union of Medical Syndicates, the parliamentary doctors approved a resolution saying that the orders were essential to private clinics and that until there were a sufficient number of lay nurses, the government should act with tolerance on all requests for permission to employ members of authorized congregations.[81]

Although the *groupe médical parlementaire* agreed that the growth of lay nursing schools would resolve the problem, the only bill to this effect came in November from Doizy and Vaillant, on behalf of the socialists. The bill never made it out of committee, despite their arguments that the issue had ceased to be one of anticlericalism. That theme was taken up by others, like Julien Noir, who wrote that although the passions of the 1880s had reduced Bourneville's efforts to "a simple anticlerical manifestation," even his detractors now recognized the necessity for nursing education, which was no longer the platform of a particular group.[82]

This survey of our doctors' activities in matters related to the medical and health professions has revealed a number of important traits. It is clear, for example, that although large numbers contributed to the work of committees that reported out bills in these areas, the initiative in proposing and overseeing them came from a relatively small group associated with the syndicats and with *Le Concours médical*. It is equally clear that this element, led by Chevandier, Dupuy, Pedebidou, Dubuisson, and others in sympathy with Cézilly's ideas, proved extremely useful in helping the profession strengthen its position in society, at least until the law of 1892. Afterwards, the increasingly narrow focus of professional goals weakened the ability of our doctors to equate such goals with the public good and the needs of a democratic society. As a result, their intervention became more limited and reactive, to the point that by the turn of the century, professional spokesmen had begun to despair of their ever becoming the political arm of the medical corps.

As the last two chapters will show, certain individuals in our group continued to offer their help on a number of issues, especially those involving the participation of doctors in the application of social laws. By then, however, physician–deputies and senators had ceased to be regarded as central actors in the medical struggle and were seen instead as just one of many tools that militants could use along the way. As evidence, one need only consider the limited role played by the physician–legislators in the revolt of students and practitioners before 1914, not to mention their inability to address the causes of discontent, such as overcrowding and illegal practice, among the rank and file. This reflected more than a refusal to become identified with the interests of a particular profession; it evolved also from a preoccupation with local matters and from what Dogan has termed the *optique arrondissementière* that characterized all deputies. Indeed, the structure of politics under the Third Republic limited the power of parliament itself to alter the social forces that regulated progress in the health professions, as we have just seen in the case of pharmacy and nursing. The persistence of these forces will become even more evident when we consider the role of our doctors in health and welfare.

6

Defense of the people's health

As we saw in Chapter 4, physicians made up a large share of the deputies and senators who were involved in the campaign for health and welfare laws between 1871 and 1914. Was this activity common to all medical men who held seats, and was it more characteristic of some political factions than of others? Most important, did it contribute in significant ways to the progress of public health legislation in France?

This chapter will attempt to answer these questions, first, by examining the role of the physician-legislators in modernizing the system of hygienic administration in France and, second, by focusing on their work in pure water and pure food laws, military hygiene, and the struggle against tuberculosis. In particular, it will try to explain why, despite their numbers in each legislature, the doctors were often unable to achieve their goals or to overcome the limitations inherent in parliament's power to enforce hygienic laws. As we shall see, the duplication and confusion surrounding the public health bureaucracy meant that parliament was often just one of several competing forces that affected the outcome of health and welfare measures. The diffusion of hygienic authority, along with the resistance of local assemblies and property owners to state intervention and increased spending, had parallels in all countries, including England and Germany. Both of the latter, however, were able to codify their sanitary legislation at a much earlier date than France did, and both succeeded in forging a stronger political and legal framework for supporting government action in this domain.[1]

Before turning to these issues, it will be helpful to survey the voting behavior of our doctors on hygienic issues and to identify the professional types that led the movement in parliament. Because of the connection between public health problems and the social questions treated in the next chapter, I will also trace the political assumptions that shaped their vision.

PUBLIC HEALTH ACTIVISTS AND THE HYGIENIC CRUSADE

A profile of medical men based on voting records poses a problem insofar as public health matters are concerned, primarily because of the paucity of examples showing a clear pattern over time. One difficulty is the rarity with which hygienic legislation reached the floor, itself testimony to the low priority assigned to this matter by the political leadership. Second, many bills that did receive a public airing were the product of years of debate, many having survived only as patchworks of amendments that had vitiated the original intent and that, when finally brought to the floor, were approved in almost cursory fashion by voice vote. Third, recorded votes did not always express a deputy's real thinking but, rather, the tactics of his group. Many moderate physician-deputies were no doubt appalled by the government's clumsy response to an outbreak of cholera in the south in 1884, for example, but only a fourth – about the same as for the whole Chamber – were prepared to join the radicals in a vote of no confidence.

There were, it is true, certain issues on which medical men exhibited an apparent professional consensus cutting across factional lines. Most, for example, strongly favored obligatory small-pox vaccination, as can be seen in their response to Dr. Liouville's proposal to this end on 8 March 1881, which 95 percent approved (64% for all deputies). The doctors also were consistent in their support of government action to promote urban sanitation and the cause of pure water: In a motion on 25 January 1888 to purify the Seine by means of a new method of waste treatment called *tout à l'égout,* 80 percent voted in favor, as opposed to 53 for the entire assembly. Two years later, 89 percent (76 % for the Chamber) endorsed a bill aimed at providing Paris with fresh water from springs in Vigne and Verneuil, against the objections of local property owners. Physicians in the Senate showed similar tendencies, as evidenced by their votes on the bill leading to the 1902 Law for the Protection of Public Health. Seventy-one percent favored a provision for the sanitary inspection of housing (session of 6 February 1897), as compared with 60 percent for all senators. Four days later, 42 percent supported a controversial article spelling out sanitary steps to be undertaken by local governments; for the whole Senate, the figure was only 16 percent.

In those instances in which public health measures touched on the interests of a particular region, such medical consensus as did exist largely vanished. This localistic mentality was visible in many areas, but especially in pure food legislation. Only 57 percent (as opposed to 64% for the whole Chamber) supported Bert's motion on 21 December 1883 to suspend imports of U.S pork until parliament could consider organizing an inspection service to guard against trichinosis. Only a fourth endorsed an amendment by Vaillant on 1 December 1904 to strengthen a bill on food fraud by inserting a precise definition of adulteration. In both cases, the proportions reflected those of other professional groups in the Chamber and were, as we shall see, tied directly to the pressures that each deputy or senator faced from political and agrarian forces at home.

Most of the members of our group were willing to compromise their principles in return for political survival, and this, as the last chapter will show, extended to the battle against alcoholism. Still, it is possible to identify a smaller element that showed consistently high levels of support for hygienic measures and that exhibited a strong professional motivation in their behavior. These individuals formed the bulk of committees dealing with health and welfare before 1914 and, as seen in Chapter 4, were responsible for most private bills in this area. In all, 104 individuals can be judged as having been "extremely" active on issues related to health, as measured by their authorship of bills and amendments, committee memberships, service as *rapporteurs,* and speeches. Of these, 31 were interested less in problems of public sanitation than in social issues containing medical and hygienic components, such as the regulation of wet nursing or aid for the sick and elderly. Together, the two groups account for 29 percent of all doctors who served in parliament.

The hygienic activists were generally of three types. The largest was the country practitioners, which included several prominent *médecins-agriculteurs* who were interested in pure food issues. Next were the urban radicals, coming mainly from Paris and the industrial districts of the north and east and including such figures as Dubois, Chassaing, Chautemps, Levraud, Georges Martin,

Table 6.1. *Proportion of physician-deputies specializing in health and welfare issues, 1876–1914*

Legislature	%
1876–77	20.9
1877–81	18.3
1881–85	16.9
1885–89	25.4
1889–93	22.4
1893–98	22.5
1898–1902	33.3
1902–6	40.0
1906–10	42.1
1910–14	46.1

Vaillant, Dron, Defontaine, and Doizy. Last were the professional and academic elites, of which the most important were Bourneville, Cornil, Roussel, Labbé, Lannelongue, and Liouville. The last group often spearheaded the drive for public health laws. All three types were active in each legislature of the period and increased steadily over time, as Table 6.1 shows. The upturn starting in 1898 mirrored a similar increase in the number of legislative texts dealing with public health (laws, decrees, and circulars), which corresponded to a growing concern in parliament generally with social issues.[2] In regard to public health activists, that same year also saw an increase in the proportion of deputies representing the northern industrial departments, which stood at around a third in all subsequent legislatures.

Certain of the more leftist members of this faction, as typified by the socialist Vaillant, considered their interest in matters of health and welfare to be a distinctive component of their own partisan values. Nevertheless, the distribution of political ideology for the group as a whole, which is akin to that for all physician-deputies, suggests the presence of other ideological motivations as well (see Table 6.2).

What were the ideas that bound this group together? It would be easy to interpret their work as simply an effort to enhance the authority of their own profession, but to do so would ignore the richness of the larger current of which this work was a part and which Paul Strauss, deputy of Paris and a leader of the movement,

Table 6.2. *Political ideology of hygienic activists in Chamber,*
1876–1914

Political ideology	%
Right	0.9
Conservative republican	12.5
Moderate republican	35.5
Radical republican	41.3
Socialist	9.5

hailed as *la croisade sanitaire.*[3] The term was fitting for a cause that
spoke the language of moral passion as much as of science and
whose disciples seemed confident of the imminent victory of medicine over its ancient foes. Science, Vigné d'Octon boasted to the
Chamber in 1896, was slowly triumphing over death, and perhaps
tomorrow it would create life itself.[4]

Because great numbers of physician-legislators saw themselves
in the vanguard of this crusade, their ideas serve to illustrate the
moral imperatives that fueled the movement in France. These
rested on several political ideas, of which the first was the notion
of public health laws as a democratic response to disease, which
had always claimed its greatest number of victims from among
the oppressed. Because hygiene now had the power to alleviate
and even to eradicate epidemics, it was a tool essential to achieving equality. Echoing a sentiment heard often among physician-
legislators, Naquet in 1904 praised Pasteur, Lister, and Roux as
having contributed far more to the victory of social justice than
had even the most idealistic partisans of violent revolution.[5]

The extension to all citizens of equal protection against disease
was seen by politicians of the Third Republic as one of the loftiest
forms of social solidarity. It is true that the philosophy of *solidarisme*
could be made to serve the political ends of the ruling classes, just
as it is true that many owners and employers accepted hygienic
laws only because they offered a savings of "human capital." Still,
the solidarist vision bore traces of an old idealism that was evident
among advocates of public health reform as early as the Revolution. "The misery and sickness of one creates misery and sickness
for the other," Dr. Peyrot of Dordogne said during a Senate discussion of lead poisoning in 1901. Today, he added, all people

should consider themselves socialists when the health of their fellow citizens was concerned.[6] Doctors invoked such arguments in all debates on public hygiene and often reminded parliament that the principle of collective responsibility for illness was rooted not in modern doctrines of solidarity but in revolutionary *fraternité*.

A corollary of this principle was nationalistic in character and strove to erase the presumed physical inferiority of French people vis-à-vis the Germans. In parliament, few discussions of health issues took place without favorable references to the quality of Germany's institutions and to its repeated victories in the war against disease. The most troubling aspect was the perceived health and vigor of the German army. Figures assembled by Labbé in 1903 revealed that though the peacetime mortality rates of French forces had fallen over the last twenty years, they still stood at 4.58 per 1,000 effectives, as opposed to 2.32 for Germany.[7] Dr. Lachaud, who specialized in military hygiene, told the Chamber a few years later that France's rates continued to be inferior to those of Germany, that its soldiers suffered from crippling attacks of typhoid fever, diphtheria, scarlet fever, and measles, and that the hardest hit were recruits from rural areas.[8]

Invariably, these warnings sounded a danger that transcended matters of combat readiness. In a report dated 1892, Dr. Langlet pointed to the large proportion of conscripts rejected for medical reasons, ranging from shortness of stature, which was common among the rural and urban poor, to a host of scrofulous afflictions, deformities, and lesions.[9] The problem did not end there, especially in an era when the draft was exposing the whole country to the dangers of barracks life. The army, said Amodru, was "the most important of our social collectivities," for each year a part of it dissolved, sending thousands of young men back to the towns and villages from which they came, and with them such infections as diphtheria and tuberculosis. There was "an incessant exchange" of this sort going on, Brouardel said in 1897, noting that polluted water supplies in the towns and villages through which the troops passed or were quartered often poisoned them.[10]

As important as these ideas were to the hygienic cause, doctors were able to invoke an even more primordial necessity in support of their views, which was the need to reverse the country's population decline in order to ensure the survival of the French "race." Robert Nye has called attention to the significance of biological metaphors and the medical concept of "degeneracy" in contemporary attempts to explain the decline and weakness of post-1871 France.[11] Such themes also influenced the thinking of our doctors, who used depopulation as one of their most effective rhetorical tools and who, like Berthelot, condemned opposition to hygienic legislation as a "murderous action" against the species itself.[12]

The basic facts were simple. The population of France, which during the 1880s hovered at around 38 million, showed only minimal growth, leading many observers to consider it only a matter of time before the death rate outstripped the birthrate. At first glance, French mortality levels did not appear to be excessively high, standing during the first decade of the Republic at an estimated 23.7 per 1,000. That was higher than rates for England, Belgium, and Switzerland but lower than those for Italy and certain south German states. Yet, as Chamberland had noted in a report in 1887, France could take no comfort from these figures, for the simple reason that its death rates were highest among infants. If France's birthrates were higher, he reasoned, its death rates would also be higher, because its levels of infant mortality were among the worst in Europe. An infant in France, Roussel had observed in 1874, had a smaller statistical chance of living for a week than did a ninety-year-old man.[13]

Most of our doctors understood that depopulation stemmed less from high death rates than from low birthrates, which had fallen from 26.7 per 1,000 in 1872 to 23 in 1888. Explanations varied, but the physician–legislators repeatedly used certain ones. Dr. Javal, deputy of Yonne and author of a bill exempting large families from personal property taxes, singled out a variety of factors, from the equal-inheritance provision of the Civil Code, which led many couples to limit themselves to one son, to the heavy burden imposed on large families by taxes on articles of consumption.[14] Nevertheless, Javal and his colleagues also regarded poor hygienic conditions as contributing to the crisis. The toll taken by diseases of infancy and childhood formed the best proof, for here the loss of life appeared to be even greater than that suggested by estimates based solely on the first year of life. The hygienist Gustave Lagneau told the Academy of Medicine in 1890 that statistically, 3 children were born to each household in France but that early death reduced this figure to 2.07. Even this mortality rate was not as high as that indicated by Langlet's report to parliament two years later. If, he said, one compared the number of males born in any given year with the number called to military service twenty years later, one would find that barely two-thirds survived. Put another way, for every 1,000 males born in 1843, only 632 survived to age twenty, which represented a mortality rate of 36.8 percent.[15]

Few physician-legislators believed that medicine in itself could solve these problems, despite its promises. The real hope, rather, lay in preventive strategies, whose basis was bacteriology. Like the miasmic theories of earlier generations, bacteriology left a deep mark on public health politics. As Claire Salomon-Bayet has argued, Pasteurianism signified both a theoretical revolution and a medicalization of society, both of which were transferred to the political plane by an accompanying legislative revolution that was "analogous to the classical structure of scientific revolutions."[16]

The vast majority of physician-legislators supported bacteriological ideas. The exceptions stand out and usually could be found among those for whom eccentricity was a badge of honor. Després of Paris, for one, delighted in mocking Pasteurian precepts, never permitting carbolic dressings in his service at Charité, where he was known to some as "the dirty surgeon." Dr. Michou, who blamed the high rates of typhoid in the capital on the Parisians' riotous manner of living, dismissed "the unbelievable show-off of microbes" among bacteriologists, saying that fifty or sixty years would be needed to determine the real value of the theory. Dr. Treille could not have agreed more. He scoffed at the notion that germs were transmitted via water (he called this "the absolute hydrous formula") and invoked his experiences as an army doctor in North Africa as evidence.[17]

More typically, Dr. Chautemps in 1890 ridiculed those who opposed bacteriology, adding that the best support for its validity was in the statistics for German and Austrian cities showing dramatic declines in disease mortality rates after the introduction of pure water supplies.[18] By then, several figures in our group were helping propagate the new doctrines in surgery – Maunoury at Chartres, Monprofit at Angers – and the sense of mission they brought to this task was shared by many. Lannelongue, for instance, related to the Chamber in 1896 how thirty years earlier Paris surgeons had operated on patients outside the city where there was "good air," not realizing that their own hands were the carriers of deadly germs. But Pasteur had changed all that: "He has shown to mankind the means of recognizing his most implacable enemies. Where there was only doubt and darkness, he has brought light."[19] This tone of reverential awe was common in parliamentary debate and transcended political ideology: "Pasteur should have a statue in every French village," the royalist physician Paul Bourgeois told the Chamber in 1895.[20]

New knowledge regarding the etiology of cholera and typhoid meant that pure water was the key to all public health systems. Jean-Pierre Goubert has stressed the degree to which all modern hygiene proceeded from the "laicization" of water during that era, when it was stripped of its religious mysteries, subjected to chemical and bacteriological analysis, and even made to celebrate the virtues of the Republic in a proliferation of public fountains.[21] "It is incontestable," wrote Dr. Langlet in 1892, "that one of the first necessities for meeting the demands of hygiene is to have water of good quality and in sufficient quantity – of good quality, because it is used for human consumption, and of sufficient quantity, because it is the natural vehicle for carrying the wastes and refuse of human life far from cities and inhabited areas."[22] Next came the task of disinfecting the dwellings of the sick. The worth of this measure was plain to see, Cornil assured the Senate, for before disinfection procedures were employed in Paris, such diseases as smallpox, typhoid fever, diphtheria, scarlet fever, whooping cough, puerperal fever, and erysipelas killed an estimated five thousand people a year.[23]

Most parliamentary doctors thus accepted the idea that the eradication of harmful microbes in drinking water and in human habitations was fundamental to public health. What uncertainties they evinced were those inherent to bacteriology itself and, as we shall see, arose most often on questions concerning soil rather than water. At the political level, conservatives sometimes extolled the new science as having sanctioned their own values by shifting the blame for disease from social conditions to disease-specific microbes.[24] Most medical men in our group, however, tended to view bacteriology as a complement to more advanced forms of political thinking. Certainly, Amodru wrote in 1901, the tuberculosis germ and its route of contagion were now known, but hygienists also understood that its underlying causes included powerful predisposing causes, such as poverty and the unsanitary milieu found in the urban and industrial centers.[25] This dual explanation for disease – microbes and a social environment that nurtured their growth – was evident in the speeches of many members of our group, who accepted Cornil's view that disease had two parents: "The first is the germ; the second is the terrain."[26]

Far from weakening the political basis of hygienism, bacteriology gave it a more precise grounding. Thanks to Pasteur, Chamberland argued, the task of reformers could be mapped out in specific terms: the rigorous disinfection of towns, streets, and houses; the removal of pathogenic germs from all products of human consumption; and new forms of hospital construction.[27] Cornil defined the essentials of public health as "ventilation, good quality of water, enough water and sewers necessary to remove human wastes, cleanliness of dwellings, preventive measures against the invasion of epidemics, such as preventive or curative vaccinations, the surveillance of new arrivals at the frontier, a maritime police, and the limitation and destruction of centers of epidemics by disinfection of dwellings and objects soiled by the sick."[28] In France, as in England and Germany, the germ theory of disease strengthened the hand of health reformers at all political levels.

In their dual role as medical men and politicians, the doctors evinced a deep tension between their hygienic idealism and the liberal ideology that characterized their social class. Few were eager to promote the cause of an intrusive state, and few liked the idea of higher taxes in order to implement public health laws. Nevertheless, the theoretical values derived from social hygienism, whether based on miasmatic or Pasteurian theory, were conducive to a more empirical view of social problems than was true for lawyers and, by contemporary standards, could indeed be seen as a corollary of republican and radical ideology. Public health, legitimized by bacteriology, was a collective enterprise necessitating the subordination of private interests to the general good. This meant that property rights must not be allowed to dominate all other considerations. The same was true for disinfection, isolation, and vaccination, even if citizens complained of assaults on their freedom. Freedom, Langlet reminded parliament, had many faces when viewed against the suffering of smallpox, which he considered a more fundamental violation of liberty.[29]

Finally, hygienism provided new and compelling reasons for extending the coercive powers of the state. Like Roussel, many doctors contended that the essential flaw of all hygienic legislation in France was its reliance on voluntary compliance. Enhanced governmental surveillance of public health thus presumed acceptance of an enlarged and costly bureaucracy, along with expanded methods of inspection and information gathering that, in the eyes of many conservatives, were alien to the true functions of government. Even so simple a matter as keeping death statistics, Cornil told the Academy of Medicine in 1906, was a task that many local administrators did not regard as being within their purview.[30]

There were many ways in which the doctors pursued their interests as hygienists, apart from their activities in parliament. For the few belonging to the Academy of Medicine, periodic debates on hygienic issues provided a prestigious forum. Others brought their knowledge to bear on elite councils of state, such as those on public assistance, protection of children, and labor.[31] They were likewise visible in numerous private associations. The influential Society of Public Medicine and Professional Hygiene, created in 1877, attracted leading architects, engineers, and doctors, including Laussedat, Liouville, Testelin, Cornil, and Javal, all of whom served among the first officers. Lourties was active in the Alliance of Social Hygiene, founded in 1907 to combat infant mortality, alcoholism, and tuberculosis, and Dr. Peyrot was cofounder of the Society of Defense Against Tuberculosis Through Popular Education and, after 1902, vice-president of the Federation of French Antituberculosis Groups. One could mention also Henri Ricard's Scientific Society of Alimentary Hygiene and Rational Human Diet, which sought to advance research on nutrition and food fraud.[32]

International gatherings provided an even broader forum. Laussedat and Liouville were among the main organizers of the First International Congress of Hygiene and Life Saving, held in Brussels in September 1876. At the meeting's conclusion, Liouville proposed a sequel in Paris to coincide with the Exposition of 1878, afterwards convincing the Society of Public Medicine and Professional Hygiene to help with arrangements. Several physician-deputies contributed their efforts by serving on organization committees, including Cornil, Bert, Roussel, Testelin, Wurtz, and Bernard-Lavergne. Liouville assumed the post of secretary of the congress, which was finally held at the Trocadéro in August 1878, attracting over a thousand delegates from across Europe to hear papers on infant hygiene, housing, diet, and the pollution of streams and rivers.[33] At Turin two years later, Bourneville headed the section dealing with school hygiene, and Liouville provoked a spirited debate by asking delegates to approve obligatory small-pox vaccination.[34] These and several others in parliament were active in subsequent congresses.[35]

An international focus was seen also in the work of the Chamber's Committee of Public Hygiene. After its first chairman, Ville-jean, had persuaded parliament to grant it special investigative powers, it sent delegations on several study tours abroad – to slaughterhouses and water filtration plants in Berlin and other German cities in 1903, for example, and to the London meat markets. Villejean, Hugon, Pourteyron, and Lachaud were among a delegation to visit navy hospitals at Brest during a typhoid outbreak that December, at the same time examining working conditions in installations manufacturing gunpowder for the navy. Another outbreak of typhoid, this one at Verdun in 1907, led the same group to make an on-site inspection of water supplies; committee delegates visited Saint-Nazaire and Cherbourg during outbreaks of yellow fever as well. Insisting that all bills touching on health and hygiene pass under its scrutiny, the committee emerged as an important focus of hygienic activity before 1914, hearing testimony from government experts, manufacturers, professional groups, hygienists, and scientists. By 1910, it had divided itself into five subcommittees working in the areas of school and infant hygiene, military hygiene, industrial hygiene, housing, and nutrition.[36]

The fervor that inspired the work of hygienists everywhere thus left a mark on the French physician-legislators and served as the moral and ideological context for many of their own efforts in parliament. We will now examine these more closely, starting with their campaign to forge new instruments of public health administration.

THE REFORM OF PUBLIC HEALTH
ADMINISTRATION

Like their predecessors of 1848, many of our doctors shared the old dream of hygienists that the state would become the prime defender of its citizens' health. The high levels of political optimism visible during the early years of the Third Republic encouraged that hope, while the progress of bacteriology provided the means for its realization. Two obstacles stood in the way, however. One was the growing resistance of the medical corps itself: As Martha L. Hildreth has observed, the Pasteurian revolution, with its stress on preventive medicine, left a divided legacy among private practitioners, as it shifted the focus away from traditional concepts of individual treatment, on which their livelihoods depended. At the same time, new and comprehensive public health programs seemed to threaten the doctor's autonomy by creating a strong, centralized medical bureaucracy.[37] In parliament, therefore, the drive to write public health laws ran up against the indifference, and eventually the hostility, of the medical profession. Except for Cornil and a few others, the deputies and senators who led the movement were rarely those who associated themselves with the syndicates or who had been active in the campaign to revise the laws concerning medical practice.

The second problem was much older and arose from the weakness of existing hygienic institutions. For what most characterized the public health bureaucracy in France was its administrative chaos. Two ministries shared responsibility over this domain – commerce and industry, which oversaw public hygiene, and interior, which controlled welfare, hospitals, and asylums. The system rested on an array of laws going back to the Revolution, which had left enforcement in the hands of the mayor.

The Republic of 1848 had tried to forge a more rational system. It created the Consultative Committee of Public Hygiene, which was to advise the government on quarantines, thermal establishments, mineral waters, smallpox vaccination, and factory hygiene. Later, it organized hygienic councils in each department and canton and in April 1850 passed a law on unsanitary housing. All these measures suffered from the same defects, which was their reliance on voluntary compliance and their lack of funding by the *conseils généraux*. In 1873, a total of thirty-nine departments failed even to submit reports on the work of their hygienic councils. As for local housing commissions created under the 1850 law, only nine were still in operation by 1878.[38]

The continuing toll taken by epidemics served as a reminder of the problem's deepening urgency. Although not the killer it once was, smallpox still claimed large numbers of victims, ranging between 2,000 and 3,000 a year.[39] The epidemic of 1870–1 had taken a severe toll, especially in the army, where 20,000 men died of it (losses in the Prussian army, where vaccination was mandatory, were 264). Typhoid was another killer. By the 1880s, the morbidity rate in the army stood at 243 per 100,000, as compared with 95 for Germany and 91 for England. Cholera also continued to pose a danger: An outbreak in the south in 1884 claimed 12,000 lives and was the latest in a cycle going back four decades.[40]

The leadership of our group stands out clearly in the long drive to overhaul the institutions designed to prevent such tragedies. Dr. Liouville, deputy of Meuse, took the first steps. In 1880, he presented to the Chamber, in the form of a petition, a report written by A.-J. Martin for the Society of Public Medicine and Professional Hygiene, urging a reorganization of departmental hygienic commissions and the creation of a new *direction* of public health under a single cabinet officer.

While the Consultative Committee of Public Hygiene pondered the matter, Liouville, observing that most other Western countries were already conquering smallpox by the use of Jenner's vaccine, approached parliament with a plan to make smallpox vaccination mandatory for newborns and to require revaccination every ten years. More than half the committee members named to review his bill were medical men, including the reporter, Louis Le Maguet, who finished his work early in 1881. Citing Benjamin Disraeli's axiom that the people's health dominated all other social problems, Le Maguet labeled smallpox one of the most murderous diseases in France and argued that there was no longer any doubt that modern medicine was capable of wiping it out entirely. The first (and only) reading of the bill took place in March 1881. Despite attacks on it, Liouville succeeded in winning over a majority, including all but two of the doctors.[41]

Although the bill eventually got shoved to the side in face of more pressing political matters, it had generated much discussion in medical circles, and soon afterwards both the Academy of Medicine and the Consultative Committee of Public Hygiene declared themselves in favor of obligatory smallpox vaccination.[42] Two further developments helped keep attention focused on Liouville's ideas. The first, coming in the wake of renewed outbreaks of typhoid in Paris, was a bill by Martin Nadaud to reform the law of 1850 on unsanitary housing. His suggestions for reform found

a sympathetic reception among such political radicals as Félix Can-
tagrel, who reported that there were 219,270 houses in France
without windows, that many of these had up to six people per
room, and that a total of 1.3 million French citizens "existed in a
state completely identical with that of animals."[43]

The second was an outbreak of cholera in the south during the
summer of 1884. After visiting the stricken cities of Marseille and
Toulon, a delegation from the Consultative Committee of Public
Hygiene urged better coordination of local authorities in attacking
the evil at its source, which was polluted water supplies. The
government's halfhearted response angered medical men like Bert,
who saw the heart of the problem as the state's lack of enforcement
powers. As an example, he cited the absence of a law requiring
doctors to report cases of contagious diseases, estimating that only
150 of every 2,000 such cases were ever brought to the attention
of authorities. Seconding these criticisms was Clemenceau, who
proposed sending a parliamentary delegation to tour the south.
A. C. Hérisson, minister of commerce, objected that this would
interfere with the work of local officials and thereby persuaded
the Chamber to vote the idea down.[44]

While the cholera was still raging in the south, Liouville submitted a new proposal, this one asking the government to concentrate all hygienic services under one ministry. But his proposal
never reached the floor. Thus, in June 1886, he and twenty other
physician–deputies joined Chamberland and Jules Siegfried in presenting a more comprehensive plan that, besides grouping health
services under one ministry, envisioned a new corps of sanitary
agents to oversee the enforcement of all hygienic policies. The bill
also proposed the creation of a National Health Council, which
would replace the Consultative Committee of Public Hygiene and
be drawn from the ranks of parliament, the Academy of Medicine,
the medical faculties, and assorted state bureaucracies for mining,
engineering, commerce, and agriculture. Each department would
have its own council of health, and each of the sanitary districts
in which it was to be divided would have its own commission of
health. Finally, a new laboratory would be built to assist the state
in carrying out research on contagious diseases. Half the costs
were to be borne by the state, half by the departments.[45]

In response, the government submitted its own bill, which went
to the same committee then reviewing the bill from Chamberland

and Siegfried, and on which doctors formed a majority. The government version, which incorporated some of Nadaud's ideas on housing, likewise called for stronger hygienic councils within the departments, but by means of the more effective use of present laws. It contained no provisions for an expanded inspection bureaucracy, for example. Because the government was reluctant to strip the Ministry of Commerce and Industry of its powers over public health, whose policies affected economic life, it also proposed to maintain the Consultative Committee of Public Hygiene in its present place and role.

Chamberland himself wrote the committee report, and although it was never discussed on the floor, it was an important first step on the road to reform. The document laid out in detail the facts of France's inferiority to other countries in regard to infant deaths and disease morbidity and mortality. Emphasized most was the need to expand the state's authority in health matters, an area in which mayors had neither the interest nor competence to carry out effective policies. It proposed that departmental inspectors coordinate the work of local hygienic councils and that they report to an enlarged public health administration, or *direction*. Seen as being less vulnerable to cabinet turnovers than a ministry of health would be, the *direction* would exist as an autonomous service in the Ministry of Interior and would be advised by a superior council of public health. Such a move would not only place under one roof all responsibility for health and welfare, but it would also improve services. Hospital officials, for example, whose resources were invariably strained during epidemics, would now have a direct interest in prevention.[46]

In January 1889, partly as a result of this report, the government transferred all hygienic services from the Ministry of Commerce and Industry to the Ministry of Interior, with the exception of those affecting workshops and factories. Following the general elections of that year, a new committee was named to review again all previous proposals, the government having added several new provisions to its own bill. The most important called for obligatory smallpox vaccination, mandatory notification of contagious diseases by doctors, and compulsory sanitation of unclean dwellings. Because of the importance of its task, this committee was doubled in size to twenty-two members, of whom nine were doctors. Over the course of seventeen meetings, it strove to reconcile the Siegfried–Chamberland bill with that of the government, especially on the matter of unsanitary housing and property rights. The final report, written by Dr. Langlet, reiterated the arguments advanced earlier by Chamberland and provided new information on the worsening state of the cities, whose slums were overflowing with immigrants from the countryside.[47]

Introduced in the Chamber by Langlet in June 1893, this bill sided with Siegfried and Chamberland on the need to enhance the state's hygienic powers. It stipulated that all communes would henceforth be compelled to provide pure drinking water. In towns of five thousand or more, no building could be constructed or occupied unless the owner had obtained a permit indicating that all hygienic conditions had been met; in extreme cases, the mayor could ban occupation outright. Departmental councils and commissions of hygiene would be revived and supported by a corps of sanitary inspectors, all appointed and paid by the state. Smallpox vaccination was to be mandatory, and all doctors, health officers, and midwives would be required to notify public authorities of contagious diseases, within twenty-four hours. Although that obligation had been written into the Medical Reform Act of 1892, the present bill applied it also to heads of families, directors of hotels and rooming houses, and all who treated patients of any kind. The list of declarable diseases was to be drawn up by the Consultative Committee of Hygiene and the Academy of Medicine. Although some deputies objected that the provisions on housing violated property rights, the majority, by voice vote, approved the bill and even agreed to forgo a second reading.[48]

Following this vote, the Senate named a review panel of nine members (including five medical men), who chose Cornil as reporter. Between September 1892 and December 1895, the group prepared its own version, changing several of the bill's features. It strengthened the right of appeal among property owners accused of maintaining an unhealthy dwelling, and, fearing objections to new bureaucracies, proposed that enforcement be carried out by existing services for abandoned children. As for centralizing the public health authority, it opted to keep the present system, although it agreed to expand the duties of the Consultative Committee of Public Hygiene.[49] Arriving on the floor in February 1897, the measure consumed five sittings in all, during which the Senate altered the bill further. The size of towns to be covered was changed from a minimum of five thousand to twenty thousand, and the article requiring the mayor's approval prior to occupation of a building was scrapped. The cause of inspection likewise suffered, as François Volland, a specialist in the legal aspects of social legislation, forced an amendment compelling prefects to obtain approval from the *conseils généraux* before organizing inspection in the smaller towns and villages. This passed with more than three-fourths of the Senate in support, despite warnings from Cornil that local assemblies would never approve the funds.

On the whole, doctors in the Senate were more conservative in their response to the bill than were their counterparts in the Chamber. Fifty-seven percent, for example, supported the Volland amendment. Others were reluctant to curtail property rights, as was evident in their vote on Article 11, which would have increased the mayor's powers to make owners clean up their property. The Senate rejected this provision by nearly three to one, with less than a third of the doctors in support. Then there was the damage inflicted by Dr. Treille, who ridiculed the plan for inspection services ("We can say goodbye to intimate outpourings! Just at the moment when two lovers are sharing tender little intimacies, the sanitary inspector will come storming in with a court order") and who assailed the bacteriological assumptions implicit in the provisions to create pure water supplies. So great were the objections that, at Berthelot's suggestion, the first reading was suspended while the committee sorted things out. Debate resumed only in December, when it returned with a greatly modified bill. Gone was the plan for an inspection service, as was true for provisions strengthening local hygienic councils and empowering municipalities to move against owners of unsanitary dwellings.[50]

Even this watered-down version was barely kept alive over the next three years for the required second reading. Helping the cause, however, was the committee's decision to enlist the aid of Senator Volland, who, in examining the facts, became convinced that the housing law of 1850 was unworkable and that circumstances now justified change. In support, one could also invoke the findings of a new commission on tuberculosis appointed by Prime Minister René Waldeck-Rousseau, which declared the chief cause of the disease to be unsanitary lodging, especially in tenement districts where rents averaged under three hundred francs a year, as was true for 40 percent of Paris housing. Finally, other physician-senators, such as Labbé, began to take a more active interest, whereas in the lower house Vaillant pressed the government to explain the Senate delay. Encouraged, Cornil and his group resolved not only to bring the proposal back but also to ask reconsideration for several items already voted down.

This second round of debate occupied six sessions, starting in December 1900.[51] This time, Treille saw the initiative slip away, especially after Labbé and Berthelot attacked him as an obstructionist. Each article was then approved by voice vote. The articles concerning housing, though now featuring safeguards to protect the rights of owners, empowered mayors to disinfect unsanitary dwellings and to ensure the purity of drinking water; should the mayor fail to act, the prefect would step in, particularly in communes whose mortality levels exceeded the national average three years in a row. Disinfection services (carried out by steam and chemical vaporizers known as *étuves*) would be created in all towns of twenty thousand and over, each of which would establish its own municipal health board (*bureau d'hygiène*). There, no new structure could be built without a sanitary permit. Overseeing implementation would be departmental councils of hygiene, each numbering ten to fourteen members and including at least three doctors, one pharmacist, one veterinarian, one engineer, and one architect. Also endorsed were compulsory smallpox vaccination and compulsory notification of contagious diseases, although responsibility for notification would be placed squarely on the doctor, thus absolving the heads of families. After a budget committee report, which placed implementation costs at 2.6 million francs (of which the state would pay only 12%), the measure was approved. From there, it went back to the Chamber and, after a report by Dr. Borne, was passed without debate.

Despite the compromises that had been the condition of its passage, the law of 1902 generated widespread resistance, ranging from property owners and municipalities to the medical profession. Writing in 1910, Villejean argued that the law had been sabotaged by "passive resistance" and that the obligatory declaration of diseases "has still not become ingrained in the behavior of doctors." He also noted that most new municipal health boards were "phantom boards" that did little. As for the inspection services, these hardly existed anywhere.[52] Julien Noir faulted local governments for their indifference. Many towns had no disinfection services at all, he pointed out, whereas in others they "are carried out in a comic-opera fashion by firemen, constables, and railroadmen who haven't the faintest idea what they are doing."[53]

The doctors in parliament worried over these failures, but they were hard pressed to offer solutions. Although they did achieve some success in opening up the membership of the Consultative Committee of Public Hygiene, whose composition in 1902 had been weighted in favor of *ex officio* members taken from the administrative elites of Paris,[54] other problems proved more vexing. Most troubling was the matter of inspection and enforcement. In November 1912, Dr. Doizy, a member of the Committee of Public Hygiene, submitted a bill calling for the creation of a corps of departmental inspectors, to be named after competitive examinations and paid for by the departments. He and Lachaud, chairman of the committee, also began pressing for a law to provide state funds to departments unable to afford disinfection services, but neither proposal made any progress.[55]

Along with these frustrations, doctors in parliament found themselves under increasing attack from their colleagues in the medical profession, who accused them of failing to protect the interests of private practitioners. Typical in its response was the syndicate of Versailles, which declared that the success of the 1902 law depended most on physicians and that those serving on local hygienic councils should be elected by their peers and well paid for their time.[56] As Martha L. Hildreth has shown, the bulk of practitioners favored decentralized programs of public health and medical assistance, which were far more open to control from the syndicates than were those designed in Paris or even by the departments. This helps explain why the municipal assemblies, bruised by their battles with the organized profession after the 1890s, often exhibited less enthusiasm for health and welfare measures than did parliament.[57]

Some of the harshest criticisms coming from the medical corps were aimed at the requirement for compulsory notification of contagious diseases.[58] In an appearance before a Senate committee in 1909, Léon Lereboullet, AGMF president, argued that the obligation damaged the doctor's practice because it resembled a "denunciation" that was contrary to the doctor–patient relationship and because it violated Article 378 of the Penal Code requiring confidentiality.[59] The profession's resistance to compulsory notification constituted a dilemma for the physician-legislators, for many agreed with Cornil that the measure was essential to public health policy. A delegation from the *groupe médical parlementaire* that appeared with Lereboullet during his Senate testimony expressed much sympathy toward private practitioners, but it was reluctant to place the burden of notification entirely on the family, which was often distracted by grief. Dr. Dron, deputy of the Nord, observed also that many families were too isolated to get word to authorities in time and that there were few sanctions that could be applied against those who disobeyed. Doizy later offered a compromise: Doctors encountering a declarable disease would present a certificate to the head of the family (or hotel or rooming house manager) indicating the disease to be reported, and the recipient would mail this to the public health authorities, who would then inform the doctor. If the doctor heard nothing within three days, he would send in a duplicate.[60] Doizy's bill went to the Committee of Public Hygiene, which heard favorable testimony from the AGMF and the syndicates. A report, written by Dr. Even of Côtes-du-Nord, endorsed the bill, but its progress was interrupted by the war.

Such were the limits on our doctors' crusade to reform French public health institutions. Despite their motives and the promise of the law of 1902, those who had fought for reform saw their efforts compromised by the Senate's refusal to resist the claims of property owners and to allocate the funds needed for implementation. The growing conservatism of the medical profession greatly complicated the problem and, as we shall see in the next chapter, continued to do so on proposals affecting social welfare. Let us turn next to the ways in which political and economic interests affected the outcome of more specific aspects of the public health crusade.

PURE WATER AND PURE FOOD, MILITARY HYGIENE, AND THE CAMPAIGN AGAINST TUBERCULOSIS

If the reformist doctor-politicians found it difficult to reshape the nation's sanitary institutions, their efforts to attack some of the more scandalous evils they observed were doubly hard because of the economic interests at stake. As was true elsewhere, the hygienic crusade in France paid close attention to matters of consumption, and of all substances ingested by human beings, pure water occupied the highest priority. In 1888, Jules Rochard wrote that although the health of a city was proportional to the quality of water it consumed, France still had not matched the Romans in the value it placed on this resource.[61]

Langlet's report to the Chamber four years later cited a recent survey showing that of the 588 towns studied, only 308 had any systems for water supply and distribution; few were favored with subterranean aquifers *(eaux de source),* which hygienists regarded as the purest, and 103 still relied exclusively on rivers. The risks were plain to see, as Bourneville observed. Thirty kilometers above Paris, the Seine was "clear, transparent, and of a pleasing taste." But around Corbeil, it began picking up urban and industrial wastes, and by the time it reached Paris it already resembled sewer water. Cornil remarked to the Senate that at the place below the city where collectors dumped their wastes, the Seine had up to 100,000 microbes per cubic centimeter. Black sediment lay on the bottom and along the banks, and when the river was low, massive bubbles of sulfurous acid and other elements were visible on the surface.[62]

The pollution of rivers hurt the cities most, especially during the hot months when shortages forced inhabitants to take their water directly from the rivers. The worst off was Paris, where one five-month outbreak of typhoid, starting in August 1882, alone claimed over 2,300 lives. How the doctors in parliament viewed the problem can be seen in their response to a government bill in 1885 proposing to purify the Seine by diverting the wastes of Paris to designated treatment locales. The means to this end was a system known as *tout à l'égout* (literally, "everything into the sewer"), an innovative design for which Paris seemed an especially promising prospect. By 1881, it already had an advanced network of sewers absorbing up to 100,000 cubic meters of wastewater a day, most of it dumped untreated into the Seine.

The plan had three steps. The first was the replacement of outmoded toilet systems with modern water closets, each connected to a sewer main and capable of supplying at least 10 liters of fresh water per person per day.[63] Second was the requirement of a sophisticated technology capable of piping wastes away from centers of population to special cleansing fields. There, the means of purification was to be the soil itself, which, if treated with the proper ratios of water to land surface (an estimated 40,000 cubic meters per hectare each year), was not only the most efficient method but also one capable of extracting fertilizers for use in agriculture. Finally, because the plan required vast amounts of water in order to effect the rapid flushing of urban wastes, it would be necessary to tap additional underground aquifers in surrounding regions, even over the objections of local inhabitants. The plan was costly, but proponents believed that the city had no choice. Even before the bacteriological revolution, hygienists such as the engineer and future prime minister Charles de Freycinet had been urging adoption of the English "principle of continuous circulation," based on the idea that stagnation was incompatible with health and that the agricultural use of wastes formed part of a never-ending "chain of life."[64]

The first of the physician-legislators to become involved in this plan were Liouville, Levraud, and Bourneville, who were appointed in 1882 to a commission studying the problem of waste removal. Later, after the government had submitted a proposal to cede state lands to the city in order to carry out the project, Bourneville was named reporter for the parliamentary committee of review. But despite the committee's approval, the bill failed to reach the floor and was resubmitted after the elections of 1885, again on a report by Bourneville. This document, cited years afterwards for its quality, extolled *tout à l'égout* as an important step forward because it would improve hygiene among workers and reclaim for human use valuable fertilizers now being lost.

Bourneville estimated that every one hundred cubic meters of sewer water contained as much nitrogen as did one thousand kilograms of manure and that each day the equivalent of three thousand tons of manure passed unused through the collectors of Paris. As to fears that sewer farming (*épandage*) would spread the germs of typhoid, cholera, and dysentery, he argued that permeable soil constituted an efficient filter, trapping toxic elements and purifying the water as it percolated through. This point formed a critical part of his report, as the plan had come under attack from the deputies of Seine-et-Oise, whose inhabitants were not eager to avail themselves of Parisian largess. The most troubling reservations came from Pasteur, who argued that certain organisms, such as anthrax, could survive for years in the ground.

During the initial floor debates in early 1888, Bourneville tried to answer Pasteur's objections, insisting that these were based on a misunderstanding of the plan. On the whole, doctors in the Chamber applauded Bourneville's ideas, with over 80 percent of them voting in favor of the bill, which was a much higher proportion than for the legislature as a whole.[65] In the Senate, Cornil assumed the task of reporter, aided by Combes, Naquet, and Georges Martin, who, like him, were partisans of *tout à l'égout*. Answering Pasteur's objections was their hardest job, because at this point one could only infer from experience the antibacterial qualities of the soil. Thus when debate started in the Senate in late 1888, Cornil explained that although no one knew the reason, scientists had proved that even the dirtiest water was purified as it percolated through the earth. In experiments at Gennevilliers, near Paris, for example, the microbic content of sewer water that was filtered through the earth had dropped from between 80,000 and 200,000 per cubic centimeter to between 40 and 600. After several days of debate, the bill passed with only minor changes. As in the Chamber, the majority of doctors in the Senate backed the plan, only a handful of them favoring a canal to the sea.[66]

Eventually, *tout à l'égout* began to prove its value. A decline in the number of fixed-tank systems and an increase in the number of water closets did contribute to greater personal hygiene among the workers, just as Bourneville, Vaillant, Cornil, and other physician-legislators had predicted. In addition, the greater use of pure water for drinking and bathing helped lower the city's mortality rates, rendering even more ironic the opposition by Pasteur, whose discoveries had inspired proponents of the project.[67]

Pure water supplies led to another hygienic campaign initiated by certain doctors in parliament. This was the attack on urban cemeteries as a danger to wells and underground streams. In general, the subject of death provoked intense debate along hygienic lines, from the practice of laying out the corpse at home to the observance of religious ceremonies during times of epidemic.[68] The church's monopoly over funerals meant that it was hard to separate one's hygienic concerns from politics, and it is not surprising to find radical doctors leading the drive to give control of funerals to local municipal councils and to end the division of cemeteries by religion. For example, the law of 15 November 1887 regarding the liberty of funerals owed its existence to Chevandier, who six years earlier had offered a bill giving each citizen the right to choose a civil or religious ceremony and barring any form of discrimination against freethinkers, Protestants, and Jews.[69]

In regard to public health, the debate centered on whether the dead were capable of poisoning nearby water, soil, and air. As early as 1852, miasmatic theorists like Tardieu had portrayed urban cemeteries as giving off putrid vapors – what Freycinet later called "cadaveric emanations." By the 1880s, experiments were suggesting that this view exaggerated the dangers, that, depending on the soil, the corpse disappeared in three to five years and, if buried at the proper depth, posed no threat to the living. Bourgoin, whom the prefect of the Seine asked in 1879 to investigate the matter, experimented at Montparnasse using rabbits and pigeons, which he left for a month in trenches dug alongside graves. The absence of any ill effects was conclusive, he believed: "And the proof was that at the end of the experiments the employees of the cemeteries argued over the rabbits, which they ate and which they found succulent."[70] Although such findings seemed to confirm the power of the soil to neutralize toxic elements – a key assumption of *tout à l'égout* – they were not unwelcome on the Right, if for no other reason than that they helped undercut the claims of cremationist ideology, which the church viewed as being materialist in inspiration. Indeed, it was the alleged danger of urban cemeteries that served as a key plank in the cremationists' platform.

Among the most outspoken of the cremationists was Bourneville, who in 1880 helped found the Society for the Propagation of Cremation. Initial members included several in our group, such as Georges Martin, Brousse, Henri Chassaing, and Cornil, the last of whom served on the governing board. Bourneville, president of the society after 1884, went on to win approval from the city of Paris to build an experimental crematory at Père-Lachaise for burning body parts from the hospitals.[71] Two years earlier, Paul Casimir-Périer, deputy of Seine-Inférieure, had submitted a bill allowing citizens a choice of incineration or inhumation as their mode of burial. Not until March 1886, however, did the issue get a hearing in parliament, and only because Dr. Blatin, radical of Clérmont-Ferrand, brought it up during a discussion of Chevandier's bill on the liberty of funerals. Blatin offered an amendment specifying that an individual could determine the kind of burial he or she wished to have. In support, Blatin charged that cemeteries represented "a veritable legal organization of poisoning of the living by the dead." Archbishop Freppel, the only representative of the clergy in the Chamber, rejected Blatin's arguments as a return to "a materialist paganism that no longer recognizes in the human body the abode of an immortal soul." A majority, 321 to 174, nevertheless, agreed with Blatin. Only two doctors voted against the procremation amendment.[72]

Whether from the dead or the living, the flow of toxic wastes into waterways continued, however, to trouble the medical men. Although the Consultative Committee of Public Hygiene was responsible for determining the quality of all local water supplies, no central agency existed to search out new reserves or to devise new technologies for tapping them. A private bill dated 1892, reported out by Dr. Ducoudray, aimed to resolve this problem by creating a special corps of engineers at the Ministry of Public Works, but the bill never arrived on the floor.[73] In 1899, Drs. Borne, Pedebidou, Peschaud, Hugon, Cazals, and Vaillant, along with nine other deputies, joined Dr. Dubois of Paris in proposing the creation of a special laboratory to conduct a chemical and bacteriological analysis of the country's streams and rivers. Such a study, they hoped, would be able to determine precise types of pollution, seasonal variations, and toxicity levels at different points along the flow. The next year, Dubois and Levraud offered an additional bill asking the government to analyze water, air, and dust in all state establishments, including schools, but neither this, nor earlier proposals, achieved any results.[74]

The doctors' interest in water purity was also evident in food legislation, although the political risks were much higher. By the turn of the century, food fraud had become big business; *La Presse médicale* complained, for example, that most French beer contained glucose, saccharin, and bitters in place of malt and hops, that milk was mixed with everything from carrot juice to chicory extract, and that bread had become a blend of flour, vegetable starches, plaster, and even clay. The pharmacist-deputy Augustin Féron of Paris also accused bakers of mixing sawdust into their batter, which they purchased from sawmills at one franc fifty a bag. Periodically, efforts were made to crack down, but the *fraudeurs* were a resourceful group. Cazeneuve, a leader in the war against them, compared the fight with the struggle between shell and armor.[75]

By law, the Ministry of Commerce was responsible for setting uniform food standards, but as Vaillant pointed out in 1904, it lacked the chemical and agricultural laboratories needed for systematic testing. At present, he said, there was not even a clear definition of meat, as there was for American pure food laws.[76] When standards did exist, there were few means of enforcement. A private bill in 1888 to crack down on food fraud charged that this industry had become "an integral part of our national production" and that the dyes, fragrances, and other substances it routinely added to meat, vegetables, preserves, and beverages had already caused numerous deaths.[77] The problem was not simply one of catching the *fraudeurs* but of monitoring the food-processing industry, of which small family firms, exempt from surveillance, made up a large part. Dr. Dron described conditions there as being extremely unsanitary, especially for apprentices in butcheries.[78]

For the physician-legislators, the inferior quality of meat ranked at the top of food fraud issues. The issue arose often during debates over army food, a sensitive matter at home because of complaints from the families of conscripts. Drs. Gustave Chapuis and Henri Chassaing singled out defects in canned meats that were purchased by the army. Gacon and Empereur focused on the lack of sanitary inspection of army livestock, the consumption of which caused gastrointestinal disorders and, in certain cases, tuberculosis. During a debate in 1908, Cazeneuve recited instances in which random inspections showed animals to be ridden with sores and parasites; Vaillant added that cattle failing to pass muster at civilian meat markets frequently ended up on the soldiers' plates. He and other doctors then joined in support of a resolution urging a national system of meat inspection.[79]

The destruction of diseased livestock had been a chief goal of hygienists during the debates in 1881 on the animal sanitary police, but cracking down was not easy. Private slaughter yards, which thrived in the villages and on the outskirts of cities, carried on a semiclandestine trade that was difficult to monitor, despite the odors they emitted. Since 1878, when the Consultative Committee of Public Hygiene had called attention to the dangers of these yards, hygienists had sought to outlaw them and to encourage the building of public facilities. In the fall of 1893, the pharmacist Alfred Leconte presented a bill to this effect, which passed the next year but then became mired in the Senate. In the meantime, private butcheries continued to flourish, despite efforts by Vaillant to ban them outright.[80]

Posing another problem was the importation of meat from countries where livestock diseases were widespread. Many doctors favored strict inspection at the frontier, but that this was not always practical became clear during the great trichinosis scare of the early 1880s. The controversy aroused considerable passions, for both political and hygienic reasons. Because it was cheaper than beef or mutton, pork had come to be the preferred choice of workers and the urban poor, who were attracted by the low prices of imported American cuts. The danger was trichinosis, a parasitic and sometimes fatal sickness that was endemic in the United States and in parts of Germany. France itself had been largely spared (only one case had ever been verified). Otherwise, scientists had had trouble even finding the parasite. Bert, who claimed to have been among the first in France to see it under a microscope, had been forced to rely on a sample furnished by Virchow in 1862. Testelin, who carried out experiments four years later, reported that he had examined five hundred hogs, two hundred hams and lard samples, and even countless rats caught in the municipal slaughterhouse of Lille – all without finding a trace.[81]

Nevertheless, the decision of Italy, Germany, and Spain to ban imports of American pork because of trichinosis prompted the government to take action, if for no other reason than the threatened inundation of French markets. There followed an outcry from the port cities and from the United States, which warned of retaliation against French wines. The government thus began backtracking, offering a bill to allow entry to pork that had been certified as "fully cured" by inspectors in the country of origin. This the Chamber endorsed in March, after voting down a counterproposal to establish a full-scale service for microscopic examination. About half the doctors supported the counterproposal. The rest believed that there was no danger or else were intimidated by committee warnings that such a move would necessitate an army of inspectors.[82] Confusing matters further was the Senate's decision to reject even this watered-down bill. The government thus repealed the ban altogether.

In December 1883, Bert attacked this decision on the floor, arguing that the threat of trichinosis was comparable to the one posed by phylloxera and that, once introduced into French herds, it would become endemic, as in Germany. He then offered a resolution compelling the government to reinstate the ban until the Chamber could reconsider the matter of an inspection service. This passed with 64 percent of the Chamber in support. Of the doctors, 57 percent were in favor; those in opposition included numerous urban radicals whose constituents had been hurt by the absence of cheap pork.[83]

Economic motives of this sort are most evident in regard to foodstuffs identified with particular geographical regions, which helps explain the visibility of certain *médecins-agriculteurs* in touting the virtues of local products against "adulterated" versions, which were always cheaper. Dr. Ricard, who spent much of his life campaigning against wine fraud, was also president of the *groupe viticole* in the Chamber. Dr. Legludic, who promoted the cause of pure milk technology and led the attack on the health dangers of margarine, was president of the French Society for the Encouragement of the Dairy Industry. Dr. Lesoeuf, equally hostile to margarine, was a butter producer in Seine-Inférieure and president of the Society of Agriculture of Rouen.

Allegations of fraud in milk and milk products intruded into an especially delicate area. After Pasteur, hygienists came to view pure milk as the best means of lowering infant mortality rates; yet, legislative efforts to guarantee milk purity were feeble, because most deputies rejected the idea of strict state inspection. As representatives of rural France, doctors were little different. For example, an amendment by Cazeneuve on 15 January 1908 that would have given local officials greater power to inspect stables and to regulate the hygienic conditions of milk production found only about a fifth of them in support, about the same as for the whole Chamber. Similar concerns over local interests dominated debates in 1887 and 1896 concerning the regulation of margarine. Whereas leftists like Naquet and Vaillant defended margarine as the "butter of the poor," Legludic and other defenders of the dairy farmers of Normandy denounced it as harmful to the digestive tract – the unwholesome product, Legludic charged, of old tallow from Chicago and the oils and grease of restaurants.[84] This pandering to agrarian interests was reflected in the modest number of doctors who were willing to brave the wrath of the food-processing industry during debates on the law of 1905 banning the adulteration of food and agricultural products.[85]

Levels of hygienic activism tended to increase in areas that lacked such political constraints. The health of the troops was one example, and it was one in which great numbers of doctors took a particular interest. Aside from their professional interests, which often sprang from their own years of service as army doctors, some were influenced in this direction by constituent pressures, judging by the letters of complaint they quoted at the tribune. In a speech in 1907, Lachaud read from mail complaining about the physical abuse of young recruits, and he angrily contrasted the filthiness of French barracks with the cleanliness and order prevailing in those of the Germans. Clemenceau had done the same thing in the Senate four years earlier, delivering a scathing attack on the minister of war and citing one letter from the grandfather of a young trooper at Rouen who had died of typhoid after being denied medical help. Later, Clemenceau and Labbé themselves went to Rouen to see what action had been taken. There they found the infirmary so crowded that the beds touched one another, and the garrison's water supply still had nine thousand bacteria per cubic centimeter.[86]

Doctors had been calling attention to such scandals since the post-1871 debate on the reorganization of the army. The saddest evidence was the war itself, whose losses to disease had evoked memories of the Crimea. Dr. Marmottan told the Chamber in 1880 that although statistics were incomplete, at least 150,000 French soldiers had died, of which only 30,000 deaths appeared to have been caused by battle wounds.[87] What most angered him was a system of hygienic administration that had sent surgeons into battle without instruments, abandoned the sick and wounded for lack of transport, and showed utter confusion in face of epidemics. In theory, army doctors had complete authority over medical matters, but such power hardly existed. All personnel, from physicians to stretcher-bearers, fell under jurisdiction of the Army Services Corps (the *intendance*). This meant that nonmedical comptrollers, preoccupied with financial and administrative details, routinely handed down orders regulating details of camp sanitation, hospital wards, transport, and ambulance services.

Marmottan blamed the *intendance* for the medical disasters of

1870–1. His solution was to reconstitute army health services as a special corps, similar to that for engineers and the artillery, which would have a fixed place within the military hierarchy and be accountable only to the commander of the army.[88] A victory of sorts seemed imminent in December 1876, when the Senate approved a bill increasing the independence of the military health services. Opposition from the army delayed the measure, however, and by 1880 it appeared to be all but dead.

At that point, Marmottan, supported by Cornil and Larrey, presented a new version aimed at appeasing those who were worried over who would make final decisions regarding men and matériel. Under its terms, the health corps was to be directed by doctors and to have its own place within the chain of command but would be accountable to a special *direction* of health affairs located at the Ministry of War.[89] The Chamber approved the idea, but opposition from the army continued to spell trouble. The government thus decided to offer a new bill which, though paying lip service to the independence of the army doctors, kept intact the powers of the *intendance*. A committee of the Chamber rejected this scheme, recommending instead that the health corps be reorganized as one of the main groups comprising the administration of the army and that its ambulance and hospital directors (all of whom were to be medical men) have full authority over military and civilian personnel operating within their sphere. Henceforth, relations with the *intendance* were to be primarily financial.[90] This version passed the Chamber in April 1881 and then went on to the Senate, where it received a favorable report from Louis Cazalas, a military doctor and pathologist at Val-de-Grâce. After modifications, it became law the following year.[91]

Doctors in parliament frequently called attention to the poor quality of health care in the ranks, and they were quick to remind parliament that losses to smallpox during the war with Prussia had been the equivalent of two divisions. Later, the introduction of compulsory vaccination in the army had all but eliminated the disease there, and Prime Minister Freycinet's efforts in the late 1880s to supply military installations with pure drinking water had produced a dramatic decline in typhoid fever.[92] Yet, soldiering continued to be a dangerous occupation. In 1902, Senator André Gotteron cited a German report comparing the health of its army with that of France. It showed typhoid continuing to be a killer among French soldiers, followed by tuberculosis, respiratory diseases, and influenza. Since 1871, Gotteron said, German losses to disease had been around 13,000 men. For France, the figure was 99,000 – "that is, the equivalent of three complete army corps on a war footing."[93]

Many doctors knew from experience that the German report had not exaggerated. From time to time, they themselves had attacked army negligence following outbreaks of typhoid at particular garrisons.[94] Gotteron's efforts to elicit the views of the minister of war served to focus attention on the whole question of military hygiene, and in March 1903 the Senate began debating three separate *interpellations* by Drs. Treille, Dubois, and Lachaud. It was Labbé, however, who best laid out the steps that France should take in order to make its army comparable to Germany's. First, recruitment standards must be toughened, so that the troops would have more resistance to disease and thus less chance of spreading it to others. Second, living conditions must be improved; at present, beds were crowded together in the barracks; water supplies were suspect in at least eighty-seven garrisons; and recruits were subjected to grueling marches and punishment details while in poor physical shape. Third, hygiene must be improved in the towns where the garrisons were located, because many soldiers came from isolated villages and had no acquired immunities. Numerous other doctors joined to support Labbé, but after four sessions the most that they could obtain was a resolution stressing the need for stricter enforcement of sanitary regulations.[95]

The toll taken by typhoid during the Moroccan campaigns of 1907 and 1912 provided further evidence for Labbé's criticisms. In June 1912, Labbé submitted a bill to make typhoid vaccination mandatory in the army. The move was essential, he observed, for between 1892 and 1912, the disease had struck a total of 28,503 French soldiers in Algeria and Morocco, killing 4,620.[96] In January 1914, the radical physician of Corrèze, Edouard Lachaud, chairman of the Committee of Public Hygiene and author of *Pour la race, notre soldat, notre caserne,* began calling attention to living conditions among the troops in eastern France, which had recently suffered outbreaks of measles and scarlet fever at the fortresses of Epinal, Belfort, Toul, and Verdun. After visiting the installations there, he told the Chamber that the barracks conditions were atrocious, from their contaminated water sources and filthy latrines to their poor construction. Doizy and Vaillant confirmed his assertions. Afterwards, the Chamber approved a motion from Augagneur asking the Committee of Public Hygiene to work with the government on ways to reduce military mortality. Specifically, its members were to inspect barracks and to prepare recommendations.[97]

The committee subsequently divided itself into subgroups, each of which visited a particular army corps. The visits were preceded by questionnaires sent out to all army doctors, asking for their advice. The final report, written by Lachaud, urged that large barracks – or those built according to designs new in 1877 and 1885 and having up to one hundred beds – be abandoned for smaller units, where disease could not spread so rapidly. The committee found that the safest structures hygienically were those built during the time of Vauban, because they were made up of small rooms having space for only eight or so beds. Second, the barracks must include more water taps and basins and, whenever possible, use only spring water. The widely used *tinettes mobiles,* or portable toilets, must also be abolished in favor of newly devised septic tanks. Finally, the army must increase its number of doctors and distribute them more evenly throughout the ranks.[98]

For typhoid fever, it was fairly easy to offer solutions. The opposite was true for tuberculosis, a disease so widespread and so complicated in its causes that simple answers were impossible. What did seem evident was that its growth was linked to universal military service, as it was carried by conscripts into crowded barracks and thence spread to other young men and their families on farms and in factories. Lachaud, author of a bill allowing draft boards to reject those showing a predisposition to the disease, told a reporter from *L'Eclair* in 1901 that every ten years tuberculosis claimed enough men in uniform to form an entire corps. Dr. Dubois, who earlier had proposed creating special sanatoria for the troops, placed annual losses at 9.4 per 1,000, which included 1.1 from death and 8.3 from dismissal. By 1914, the latter had risen to 16, a matter of grave concern to those who saw early dismissal as only spreading the disease.[99]

The most common estimate for the number of tuberculosis deaths in the country each year was 150,000, although this was probably high.[100] Figures assembled in 1912 by the Permanent Committee on Tuberculosis of the Academy of Medicine reported that the mortality rate had declined but still stood at 217 per 100,000 inhabitants, as opposed to 168 for Germany, 166 for Italy, 162 for Spain, and 146 for England.[101] Cities were known areas of danger, the annual death rate in Paris being 389 per 100,000 in 1905. In addition, there was increasing evidence that the disease was far more widespread in rural areas than previously believed.[102]

Although some physician-legislators viewed tuberculosis as "a French disease" rooted in alcoholism,[103] others recognized that the blame lay with conditions over which the individual had little control. In his report to parliament in 1901 on the subject, Dr. Amodru included overcrowding and unhealthy housing among tuberculosis's predisposing causes. Vaillant, claiming that up to half of all working-class families were infected, listed long hours, overwork, and low wages. German hygienists and insurance specialists, he said, had already established a correlation between the disease and specific occupations, and the proof was in the nature of cures recommended by modern medicine, which consisted of removing the sickened worker from his milieu. Dr. Charles Borne supported these arguments, noting that silica-producing jobs were especially risky, from stonecutters and millstone makers to iron-mongers and tool sharpeners.[104]

Robert Koch's earlier discovery of the contagiousness of tuberculosis had prompted a number in our group to become active in the growing crusade against its spread. Following an international congress in Paris in 1888, Cornil and Lannelongue served on a permanent committee charged with reporting on the best means to protect oneself. The committee stressed that tuberculosis was spread by microbe-laden dust and, to a lesser extent, by contaminated milk and meat. The dangers of spitting, Cornil warned later in the Academy of Medicine, were so great that it was essential for the sick to have porcelain spittoons that could be disinfected with boiling water. He also emphasized the duty of doctors to discourage tuberculosis-infected individuals, like those with syphilis, from marrying.[105]

Thereafter, several from our group served as delegates to periodic congresses.[106] Others were active in philanthropic societies or, like Peyrot, Lannelongue, Lachaud, Pedebidou, and Petit-jean, in the extraparliamentary commission created by Waldeck-Rousseau and transformed by Combes into the Permanent Commission on Tuberculosis. The latter, presided over by Léon

Bourgeois, pressed for the building of sanatoria for soldiers, sailors, and state employees.[107]

Finally, doctors belonging to the Chamber's Committee of Public Hygiene took up many of the same themes, as can be seen in the recommendations contained in Amodru's report in 1901. While backing the idea of sanatoria, the committee urged in the interim the enforcement of a ban against spitting in public buildings (which should henceforth be equipped with hygienic spittoons) and recommended that they be cleaned only with mops and water, to keep down the dust. All state workers should have a personal health card to ensure the keeping of accurate statistics, and the government should do all in its power to encourage urban dispensaries, mutual-aid and insurance societies, and tuberculosis education.[108]

Despite these activities, the role of the physician–legislators in the fight against tuberculosis was not nearly so pronounced as it was in other areas of public health. On certain fronts, as in the parliamentary movement for housing reform, their contributions were minimal, or certainly less significant than those of the engineers, architects, and industrialists who belonged to such reformist groups as the Société française des habitations à bon marché.[109] Preoccupied with rural misery, few doctors were willing to countenance the cost that true prevention and cure would have required. One estimate in 1900 suggested that the building of sanatoria would require an initial outlay of 400 million francs, with about half that amount to be spent every year thereafter, excluding aid to families. Yet, as Roux told the Academy of Medicine, even if sanitoria had been built by the dozens, they would not have been able to accommodate the great numbers of sick.[110]

Despite these failures, it is clear that the medical men in parliament who took an active part in legislative activities pertaining to public health constituted a significant force in the hygienic crusade before 1914. Though swayed by the same pressures affecting all deputies and senators, they managed to achieve several notable gains, even if these rarely came close to achieving their original goals. As examples, one could mention their role in the pure water campaign, including the battle over *tout à l'égout,* and in the fight to improve army hygiene, which owed much to the efforts of Marmottan, Labbé, Lannelongue, and Lachaud. Most important was their work in improving hygienic administration, which would not have been realized without the efforts of Liouville, Langlet, and Cornil. For all its flaws, the law of 1902 was an improvement over the anarchy that, had reigned earlier; its main provisions, from smallpox vaccination to obligatory disinfection, were long overdue ones that, as Salomon-Bayet has observed, validated Pasteurian precepts in law and constituted an important step forward along the road to hygienic security in France.

7

The social question

Besides their work on public health and sanitation, the hygienic activists in parliament focused much of their energies on problems of social welfare. Although most thought of themselves as part of a larger group of reformist deputies and senators who favored the idea of self-help for the worker,[1] many were also willing to accept limited state intervention in areas that could be tied to the physical amelioration of the masses and to the reversal of population decline. Because of their technical knowledge and professional skills, they were thus in a position to exert a strong influence over the social laws of the period. In a speech in 1888, Dr. Théophile Roussel remarked on this growing bond between medicine and the public powers, citing as evidence parliament's dependence on the Academy of Medicine during the preparation of all "medical laws."[2]

That the secular and scientific outlook of the regime made it receptive to a "medical mode of social analysis," in Robert Nye's words, cannot be doubted. As Nye shows, the tendency to apply medical criteria to society incorporated an even grander biological metaphor of "degeneracy" as a model for explaining national weakness and decline. The physician-legislators helped popularize this way of thinking, but that was only a small part of their influence. What follows will try to draw out the essential features of their social vision, starting with an analysis of their most pronounced failure, namely, the crusade against alcoholism. Next is a description of their efforts on behalf of social and medical assistance, along with their drive to enact protective legislation on behalf of infants, children, and the elderly. The last section traces their work on factory hygiene and safety.

ALCOHOLISM AND THE REFORM OF
INSANITY LAWS

Of all issues affecting health, that of alcoholism elicited the most muted response from parliament, which knew the value of the alcohol industry to the treasury and which understood the degree to which its power had penetrated all walks of life. Jean-Vincent Laborde, editor of *La Tribune médicale* and a leader of the French Antialcoholic Union, told the Academy of Medicine in 1898 that any hopes he might ever have had in parliament's willingness to attack the problem had long disappeared: "We are justified in saying today that the public powers, to use the modern expression, have become bankrupt on this matter."[3] Maurice Debove, the feisty dean of the Paris faculty who in 1905 became president of the newly formed National League Against Alcoholism, was equally skeptical, complaining to the Academy of Medicine that most legislators had adopted the maxim that "fear of the tavern keeper is the beginning of wisdom."[4] Some critics even believed alcohol to be the essential lubricant of republican politics, noting that candidates frequented the taverns in order to ply voters with drinks and that they were quick to acclaim this "all-powerful god, on whom they depend absolutely." The bistro, mused one observer, had two annexes – "the hospital and the Palais-Bourbon."[5]

As men of medicine, the physician-legislators occupied a delicate position on the matter. Most viewed alcoholism as a crisis of epidemic proportions, and few doubted that there were links between it and other social maladies. Among these, Dr. Gadaud placed suicide, crime, divorce, declining birthrates, and insanity, giving special emphasis to the last.[6] The disease was seen as taking its worst toll on the lower social orders. Charles Aubry, physician-senator for Algeria, declared that it was "a known fact" that alcoholism wreaked its greatest havoc among weak and oppressed peoples, such as the tribes of equatorial Africa and North America.[7] While admitting that no corner of France had been left untouched, Lannelongue painted a bleak portrait of its grip on urban workers, noting that it was costing them and their families over a billion francs a year.[8] Some doctors even depicted the worker's tendency toward violence as less the product of his social condition than his abuse of alcohol, and the Paris uprising of 1871 was invoked most often as evidence.[9] That idea offended leaders of the Left, but even the socialist Vaillant warned of the damage done to the proletariat by alcohol and other forms of "aromatism, poisoning by essences, epileptic and convulsive toxins, breeders of degeneracy, of misery, of dementia, of insanity, of crime."[10]

Although many believed alcoholism to be hereditary, and hence a threat to the biological survival of France, doctors tended to explain the problem in ways that were consistent with the regional interests they represented. For most, these centered on the wine industry of the south and southwest, but others had to answer to the northern makers of industrial alcohols, who extracted their product from sugar beets and grains and whose distilleries accounted for over two-thirds of all taxed beverages sold. The fifty-three largest were found in the north and northwest, areas that also had the highest rates of alcohol consumption in the nation, as doctors from the Midi never tired of reminding parliament. Yet, no one knew the real levels, here or elsewhere, because official figures ignored the vast amounts of home brew turned out illegally by the *bouilleurs de cru*.[11]

As seen earlier, the doctors' campaign platforms never spoke of alcoholism, and only a handful had ever associated themselves with the temperance leagues or, after 1906, with the small and ineffectual caucus of the Chamber that called itself the *groupe antialcoolique*. The dangers of even raising the issue could be seen in the case of Lannelongue, who warned parliament in 1895 that France must confront the menace of alcoholism in the interest of its own survival. His speech, received with an air of "religious silence" by the deputies, drew applause from hygienists across the nation. But not so in his native Gers, one of the largest wine producers in France. The next year, when he announced a bid for the Senate, the wine interests went after him with a vengeance, pointing to a casual aside he had made in his speech that all alcohols, whatever their origin, contained some toxic substances and that if brandies made from wine contained fewer poisons than industrial alcohols, they were not completely pure either. From this, it was deduced that Lannelongue had said that wine brandy contained poisons and that, by extension, the winegrowers of Gers were poisoning their fellow citizens. Lannelongue was defeated, *La petite gironde* comparing his fate with that of Dr. Stockmann, hero of Ibsen's *Enemy of the People*.[12]

What strategies, then, did doctors use for explaining the problem and its solution? Few were willing to attribute alcoholism solely to the character flaws of the workers, although some thought this to be the case.[13] By contrast, Dr. Amagat of Cantal believed that there were no intrinsic reasons that France should be a nation of drinkers but that, of all causes, few had paid adequate attention to the impact of prolonged poverty or to the relationship of alcoholism to other types of poisonings and diseases.[14] Naquet blamed insufficient diet, arguing that workers lacked enough nitrogenized food to repair their bodies and were thus forced to substitute alcohol, which provided caloric energy and a fleeting illusion of strength.[15] In later years, Vaillant, Guesde, and other socialists continued to advance this thesis, contending that low salaries under capitalism precluded adequate nutrition for workers, who, in order to recover lost energy, resorted to alcoholic stimulants.[16]

More characteristic was a theory embraced by large segments of the medical corps, which placed the heaviest blame on the advent of cheap industrial alcohols. In reports dated 1871 and 1886, the Academy of Medicine called attention to an increase in consumption of cheap industrial alcohols, which had occurred at the expense of wine. Though badly hurt by the phylloxera blight, wine was still "the drink par excellence, of which we must especially encourage consumption."[17] In taking this position, the Academy of Medicine endorsed the views of Etienne Lancereaux, the nation's best-known expert on the subject, who believed that alcoholism had been unknown before mid-century and had developed only after the population stopped drinking "healthful" beverages, such as cider, beer, and wine, and began imbibing grain and other industrial alcohols mixed with essences.[18]

To doctors who hailed from the winegrowing Midi (or were themselves *vignerons*), such theories had strong appeal and supported their efforts to help their districts recover from phylloxera. Far from being viewed as a cause of addiction, wine was eulogized as "a precious food and useful stimulant"; as a tonic and restorative for anemia, shattered constitutions, and nervous disorders; as a pure and "natural" product that, in the words of Dr. Moinet, senator for Charente-Inférieure, stood as a "beneficial liquid praised throughout the centuries."[19] True, it was not good to drink to excess, but in any case, the effects of wine were far different from those of industrial distillations. "Our fathers," said Gadaud, "experienced light intoxication, [were] inoffensive and often witty, because they drank only natural wine or brandies distilled from natural wines. Our contemporaries exhibit a somber, dangerous, brutal inebriation because in general they consume adulterated wines or brandies distilled from all sorts of substances that are absolutely foreign to natural wine."[20] Labbé also saw the culprit as the toxic offshoots of northern industry: "What we see now is not the drunkenness our fathers knew; it is a sad drunkenness, a malicious drunkenness, and, it can be said with some truth, a wildly mad drunkenness."[21] Michou of Aube went so far as to identify amyl acid as the specific agent of this reaction, describing it as a poison not found in naturally fermented beverages, which made the drinker feel moody and sad. Consider, he told the Chamber, the winegrowers of Bourgogne when they celebrate "the divine liquid of their *crus*" at their banquets: "They are gay, they laugh, they dance, they sing. Our drunkards of Paris do not sing, do not dance, they fall down as if dead."[22]

Among the hundreds of aperitifs made with distilled alcohol, there was one that doctors singled out for special blame. That was absinthe, the "green fairy" of legend, touted by artists for its hallucinogenic powers. Because of wine shortages produced by phylloxera, it had also become the drink of growing numbers of workers. Roussel had warned of it in a speech in 1872, noting that consumption had grown to alarming proportions in the army and that of all forms of alcohol, it was the most destructive of mind and body.[23] The problem was most visible in the cities. Vaillant told the Chamber in 1900 that a fourth of all absinthe and bitters sold annually in France was drunk in Paris, much of it by women and children.[24] Dr. Guyot of Lyon, another area of high consumption, described France's "sacred hour of the aperitif" as a ritual of tragic proportions.[25]

Manufactured from wormwood, anise, fennel, hyssop, and other herbs, absinthe had a higher alcoholic content than wine did and was thought to cause a very deadly form of alcoholism that attacked the central nervous system. Citing the research of Valentin Magnan, director of the Saint-Anne asylum of Paris, Gadaud pictured absinthe as being responsible for a variety of mental disorders, including epilepsy.[26] Vaillant assailed it as a major cause of abortions, miscarriages, and stillbirths and in 1900 won the Chamber's backing for a move to ban the manufacture of all drinks containing essences that the Academy of Medicine declared to be dangerous. The evasiveness of the academy's response (it finally ruled that *all* essences were unhealthy) angered him; it was, he said, as if the academy had been asked which dogs should be destroyed and, instead of answering mad dogs, had said that all dogs should be killed "because they all can turn mad." He thus continued his campaign for a ban in an amendment to the 1904 bill concerning food fraud and in a separate motion in 1905.[27]

As part of a larger drive among temperance forces, Vaillant's efforts prompted a review by the Committee of Public Hygiene, for which Henri Schmidt, a pharmacist for Vosges, was made reporter. Schmidt favored banning the drink but met a lukewarm response from the majority, including Dr. Villejean, the chairman, who complained that he would not take responsibility for creating a budget deficit of eighty million francs from lost absinthe taxes. After hearing testimony from its manufacturers, the committee decided against a ban.[28] The next year, the Senate named its own committee. Five were doctors, of whom one, Charles Borne, though long recognized as a champion of public health, emerged as the chief defender of the absinthe makers. That was not surprising, in light of the fact that his own department, Doubs, was the home of Pernod, one of the biggest producers. After hearing testimony from experts that only one ingredient in absinthe was actually harmful (an elusive element called thujone), the committee decided simply to recommend a ban on this substance.[29] Undaunted, Schmidt kept alive the possibility of a total ban by offering a new bill. Discussion dragged on until the outbreak of war, when in a burst of patriotism and as a measure of national defense, the government prohibited all sales of absinthe; this was a victory for those who believed that essences lay at the heart of France's drinking problem, but it had little impact on blunting the progress of alcoholism.[30]

Besides attacking essences, doctors also extolled efforts to lower consumption by taxing beverages according to their alcohol content. That line of attack, plus stiff penalties for public drunkenness, had been the main strategy advocated by Roussel in a law in 1873 to combat alcoholism. Though some critics believed that higher taxes achieved their goal only briefly (or even increased the production of cheap alcohol and hence addiction), the wine interests supported the idea, some even advocating the abolition of all taxes

on wine, beer, cider, and other *boissons hygiéniques*. A bill presented
in 1894 by Dr. Justin Cot, a *vigneron* from Hérault, proposed to
exclude at least these drinks from the municipal excise tax (the
octroi). Arguing that the workers drank distilled spirits only because taxes had put wine out of their reach, Cot promised that if
his bill became law, "the consumption of wine would double in
the cities to the greatest benefit of hygiene and public morality."[31]
Armand Gauthier, physician-senator for the wine-rich Aude, made
similar arguments, stating that the removal of taxes on wine would
provide the workers with a cheap and healthful drink while driving
out pernicious industrial alcohols.[32]

These arguments were welcomed by the physician-deputies of
the cities, many of whom wished to promote the cause of cheap
table wine for their working-class constituents. The problem, at
least in the eyes of southern conservatives, was that some urban
radicals wanted to scrap the *octroi* on other items as well and to
remedy the deficit with a state monopoly over alcohol. A motion
by Vaillant in 1898 to eliminate the *octroi* on wine, beer, food,
fuel, and oil saw the doctors almost evenly divided – twenty-six
for and twenty-four against. The same pattern appeared later in
response to a resolution by Jules-Louis Breton to establish a state
monopoly over the manufacture and sale of alcohol, which
twenty-two supported and thirty opposed.[33] These votes reflected
regional interests, as was true for all questions of this sort. Thirty-
three doctors, mostly from the south and southwest, supported a
bill in 1896 to increase taxes on raisin wines and similar "artificial"
drinks; allied against it were physician-deputies from the industrial
north, from areas having large numbers of home brewers, and
from the cities.[34]

In debates on alcohol, the wine lobby was usually able to convince a majority in parliament that its product was worthy of
special protection against all substitutes. As with butter and margarine, regional influences exercised the dominant voice, although
public health was invoked to support particular viewpoints. In
this, a doctor could be useful, as each winegrowing region saw
fraudeurs at work in the other, whether by adding alcohol to its
wines *(vinage)*, watering them down *(mouillage)*, or clarifying
them with plaster *(plâtrage)*. Dr. Michou of Aube, proclaiming
himself "an archprotectionist when it comes to the health of my
fellow man," denounced *vinage* as an affront to hygiene, business,

and patriotism. Dr. Lavergne of Tarn, on the other hand, saw "honest" *vinage* as adding to the stock of cheap, healthful, and "democratic" wines: "I ask you to retain for the poor a healthy drink, twenty times healthier than what is found today."[35] Only a few doctors ever questioned the myth of wine as a "natural" product. In a distinct minority was Bourgoin of Ardennes, who praised water as the only true healthful drink. Nature, he once told parliament, "has never produced an ounce of wine," and what was sold as such was merely, "the product of a decomposition, whether it comes from grapes or raisins."[36]

Physician-legislators from the Midi – often in league with their alcohol-producing enemies of the north – denounced private distillers as tax cheats and poisoners. Others, like Labbé of Orne, excluded them from any blame. Those in his department, he said, were "humble property owners" whose loss of distillation rights at a time of agricultural crisis would result in the victory of a northern coalition that was seeking to crush the small farmer.[37] A Senate ballot in 1896 to preserve the rights of the *bouilleurs de cru* found eleven doctors for and fourteen against, the latter coming mainly from the south and southwest, the former from departments where home brewing was a significant industry.[38] In the Chamber, medical men were just as divided: A vote in 1900 on a motion by Vaillant to suppress the rights of home brewers found twenty-one in favor and twenty-three opposed, the same patterns applying.[39]

The ability of the medical men in parliament to combat the growth of alcoholism was thus weakened by regional political pressures and by their own assumption that wine was not a factor in the disease. During the early days of the Republic, some had reassured themselves with the thought that education and the physical improvement of the masses would eventually provide a defense. By 1914, however, alcoholism appeared to have only tightened its grip, frustrating those who wished to believe that the Republic was still capable of working miracles. "We know, gentlemen," Dr. Aubry told the Senate in 1911, "that there exists on the face of the earth 300 million or 400 million Muslims who systematically abstain from alcoholic beverages because their religion forbids it. Will reason, science, and the progress of civilization be impotent where religious faith and fanaticism have produced the most marvelous results?"[40]

The electoral pressures that dominated all discussion of alcoholism were less evident in matters of mental disease, which many considered its chief fruit. Lunatics crazed by their thirst for drink or given to absinthe-induced fits were not, it is true, uncommon images in the speeches of physician-legislators and support Nye's thesis that thoughts of social defense against deviance informed much of the reformist rhetoric in this domain. There can be little doubt, moreover, that the emerging psychiatric profession in France was influenced by the regime's positivist and anticlerical values or that, as Jan Goldstein has found, these values helped shape the prevailing views on the causes and cure of insanity.[41]

One is struck, nevertheless, by the human concerns that motivated those in our group. Most conceded that *aliénation* (from reason, as Philippe Pinel believed) had causes other than alcoholism, including the psychological shock that accompanied rural migration to the cities. The practice of medicine had also allowed many of the physician-legislators to see close up the diverse faces of the disease: "Vagrants in the cities, vagabonds in the countryside, shut up in prisons, sequestered in families, objects of derision and bad treatment, they live often abandoned, without the public authorities concerning themselves with them," Dr. Germain Dupré told the Senate in 1886.[42] Testelin reminded his colleagues that much of the abuse of the mentally ill, as among the elderly, occurred at the hands of family members. Roussel added that mental disease, unlike other forms of sickness, often altered the feelings of affection that family members held for the afflicted, who instead became objects of pity, loathing, or fear. "There is no treatment for mental disease within the family," he declared; "the efforts undertaken for keeping it in the milieu where it was born are one of the most important causes for its incurability."[43]

Among the most helpless victims were children – *des enfants idiots, imbéciles, crétins, et épileptiques,* in the alienist parlance of the day – who, as Roussel said, had been forsaken because society saw them as having no social value. Someone who knew this firsthand was Bourneville, whose services for retarded children at Bicêtre were among the most advanced in France.[44] That was just one of his passions along these lines. Reports of witches or demonic possession usually brought him or a member of his staff to investigate – always with an eye to exposing fraud or to using natural causes to explain any curious mental phenomena. The plight of psychiatric patients especially disturbed Bourneville, as was evident in visits he made to various hospital wards throughout the country between 1886 and 1888. At Tonnere, he found patients being kept in two basement *cabanons,* or prisonlike cells, each having barred windows and an opening through which food was passed. At Lons-le-Saulnier, the cells resembled caves and had doubled-bolted doors and barred windows overhead, from one of which an inmate had hanged himself a few days earlier.[45]

The primary institution for treating the mentally ill was the asylum, of which there were two types. The first was private, which took in its own boarders and, in cases when it held a contract with the state, those committed by the departments. The second was public, of which there were a total of fifty-one distributed over fewer than half the departments. Both types were regulated by a law of 1838, which stipulated that each department must have an asylum or provide access to a private or public one. Commitment was determined by *placement volontaire,* by which a family could confine one of its members with only a doctor's certificate, or by *placement d'office,* which required a declaration from the prefect or other authorities that the person posed a threat to public safety. Whatever the form of commitment, the courts played little part.[46]

While praising the 1838 law as an enlightened reform, many doctors in parliament favored revising it. Bourneville, for example, stressed its neglect of retarded children, along with the absence of standards in recruiting and evaluating medical personnel. For Roussel, its weaknesses ranged from the possibility of arbitrary confinement and loss of property, long a concern of the Left, to lack of surveillance over private institutions, which were plagued by periodic reports of brutality toward patients.[47] During the 1870s, Roussel tried without success to persuade the National Assembly to appoint a permanent commission to oversee all asylum patients. He resumed his efforts in 1883, having been appointed by the Senate, along with five other doctors, to a committee charged with revising the law.

Roussel served as reporter for this committee, which for three years heard testimony from specialists and itself toured asylums in England and Belgium.[48] Its final recommendations proposed that each department have its own public asylum and that state surveillance of patients be extended to those placed among families. In addition, special facilities should be built for patients afflicted with cretinism and other forms of extreme retardation, so as to reserve asylums for those judged to be curable. Of special importance, the committee envisioned greater involvement of the courts, which would review the patient's dossier and, after hearing medical advice, decide on the question of internment or release. As an added safeguard, each department would have a commission of surveillance, modeled on the English "committees of lunacy" and composed of local doctors, lawyers, businessmen, and administrators.[49]

After two readings, the bill was approved. A series of amendments had weakened its main articles, however, although the Senate did agree to maintain the principle of judicial primacy. But this was against the advice of Combes and several other physician-senators, who argued that only doctors were qualified to decide the fate of patients.[50] The measure then went to a committee of the Chamber, where a report by Bourneville affirmed the role of the courts and added several new provisions to strengthen services for those having extreme forms of impairment.[51] Thereafter, the campaign fell on hard times, despite the persistence of several physician-legislators.[52] One was Ernest Lafont, who produced two additional reports (in 1891 and 1894). Another was Fernand Dubief, a former asylum director, who, with the help of eight other physicians, hammered out a new bill in 1898. Undeterred by repeated failures to win government backing, Dubief kept resubmitting it after each election. Finally, in January 1907, in the wake of new scandals involving arbitrary confinements, the bill arrived on the floor.[53]

Dubief's bill gave the courts a preponderant role in internments and provided safeguards to protect the patient's property. It mandated the construction of special quarters for alcoholics, epileptics, the extremely mentally deficient, and the criminally insane, and it stipulated that all private asylums would be subject to state surveillance.[54] Approved by voice vote, the bill then went to a Senate committee chaired by Léon Rolland, former chief physician of the public asylum of Tarn-et-Garonne. A new review then got under way, but the sickness of Rolland, combined with the defeat of Dr. Paul Gérente, the reporter, caused new delays. The intervention of Paul Strauss got the bill past a first reading in December 1913, and it would probably have survived a second had the war

not intervened. It was already beginning to generate fresh opposition, however, this time from the Academy of Medicine and
Gilbert Ballet, an expert on "neurasthenia" and defender of the
psychiatric profession, who reassured parliament that accounts of
arbitrary confinements had been greatly exaggerated.[55]

The law of 1838 thus remained in effect. Nevertheless, the efforts
of physician-legislators to convince their colleagues that mental
illness was a disease and that its victims deserved the assistance
and protection of the state reflected an important dimension of
their work as legislators. It is true that they employed the standard
nosologies of the era and occasionally perpetuated some of their
worst assumptions. Dubief, for example, told the Chamber in
1907 that epileptics required isolation because their shrieks tended
to infect others who were predisposed to the disease. Yet, he also
believed that epilepsy did not necessarily imply mental illness, a
point that Roussel had made to the Senate twenty years earlier. It
was just such concerns about the stigma attached to mental disorders that led Dr. Gérente, Senate reporter for the bill of 1909,
to propose substituting the term *affections mentales* for *aliénation*.
Such efforts were not without value in a society in which many
continued to view mental illness as a sign of flawed character,
divine retribution, or demonic possession.

SOCIAL PROTECTION AND ASSISTANCE: CHILDREN, THE INDIGENT, AND THE ELDERLY

Although a few physician-legislators argued that a social defense
against illness could never be achieved by "homeopathic doses"
of welfare, a majority accepted the concept of *assistance sociale* as
the natural complement of revolutionary *fraternité*. In presenting
a bill to aid children of the poor, for instance, Dr. Rey described
those who were most deserving of help as falling into three categories: the indigent, whom sickness had rendered temporarily
incapable of working; the elderly and victims of incurable diseases,
who would never be able to work again; and children.[56]

Of these, the most biologically vulnerable were infants, who
perished by the tens of thousands from gastroenteritis and respiratory diseases. Roussel estimated in 1874 that France lost over a
fifth of its newborns each year, but no one knew the true extent

of the tragedy. In 1890, Gustave Lagneau placed the death rate during the first year of life at 16.8 per 100, observing that this figure encompassed widely disparate levels for legitimate children (15.1) and for illegitimate ones (28.6). A detailed study focusing on 681 towns and cities during the years 1892 to 1897 confirmed these findings and showed that in the largest cities, 18.4 percent of all newborns died before their first birthday. The rate was even higher in industrial areas, standing at 28.3 in the Nord.[57]

Of all political leaders, the individual who did most to focus the nation's attention on this tragedy was Dr. Roussel, who believed that modern society, for all its defense of human rights, had forgotten the newborn. In March 1873, he presented to the National Assembly a bill "relative to the protection of infants and in particular of nurslings." His proposal represented the culmination of several years' debate in the Academy of Medicine, which regarded high infant death rates as the fatal result of artificial feeding. The central problem was the impurity and indigestibility of milk and pabulums, which had been compounded by the growth of wet nursing as greater numbers of women took jobs in shops and factories.[58]

Reporting out his own bill, Roussel detailed a variety of infant killers, ranging from "hereditary degeneration" caused by alcoholism to the lack of compulsory smallpox vaccination. At the top of his list, however, were certain "vicious and injurious practices kept alive by ignorance on infant care and, in particular, on infant feeding." These, he charged, were widespread in the wet-nursing industry, which existed in two forms. In the first, which was seen mainly among the rich, the wet nurse performed her task in the home of the parents, even if it meant ignoring the needs of her own child. In the second, which applied to poor urban families, the wet nurse took the infant into her own home (often in surrounding rural areas), where its treatment was determined less by moral and maternal influences than by "material exigencies." Children thus placed, Roussel said, died with much greater frequency than did those who were breast-fed by their mothers; this fact assumed tragic proportions when one realized that in Paris wet nurses tended more than half of all newborns.[59]

Roussel's bill, approved in December 1874, stipulated that infants under two years of age who were placed with a paid wet nurse or guardian would henceforth be subject to surveillance by state officials. The task was to be carried out by the prefects with the aid of voluntary commissions made up of local politicians, doctors, departmental inspectors for assisted children, and representatives of infant-welfare groups. Subject to inspection were all wet nurses, placement offices, and intermediaries. Each wet nurse had to produce documents providing that her own child (if still alive) was over seven months old; if not, she must show that it was being cared for by another qualified wet nurse.

Despite the optimism that accompanied the bill's passage, it soon became apparent that inadequate funding and lack of inspection were undermining it. Speaking before the Academy of Medicine in 1885, Roussel observed that it was a "dead letter" in nine departments and that in twenty-eight others medical inspection had not even been organized. Yet, he added, in those places where inspection existed, infant mortality rates had declined. He thus pressed for a more rigorous application, saying this would save an additional eighty thousand infant lives a year. Specifically, he urged that departmental funding be mandatory, that the power of inspectors be strengthened, and that certain dangerous infant feeders be banned during the summer months. Five years later, he again stressed the need for these changes and added others, such as extending the law to families who sent out their infants to be cared for by relatives.[60]

Eventually, infant mortality rates, like wet nursing, did begin to decline, albeit slowly. It is no doubt true that this decline owed much to the technology after the 1890s of sterilized and condensed milk.[61] Yet, Roussel's work was not without an impact, even if not on the scale he had hoped. Where the provisions of the law had been applied, he declared in 1890, "its good effects on the rearing of children, on the education of wet nurses, on the propagation of hygiene in those milieus where it is lacking, and finally on infant mortality, have made themselves evident."[62] Every report from the Academy of Medicine on the subject arrived at similar conclusions, including those by Charles Porak in 1902 and René Blanche in 1908.[63] What most prevented the law from achieving its maximum benefit was the absence of funding, which would have allowed monthly medical visits to wet nurses in order to monitor their health and to safeguard that of the children under their care.[64]

Doctors in parliament who addressed the issue of infant mortality were unanimous in praising the virtues of breast feeding. Most realized, however, this was not always possible or likely and thus sought to ensure that artificial methods were as safe as possible. Some urged local governments to create dispensaries that could provide pure milk at low prices and could offer advice to mothers, wet nurses, and even doctors.[65] Others concentrated on the danger of infant feeders. Part of the problem lay in the poor quality of nipples, which were made of rubber and assorted elastics that trapped microorganisms in their porous interiors and that could not sustain boiling. In 1913, Dr. Doizy and others on the Committee of Public Hygiene proposed to ban the sale of all nipples not made of pure rubber.[66] His bill followed on the heels of a successful campaign to outlaw a particular type of infant feeder known as the tubed bottle *(biberon à tube)*. Popular because it could be left alongside the crib, it was, in Cazeneuve's words, "an instrument of death," because the interior of the connecting tube provided an ideal culture for microorganisms and could not be easily sterilized. Condemned by the Academy of Medicine, the tubed feeder came under attack in the Senate in 1906 with a government bill to outlaw its import or sale, which passed with little trouble. In the lower house, the Committee of Public Hygiene, rejecting pleas of manufacturers to delay implementation and to award them an indemnity, charged Dr. Durand, radical of Aude, with the task of preparing a report. This he did promptly, recommending the whole of the bill, which passed with no opposition in 1910.[67]

For many doctors, improved infant feeding was only one aspect of the crusade to preserve life. Also to be reversed were certain social attitudes that they saw as out of keeping with the progress of civilization, in particular those touching on infanticide, abortion, and abandonment. About infanticide, no one could speak with certainty regarding the numbers. About abortion, estimates ranged between 40,000 and 100,000. Dr. Reymond told the Senate in 1913 that in his own obstetrical ward at Nanterre the number of births was far smaller than the number of botched abortions. Moreover, the latter were only "an infinitely small part" of the number of successful attempts, for the advent of antisepsis had greatly reduced the risk of abortion, unless performed by the ignorant and inexperienced. In any case, statistics told little, for "nothing of what has been said approaches the truth, nothing."[68]

What doctors knew for sure was that the harsh sanctions carried by the Penal Code were of limited deterrent value. The solution, Dr. Reymond said, was to focus less on repression than on helping women enjoy motherhood. This meant the creation of confidential childbirth clinics, municipal day nurseries, and infant-feeding programs. Above all, the state must provide financial support to indigent mothers, which would require a general revamping of local welfare services. A government bill of 1892, for which Roussel served as reporter, aimed to reform these, but it was only in 1903, shortly after his death, that the measure reached the floor. Introduced by Strauss, the bill offered financial assistance to any indigent mother who was willing to keep her child and to breast-feed it herself or to provide it with a qualified wet nurse.

In preparing these recommendations, Roussel had been faced with two conflicting strategies for saving the lives of unwanted children. One, favored by many Catholics and conservatives, was the reestablishment of the *tour,* a depository attached to a hospital or hospice where a mother could leave her baby with no questions asked. Few medical men in parliament liked this idea, and a private bill of 1881 to reestablish the *tour* prompted only skepticism among those reviewing it in committee. Dr. Poujade, for example, observed that the institution was often seen as a clerical device whose goal was not to save the life of the infant but to procure it for baptism.[69] Roussel, too, opposed "the exhumation of an institution long dead" that was incompatible with the goal of preventing abandonment. To the argument that its absence drove women to commit infanticide, he answered that the *tour* itself was a veritable *"machine à dépopulation,"* citing a report from Seine-Inférieure showing that in 1858, the last year in which the *tour* existed, a total of 414 of 444 "exposed" infants had died during the first few days.

By contrast, he said, modern welfare principles advocated (1) temporary help to indigent mothers, (2) an open-door policy for the admission of infants (*l'admission à bureau ouvert*), without intensive questioning or investigation, and (3) *maisons de maternité* for assuring young unmarried women of absolute secrecy before delivery.[70] Such were the ideas that had inspired Roussel and that Strauss defended before the Senate; as approved by both houses and enacted into law (17 June 1904), the bill established the principle of state responsibility for mother and child, creating in each department a system whereby the mother – whether single, widowed, divorced, or abandoned – could surrender her infant without witnesses or inquiries. An official was to assure her, however, that if she kept the child she would receive immediate aid and assistance from the state.[71]

Medical men were among the most outspoken advocates of laws to prevent abuse of children. A bill offered by Roussel in July 1882 placed under state protection all minors whose parents had put them in peril of their lives, health, or morals. The courts would rule on the voiding of parental rights, and the prefect, assisted by a local "committee of education and patronage," would decide on the child's placement. The bill passed a second reading in July of the next year, with all the doctors in favor.[72]

Of equal importance was the working child. Though not always in agreement on the age at which children should be allowed to enter the factory, most of the physician-legislators agreed that conditions in the workplace posed a threat to the children's physical development, an idea they repeatedly stressed during debates on child labor laws. As Roussel put it in 1874, the year that parliament established twelve as the minimum age, the human body was the result of "a progressive organic elaboration" that could not be disturbed without dire consequences, no matter what the laws of economics decreed.[73]

Besides infants and children, the indigent sick also ranked high on the list of those entitled to protection. In theory, this right had been recognized since the Revolution. By 1870, however, only forty-four departments had any form of medical assistance to the poor, and there were great disparities in the amounts that local assemblies were willing to allocate to them. For the most part, the cities were better off than the rural areas. According to figures cited in 1893 by Henri Monod, director of assistance and public hygiene, 18 million citizens lived in regions having no medical assistance of any kind. Of this number, an estimated 400,000 became seriously ill each year and, if unable to pay their own way, were forced to rely on the doctor's charity.[74]

In 1872, Roussel and Morvan, physician-deputy of Finistère, presented to the National Assembly a bill to create programs of medical assistance in all departments in which they did not presently exist. In their *exposé des motifs*, they depicted rural dwellers as having been abandoned to their fate during sickness, which afflicted them far more frequently than it did the rich. A government study in 1867, for example, had revealed that in departments having programs of assistance, one of twenty-five who were registered on the rolls of the needy became ill. Outside the cities, it was one of sixteen, and if one counted all poor people, not just those on the needy rolls, the ratio was closer to one of eight. The plan they offered proposed to make local funding compulsory for medical assistance. The *conseils généraux* were to decide on how it would be organized – whether the *landais* system, in which the doctor was chosen by the patient and paid by the department according to the number of visits, or the cantonal system, in which a salaried practitioner carried out the task. Doctors were to participate in drawing up the lists of poor people and would be represented on local boards chosen to oversee implementation.

The committee of parliament that reviewed the bill set out to explore all aspects of the issue, mailing questionnaires to mayors, municipal councilors, doctors, and local hospital commissioners. In the end, it chose to limit its task to expanding local relief offices and to creating new programs of medical assistance based on the Roussel–Morvan model. A bill to this effect survived only one reading, however, before the term of parliament expired.[75] Persistent as usual, Roussel submitted it again after the elections of 1876. This, along with a similar bill offered by Richard Waddington, was then taken up by a new committee, which worked out a scheme for home treatment of the indigent sick. Though cheaper than hospital care, the plan drew fire from the budget committee, which warned that it would cost up to twelve million francs. When debate started in early 1877, these financial concerns proved decisive, despite the eloquent pleas of Waddington, Roussel, and Dr. Laussedat of Allier.[76]

After a decade, political interest in the matter began to revive, owing mainly to the agricultural crisis and its accompanying rural misery. These themes surfaced often during the elections of 1889 and were prominent in the platforms of numerous physician-candidates.[77] Further helping the cause was the creation of the Superior Council of Public Assistance in 1888, whose initial membership counted several prominent physician-legislators, including Roussel and Bourneville.[78] Under the guidance of Henri Monod, the council prepared a new bill under which the indigent sick were to be cared for at home, with the bulk of the costs to be borne by local governments. Each commune or group of communes would be required to have a relief agency *(bureau de bienfaisance)*, which would meet quarterly to draw up the list of qualified recipients and whose decisions would be subject to approval by the municipal council. Local doctors carrying out the law would be allowed to attend these sessions and to participate in drawing up the lists. This last article clearly reflected the lobbying efforts of the medical syndicates, as did the council's stated preference for the *landais* system of payment per visit, which suited the needs of private practitioners but was more costly and less efficient than the cantonal method.[79]

This bill then went to a committee of the Chamber chaired by Michel Labrousse, physician-deputy of Corrèze and a member of the Superior Council of Public Assistance. There were four other doctors on the committee, including Rey, the reporter, and Langlet, both of whom in the past had expressed support for the work of the medical syndicates. Completed in early 1892, the bill went on to the Chamber, where it passed in two readings.[80] Roussel guided the measure through the Senate, reminding his colleagues that France lagged behind other countries in social legislation and urging them to approve the bill. In response to the syndicates' demands, Cornil and Lourties proposed increasing the influence of doctors in those local commissions that would oversee implementation but withdrew an amendment to this effect after Roussel assured them that the medical corps would be consulted. After two readings, the Senate voted in favor, despite charges from the Right that the government was backing it only as a means of currying favor with voters for the upcoming elections.[81]

The law of 1893 was seen by many doctors as a reflection of the spirit of *fraternité* that had motivated reformers from the earliest days of the Republic and that had sought to democratize health care among the rural masses. Yet, the departments voted sums for implementation with the greatest reluctance, and many town governments, cowed by the hostility of property owners toward new taxes, neglected to prepare the list of poor people or else made it an object of political favoritism. Then there was the behavior of the private practitioners themselves, who waged a long campaign to impose the *landais* system on the departments. This was more profitable for them but, in the end, made the welfare of the sick a secondary concern.[82]

Whatever successes the law of 1893 may have had, it failed to address another pressing need. This was the plight of the elderly, who remained an unseen presence in society, many of them forgotten in the towns and villages that their children had long since abandoned.[83] By the 1890s, parliament was only beginning to consider pension schemes for workers in mines and factories.[84] Most people thus remained at risk, and the number of elderly citizens without means of support continued to grow. In 1895, Dr. Rey, then a member of the Superior Council of Public Assistance, and his fellow deputy of Lot, Albert Lachièze, presented a bill providing state aid to the indigent elderly and to the infirm and incurable of all ages who were no longer able to work. The authors argued that although old people in the cities could take advantage of numerous forms of charity, those in rural areas were condemned "to a humiliating mendicity in order to keep from dying of hunger." They thus proposed to create programs of home assistance by means of monthly pensions, which would range between five and twenty francs. Funding and administration would be determined by the same principles laid out in the Medical Assistance Act of 1893.[85]

Although it failed to win a reading before the term of parliament expired, the measure did serve to generate new interest in the problem. That December, the Chamber voted to ask the government to include funds for old-age assistance in the regular budget. Seeing this as a positive step, Rey and Lachièze presented their bill again after the elections of 1898, contending that many communes still left their elderly destitute. A report by the Committee on Social Insurance incorporated most of their ideas, though it proposed to lower the state's share of costs.[86] The matter finally reached the floor in May 1903, where Vaillant argued in favor of a socialist counterproposal to guarantee full social security against accidents, unemployment, and old age. Few doctors were willing to go that far; as it was, those representing poorer rural districts were fretting over the new taxes. In the end, however, they and almost everyone else in the Chamber voted in favor of old-age assistance, mindful, no doubt, of the upcoming elections.[87]

Most doctors in the Senate supported the measure as well. One holdout was Lourties, who argued that old-age assistance would weaken the impulses of private charity. Another was Guyot, who warned that state assistance would cause workers "to give to the barkeepers what they would have given to a savings fund." Only four doctors voted for Guyot's attempt to kill the measure, however, although most did agree with the majority in accepting certain changes. Whereas the Chamber's version had said that age seventy presumed invalidity and thus entitled those without resources to assistance, the Senate's version required the elderly, like the infirm and incurable, to justify their eligibility by convincing officials that they were no longer capable of earning a living.[88] These changes were to have a powerful deterrent effect on later application because of both the indignities they imposed and the bureaucratic caprice they permitted.[89]

For those who had spent the bulk of their existence in the nation's mines and factories, the quality of life during their declining years was directly related to conditions in the workplace. Surveying the state of hygiene in the manufacturing centers of Europe during the 1860s, Freycinet had concluded that industry was almost by definition unhealthy, that it had polluted the air, water, and soil with its gaseous and liquid wastes, and that the workers who carried out the vital functions of this "living being" in confined, noisy, and overheated spaces suffered "organic deformations and often even a weakening of intelligence."[90]

How did medical men in parliament respond to this aspect of the social crises? Earlier chapters have already described their views on social peace and solidarity, along with their votes on a range of political and social issues that they believed to be tied to the workers' biological amelioration. Our final section will examine in greater detail the doctors' part in attacking the specific causes of job-related illness and injuries.

INDUSTRIAL HYGIENE AND SAFETY

That the workers stood to gain most from programs concerning pure water, housing, and disinfection was a sentiment shared by all of the doctors in parliament. As a group, however, they could boast only a modest record in dealing with specific issues pertaining to health and safety on the job. The number of bills and reports the doctors prepared was not exceptionally high, and with the exceptions noted next, neither in committee nor on the floor did they exert a decisive influence in bringing about the few laws that parliament did enact in this domain.

Not all of this was the fault of the doctors. In both houses, the naming of committees to prepare reports on labor bills was a delicate process, particularly when supporters of business interests sought to secure places for themselves. These same elements tended to view the physician–deputy with suspicion, fearing, most of all, that he would seek to impose costly and impractical medical criteria to ameliorate industry's internal problems, which he only dimly understood. One often sees evidence of this attitude, as in the debates in 1891 on working conditions for women and children. Opposing a provision requiring physical examinations for minors employed in industry, Charles Balsan, a textile manufacturer in Indre, contended that doctors would approach their task from an excessively narrow point of view, unable to grasp the diversity of industrial practices. Most, for example, would automatically disqualify a child with a weak chest, though the same child might be able to perform a variety of light duties on the factory floor.[91]

Before 1890, select committees of parliament dealing with labor issues included only a sprinkling of medical men, rarely more than their proportions in each legislature would dictate. The same applied afterwards to the permanent Committee of Labor, on which doctors usually accounted for about 12 percent of the membership. While identifying themselves with radicalism, most of them represented rural constituencies, two notable exceptions being Dron of Lille, an articulate spokesman for working-class welfare, and Théodore Barrois, also of Lille, who was tied by wealth and marriage to the industrial interests of his region.[92]

It was the Committee of Labor that claimed jurisdiction over most of the proposals related to factory conditions. Among these was the first law on industrial hygiene in France, dated 12 June 1893, which sought to establish standards of cleanliness, ventilation, lighting, and safety. Except for those who sat on the committee itself, no doctor played a significant part in the passage of this measure. On the other hand, medical men had a fairly strong presence on the Committee of Social Insurance, formed in 1893. There they constituted just under a fifth of the membership, easily making their influence felt on a range of medically related topics, such as labor accidents, occupational diseases, maternity leaves, and aid to nursing mothers. Although two physicians (Cosmao-Dumenez and Lesage) served terms on both committees, the most influential were the ones having greatest seniority, like Dubuisson and Clament, who served four terms each, or Delbet and Defontaine, who served three. The latter, elected deputy of the Nord in 1893, was, like Dron, deeply concerned about conditions among miners and textile workers and was one of the few doctors on the committee having any prolonged firsthand knowledge of the health dangers they faced on the job.[93]

Seeking to stake out its own claims in this area was the Committee of Public Hygiene, dominated by doctors. It heard testimony from experts on factory hygiene, inspected conditions among workers in powder-manufacturing plants, and reported out bills to ban lead-based paints. By 1910, it had organized its own subcommittee to review all matters of this kind brought before it, and it could also call on the expertise of numerous members who had served on the committees for labor or social insurance, such as Cazeneuve, Amodru, Ricard, and Defontaine. Younger and less prestigious than other standing committees of the Chamber, however, it tended to regard itself as a poor relative when it came to reviewing legislation dealing with the regulation of industry, food processing, military hygiene, and other areas in which powerful entrenched interests believed their rights to be threatened.[94]

The doctors in parliament also maintained a presence on those elite councils that advised the cabinet on working-class affairs. Dubief, who served a term as chairman of the Committee of Labor, also sat on the Superior Council of Labor, as did Dron. Most physicians whom parliament elected to these bodies, however, reflected the social conservatism that dominated their membership. Guyot, for example, who opposed obligatory aid to the elderly poor, was the choice for the Superior Council on Old-Age Pensions. Lourties, who agreed with him, sat on both the Superior Council of Labor and the Superior Council for Mutual-Aid Societies. None of our doctors belonged to the Consultative Committee of Arts and Manufacturing, however, whose duties included implementation of an 1810 decree aimed at protecting areas adjacent to dangerous and unhealthy industries and whose pro-industry bias was the most pronounced of all. Levraud, one of six physician-deputies to serve on the Council of Health and Hygiene for the Seine, told the Chamber in 1902 that when he and his colleagues had toured local industries on behalf of the

Consultative Committee of Arts and Manufacturing, their reports had not been allowed to mention any hazardous or unsanitary conditions found inside the plant, and any attempt to initiate reform had always met with a hostile reception.[95]

There was another reason that doctors did not emerge as champions of working-class hygiene, aside from the fact that their own districts usually lay outside the nation's mining and manufacturing areas. The centers of economic power in the rural departments that sent them to parliament tended to fear health and safety legislation that could be extended from industry to agriculture or from big business to small. Banning night work for women in the dark, satanic mills of the north was one thing; doing so for the "robust *campagnardes*" of the sunny Midi was something else. Dr. Lavergne of Tarn, for instance, thought it unfair to subject village industry and small family enterprises to the same regulations imposed on big mines and factories, even though Roussel and other reformers had often complained of family workshops as being the most unsanitary of all.[96] As we have seen, a majority of physician-legislators favored banning night work for women, which they denounced as a menace to health and family. Yet, many were eager to make exceptions for their own districts. Indeed, it was Dr. Delpierre, radical of Oise and a member of the Committee of Labor, who in March 1912 proposed an amendment, supported by over half of the doctors, to exempt small industries from the ten-hour day.

A different sort of behavior marked those doctors who represented urban and industrial districts. Outspoken in committee deliberations and in floor debates, they formed a small but influential nucleus of physician-legislators who produced a variety of bills related to worker health and safety. Most were militant radicals, although there was also a scattering of socialists, such as Doizy of Ardennes and Léon Thivrier of Allier, both from mining areas. Others were found in the cities, mainly Paris, and included several who had gained exposure to the problems of urban hygiene while serving on the municipal council. Elsewhere, one could cite the names of Augagneur at Lyon, Flaissières at Marseille, and Testelin, Dron, and Defontaine at Lille.

None of these men formulated any coherent ideas regarding health care for industrial workers, but certain themes recur in their speeches. Among the most important was the relationship between capitalist modes of production and illness, a link that could be traced along very specific lines, from lung ailments to sexually transmitted diseases.[97] For a few, like Vaillant, the matter went deeper. The lot of the workers under capitalism, he argued, was "a state of continuous sickness" brought on by poverty and overwork:

In normal life there is a physiological equilibrium between what the organism takes in and puts out. Fatigue and overwork destroy this equilibrium, and from the time that fatigue sets in, a profound trouble is present in the organism, whose elements cannot be repaired normally. ... Man is no longer anything but the shadow of what he should be. Industrialism kills him, and an unprotective society is its accomplice.[98]

Few doctors were willing to contemplate the destruction of capitalism as a solution. Instead, most envisioned systematic reforms, preceded by the gathering of detailed information of the workers' living and working conditions. This theme had been sounded on the Left since the earliest days of the Republic, and it was one of the motives prompting Camille Raspail in 1886 to begin pressing for a ministry of labor, whose functions would include promoting hygiene in the workplace. The next step was to carry out research on diseases associated with specific occupations and industries. This is what Roussel had done, starting in the 1840s, in linking white phosphorous to the poisoning of match workers, whose "horrible necrosis" had so shocked Raspail during his years of medical practice.[99] Vaillant wished to go further, suggesting in 1912 that France follow the example of Germany in studying the entire physiology of labor, including the requirements of diet, rest, and energy expenditure within each occupation.[100]

The last step was to enact legislation to protect the workers against the particular dangers associated with their trade. This meant replacing toxic substances with nontoxic ones, or, if this proved impossible, banning them outright, even at the risk of violating freedom of commerce. For a majority of physician-legislators, the banning of a toxic substance entitled its maker to no financial compensation. As Cazeneuve argued before the Senate in 1909, the state could not be held liable when it penalized industries that posed a threat to human beings, for were this the case it would have to indemnify all those who found their profits hurt by any form of public health progress.[101] Naturally, this was easier said than done, as was apparent in the campaign to extend the benefits of the 1898 law on labor accidents to occupational diseases.

The person who took the lead in this campaign was the socialist Breton, whose backgrounds in chemistry aided him in exploring the various technical issues associated with the problem. In December 1901, he offered a bill allowing victims of occupational diseases to claim the same benefits as those enjoyed by injured workers under the law of 1898. This proposal, resubmitted in three subsequent legislatures, prompted the government to prepare its own version, based not on the principle of linking occupational diseases to accidents but on the principle of obligatory insurance.[102] What followed was a stalemate, despite Breton's persistence on the Committee of Social Insurance, of which he became chairman in 1910. Throughout this time, physicians outside the committee said little on the issue, sensitive to charges from the Right that their profession was growing fat on the law of 1898 and that its representatives in public life were using any means possible to expand its influence. Inside the committee, however, medical men continued to work with Breton, undeterred by such accusations or by complaints from industry that sickness insurance would ruin them.[103]

One of them, Gilbert Laurent, produced a report in 1910 mandating compensation for workers in two of the worst industries, lead and mercury. When the bill finally reached the floor, he defended it vigorously, arguing that prevention was cheaper than cure and that the proposed law would lower the costs for employers while improving the conditions for their workers. Such pragmatism failed to convince all the deputies, however. Paul Beauregard, economist and translator of David Ricardo's works, questioned whether there was any such thing as an occupational disease and declared that many ailments ascribed to lead or mercury were actually the advanced stages of alcoholism. His most impassioned attacks were directed against medical practitioners, whom he assailed for having inflated the need for their services under the law of 1898.[104] This bill survived only a single reading before the war. Disappointed, its supporters could take at least some satisfaction from passage of a government bill, endorsed by the Chamber in 1903, that banned the use of lead-based paints in building interiors and, after three years, on exteriors as well. Against the advice of Dr. Pedebidou, however, and of 37 percent of the physicians who voted, the Senate decided to remove the provision regarding building exteriors and to award an indemnity to lead manufacturers.[105] Back in the Chamber, all but five doctors voted to reaffirm the original version, which was then sent back to the upper house. The impasse was finally broken when Pedebidou, on behalf of a Senate conference committee, and Breton, on behalf of one in the Chamber, agreed on a compromise. Under its terms, the indemnity would be eliminated, and in return there would be a delay of five years in enforcement in order to give the lead industry time to adjust.

Any suspicion that the doctors in parliament were seeking to advance the material interests of their own profession cannot be verified from their involvement in the issue of occupational diseases. It is true that certain physicians on the Committee of Social Insurance, such as Dubuisson and Laurent, had ties with the medical syndicates, but they did not appear to be motivated by goals other than those they expressed on behalf of the workers' health and safety. It is less easy to make this assertion when examining their efforts to enforce the Workman's Compensation Act of 1898, although in this case their actions stemmed largely from the pressures placed on them by an increasingly powerful medical lobby.

The origins of this law go back to a bill presented by Martin Nadaud in 1881, which sought to introduce the concept of le risque professionnel. This would have awarded to workers in mechanized industry the right to compensation for injuries sustained on the job, unless it could be proved that they had deliberately caused them. In the final version, passed only in April 1898, workers were to be compensated according to the extent of their injury, with a permanent incapacity, for example, entitling one to an annual pension equal to two-thirds of his salary. Reports were to be sent to local authorities within three days after the accident and to be accompanied by a doctor's certificate describing the victim's condition. Employers were responsible for up to one hundred francs in medical costs; if the worker chose his own physician, costs were not to exceed a sum fixed by the local justice of the peace, conforming to the scales established under the Medical Assistance Act of 1893.

Shortly after the law's implementation, Dubuisson proposed an amendment designed to protect the interests of doctors, by affirming the right of accident victims to choose their own. At present, he said, many industries were telling employees that if they wished to claim any benefits under the law, they must use company doctors or those hired by the insurance society with which it was affiliated. The Committee of Social Insurance, to which Dubuisson belonged, accepted the amendment and included it among a group of proposed changes that were reported out and passed in the spring of 1901.[106]

The bill faced a tougher challenge in a committee of the Senate. The reporter, Alphonse Chovot, a member of the High Court of Justice who had reported out a number of bills on labor accidents, was, like many of his colleagues, cool to the demands of private practitioners, whether on the issue of free choice or the wish to see payment rates freed from those established in 1893. In an open letter to physician-senators, *Le Concours médical* appealed for help. When the bill reached the floor in June 1904, Drs. Gustave Gauthier, Pedebidou, Piettre, and Lourties delivered a vigorous defense of the medical profession, reminding the Senate of the historic heroism and selflessness of its members in serving the poor. A resolution presented by Treille and thirty-two other physician-senators affirmed the right of free choice and stipulated that medical fees under the 1898 law would henceforth be determined by the justice of the peace, conforming to "local custom." At the end of debate, the Senate approved it by a vote of 141 to 118, with only four doctors joining the opposition. *Le Concours médical* eulogized those who had spoken out and declared that the session had been "a good day for the medical corps."[107]

Although the Senate subsequently changed its mind, ruling that fee scales under the 1898 law would be set by the minister of commerce and industry, the medical syndicates were not entirely displeased. Assured a place for their own delegates on the special commission that would advise him, they appealed to "this highly placed colleague" (Dr. Fernand Dubief) to defend them against the insurance companies. Both Dubuisson and Pedebidou personally intervened with him to argue the case; at the same time, *Le Concours médical* warned that if doctors were unhappy with the final rate schedule, they would work in every department and canton during the upcoming general elections to promote candidates who took their sides.[108] As a result, the final *tarif Dubief,* issued in October 1905, tried to mollify private practitioners on two main points: the freedom to choose one's own doctor and the setting of fees by justices of the peace according to local precedent.

How strong an influence did the medical lobby have over the physician-legislators on social issues before 1914? Certain individuals, such as Dubuisson, Pedebidou, and a few others holding senior committee positions, were able on occasion to act as advocates for professional interests. Although the *groupe médical parlementaire* remained as ineffectual as ever, leaders of the syndicates also appear to have enjoyed increasingly better relations with conservative physicians in the Senate, who, for different reasons, shared their growing distrust for social laws. It is harder to characterize the sentiments of the doctors in the lower house. For many, no doubt, the growing rigidity of the medical corps in regard to social issues made it hard for them to espouse the kinds of professional idealism that had been common during the early days of the Republic.

In addition, the physician-deputies could not ignore the growing sentiment in political quarters that doctors were overcharging and making excessive numbers of house calls in implementing the law of 1898. These topics arose frequently in the Committee of Social Insurance, particularly on bills to extend coverage to workers on nonmechanized farms.[109] Several doctors on the Left, Augagneur among them, contended that the guarantee of free choice as an automatic benefit drove up the cost of medical services and hence worked against the interests of sick. Even Doizy, long considered a friend of the profession, admitted that some doctors were abusing their positions; the best solution, he told the Committee of Social Insurance in 1913, would be the creation of local arbitration committees.[110] So sensitive had the issue of medical rights versus medical responsibilities become by 1914 that a proposal by Henry Chéron, minister of labor and social welfare, to form a commission to study the participation of the medical corps in applying social laws drew an immediate hostile reaction from medical spokesman, who denounced Chéron as a "socialist utopian" who was trying to "domesticate" French doctors.[111]

This survey of the doctors' record on social issues has permitted us to identify several characteristics distinguishing their outlook. Taken with their labors on behalf of public health, these suggest a variety of professional influences at work in their political careers and a distinctively medical bias in their mode of social analysis. Although they held many of the same assumptions found among other bourgeois reformers, the doctors tended to focus most heavily on the practical aspects of social amelioration and were generally less concerned with the procedural and institutional barriers that preoccupied others in parliament, particularly those whom Senator Henri Tolain once described as having been nourished on "juridical milk."

This vision exhibited all the weaknesses one would expect from individuals working in a forum that was called upon daily to mediate social appetites. At its core, moreover, were certain assumptions that in themselves would have prevented any objective assessment of social issues. The condition of women is one example. Despite the laudable efforts of certain doctors to promote the cause of maternal assistance, it is clear that their primary concern was the survival of the children. That, too, was admirable, but it serves as a reminder of the doctors' essential lack of understanding concerning the forces that affected the physical and social well-being of women. Few, for example, were prepared to challenge the famous prohibition against *recherche de la paternité* in the Napoleonic Code, which, in the interest of protecting the family, had barred an unmarried woman from pursuing in court the father of her child. Few, in fact, were willing to ground their defense of women on much more than the sanctity of their reproductive function, and this was true even of those who showed the most sensitivity on the issue. Witness the comments of Paul Lafargue, son-in-law of Karl Marx, during the debates in 1892 on pregnant women in industry:

> We must look at the question from another point of view and consider that any female citizen, married or not, who gives to the world a child and who nurses it, accomplishes a sacred task and fulfills a social function *(laughs)*.
>
> Ah, you laugh, gentlemen! But what other function is more important and greater than that of giving children to humanity and of reproducing?[112]

Characteristic of that era, such flaws should not prevent us from appreciating the other contributions of medical men, whether those regarding children, the indigent sick, the elderly, or the

mentally ill. Nor should we forget that whatever their imperfec-
tions, the laws that they helped bring about had a positive impact
when applied and often served as a basis for more substantive
reforms in later years. Such was the piecemeal fashion in which
progress was defined in the regime's legislative struggles.

CONCLUSION AND EPILOGUE

This analysis of France's physician-legislators has provided a detailed look at the ways in which medicine and politics have interacted in the past, whether in shaping the assumptions that govern each area of activity or in defining the influence that both bring to bear over the process of change. What exactly have we learned? In regard to France, we are better able to understand how an important segment of the professional and political elites was constituted. As seen early in the book, medicine recruited heavily from the ranks of rural property owners and the small-town middle classes. Largely excluded from national political life before the birth of the Third Republic, the members of these social classes viewed medicine as a means of enhancing their place in society, and although they were not among the wealthiest elements of the provincial bourgeoisie, they were at least able to endure the financial sacrifices required for a medical degree. Such patterns were most evident in the rural south and southwest, where a degree in medicine enhanced one's chances for a good marriage and where strong medical traditions assured the doctor an influence in local life. Those who entered parliament were thus not professional and social failures but members of the local elites. Some of these were newly formed elites; others had existed for generations as modest medicopolitical dynasties.

It is also clear that although similar social tendencies existed among other bourgeois professions, medicine exerted distinctive influences on those who studied and practiced it. Its power was manifest at three levels: as a body of professional theory, as a method of training, and as a unique life experience and social identity. No doubt, much remains to be learned about the ways in which work alters or affects one's assumptions and behavior. Nevertheless, the physician-legislators demonstrate that this tendency exists and that our knowledge of the past would be enriched by paying more attention to the views and perspectives associated with different professional groups. Among our doctors, it is not an exaggeration to say that medicine, far from being incidental to their political careers, was their soul and substance. Not only did it provide stepping-stones to places of social authority; it also offered up countless opportunities by which the doctors could capitalize on that authority. Again, the pattern is most striking in rural areas, where the doctor enjoyed immense prestige, and was often seen as the representative of science and culture. What he most stressed in running for office, however, was his role as a man who had come from the people and whose years of medical service had afforded him a rare glimpse of the problems they faced.

If medicine provided a means by which one could achieve political office, it also helped account for the great numbers of doctors who associated themselves with the vanguard of democracy. Once again, the views of doctors had much in common with petit-bourgeois radicalism; yet, those in parliament displayed other traits that were occupationally specific, that is, derived from their distinctive training in the hospitals, their work among the rural poor, and their cumulative experiences in professional practice, especially as these related to the clergy and other traditional forces. The church, of course, opposed the materialism associated with scientific medicine, and through much of the century it exerted a powerful influence over the local political apparatus that set the conditions for its existence. That the doctors, having breached this structure as municipal councillors and mayors, proceeded to promote local programs of health and welfare as a moral imperative of science and as an expression of an almost Jacobin patriotism, added to their reputation as mavericks and radicals in the eyes of the Right.

An essential *esprit médical* thus marked most physician-legislators from their earliest forays into politics, and it continued to do so during the years in parliament. Our study of their record at this level has produced several important findings: We have seen that the doctors exhibited higher levels of radicalism on most political, social, and economic issues than did parliament in general or lawyers in particular. We have also seen that despite their weaknesses on issues involving the workers, the doctors followed an intensely programmatic agenda, as defined by such modern theorists as

Oliver H. Woshinsky and as measured by their authorship of private bills, committee membership, and service as *rapporteurs*. These activities, which usually focused on issues of health and welfare, grew naturally from their professional interests and, when joined to their presence on administrative councils and other advisory bodies, accorded well with the political role once envisioned for doctors by the social hygienists of the late eighteenth and early nineteenth centuries. The doctors' attitudes toward the medical corps itself were more ambiguous. Although repeated attempts to organize a *groupe médical parlementaire* ended in failure, Cézilly and the medical syndicates did on several occasions manage to advance their professional interests via a select group of doctors in the Chamber and Senate. The reform of 1892 is one example. Still, as this book has made clear, doctors did not run for office as representatives of their profession, and once elected, their work was too constituent oriented to allow them to assume such a role. Even if they had been inclined to follow this course, the growing perception after 1892 that doctors were committed to their own interests over all else would have made it difficult for them to equate professional rights with the good of the people, which had long been a source of strength among medical reformers.

Within the constraints imposed by constituent pressures and against heavy odds, the physician–legislators assisted the country in making at least some progress toward the kinds of social goals that other industrial societies had already achieved. Motivated in part by a reformist and humanitarian impulse that characterized an influential segment of the French bourgeoisie, they brought their skills to bear on a host of specific problems confronting the society. As examples, one could cite the names of Chevandier, Naquet, Bert, Cornil, Lannelongue, Pedebidou, and Dubuisson in medical education and medical practice; of Bourneville in nursing; of Bert, Liouville, Langlet, Cornil, Bourneville, Doizy, Gadaud, Dubois, and Vaillant in public health and hygiene; of Lannelongue, Marmottan, and Lachaud in military hygiene; of Roussel, Rey, Dron, and Doizy in social assistance and the protection of children; and of Dron, Raspail, Vaillant, Laurent, Doizy, and Dubois in factory hygiene and safety. These men were only a few who proved capable of articulating a social goal and mobilizing the political skills needed to see it assume concrete legislative form. This, after all, was the most essential of a politician's functions, one often left to others by the regime's better-known orators and power-brokers.

As with other features of French life, World War I marked a turning point in the political orientation of medical men, although this process had been under way before the war began. What was different was not so much a decline in the doctors' commitment to partisan politics; the general elections held in May and June 1914, shortly before the assassination of Archduke Francis Ferdinand at Sarajevo, saw physicians more involved than ever, accounting for 170 of 2,902 candidates, or close to 6 percent of the total. Even excluding an additional 35 pharmacists who ran, the figure represented the highest rate of medical participation in general elections since the birth of the Republic. The final vote showed 56 doctors among the winners: Following a pattern established over previous years, this indicated a continuing drop in the ratio of winners to losers but still meant that a third of all doctors who ran managed to win.

Thereafter, the proportion of medical men in each of the interwar legislatures fell off only slightly, with that of 1919 containing forty-four doctors and five pharmacists. Adding a handful of dental surgeons and veterinarians, we find similar numbers and proportions right up to 1940: Medical men constituted 7.7 percent of the legislature of 1924–8; 9.7 percent of that of 1928–32; 9.7 percent again of that of 1932–6; 7.5 percent percent of the Popular Front Chamber of 1936–40. In more recent times, the proportions of doctors among the deputies have at times matched and even surpassed those of the early Third Republic. By the 1970s, for example, physicians and dental surgeons constituted 10.5 percent of the National Assembly, and veterinarians and pharmacists made up another 5.4 percent.

What changed after 1914, rather, was the medicopolitical vision itself. Certainly, this reflected a conservative drift among the older republican groups on the Left, especially as they became outflanked by socialists and communists; but it also revealed an increasingly cautious, even reactionary, orientation within the medical profession. This was a natural response as medicine gained in professional stature and began seeking to secure its rights against a more socially active state that seemed to threaten the doctor's autonomy. Those doctors elected to the Chamber of 1914, for example, included numerous younger men for whom the great social and hygienic ideals of the early Republic had lost much of their force. Few of those in the Chamber of 1919 joined the parties of the Left; on the contrary, over two-thirds sat with the moderate and conservative groups forming the *bloc national*. In the Chamber of 1936, 45 percent were found among parties of the extreme Right. This was not unusual by this time, for doctors were showing up in increasing numbers in the disaffected factions of the Right, including the Action française. Nor is it surprising that many medical men should appear among the partisans of the New Order in 1940. After all, some might reason, the Vichy regime could boast a better record than could the Third Republic in many areas of public health, including the struggle against alcoholism. It was also responsible for making a self-regulating Order of Doctors at last a reality.

As for the old-time physician-legislators who were still alive in 1914, the war changed the world for them, too. Twenty-nine joined up as medical officers, dividing their time between their duties at the front and the Palais-Bourbon. Most were the younger members of our group, but for a few age was no barrier. For example, Amodru, at sixty-five, took charge of auxiliary hospitals in the Paris region and helped create special *formations sanitaires* for the wounded. Jean Gouyon-Beauchamps, aged fifty-nine and only recently elected for Dordogne, served until collapsing and dying of a heart attack in 1916. Several others, many of them decorated, ran hospitals for the wounded, including Fesq at Clérmont-Ferrand, Guiraud at Limoges, Hugon at Puy, and Claussat at Toul. Eugène Chassaing, deputy of Puy-de Dôme since 1909, won the croix de guerre for his work on organizing a system of air evacuation for the wounded.

A few made the supreme sacrifice. Dr. Reymond, the senator for whom the new age of aviation had become an obsession (he was the first in France to visit his constituents by airplane), joined the infant air corps and was shot down and killed on 21 October 1914 while observing the enemy. Almost as heroic in the eyes of their countrymen were those in occupied areas who stood up to the invader. Dron remained in Lille for the duration of the war and was finally arrested by the Germans on a charge of spying. Defontaine, now sixty, was seized at the outset of the war and died four years later, after his health deteriorated while in captivity. The great surgeon Samuel Pozzi, who had taken charge of the wounded at the Hôtel Astoria in Paris, met a more violent end. Mortally wounded at the hands of a deranged patient in June 1918, he is reported to have told the doctors that they would find two bullets in his abdomen and one in his kidneys, that he was going to die, but that they should go ahead and operate because "surgeons ought always to try."

The list of tragedies goes on. Cazauvieilh of Gironde lost one of two sons, also a doctor, to the war. Chautemps had one son killed, then another, and then a third wounded before he himself succumbed, shortly after the armistice. Drs. Hugon and Goy lost sons, as did Dubief, whose patriotism was able to sustain him for only a short time before grief overcame him. Pedebidou, called to the colors as a military doctor during the war, continued afterwards to devote his efforts to the care of veterans, until he himself died in a train accident near Poitiers.

Some members of the pre-1914 generation remained active in politics during the interwar period, although by the 1930s their ranks had thinned. Pierre Even of Côtes-du-Nord and Léon Sireyjol of Dordogne were still in office when the debacle of 1940 came, and both voted to give emergency powers to Marshal Philippe Pétain. The very last was Dr. Chassaing, thirty-three years old when he first entered parliament. Between 1930 and 1944 he sat in the Senate, later winning a seat in the National Assembly of the Fourth Republic, which he kept until 1955. By then, the doctor of legend, the radical who had preached *la république sociale et médicale* and whose power had caused priests and aristocrats to tremble in rage, had long vanished from public life.

APPENDIX A: PROFESSORS OF MEDICINE IN PARLIAMENT

1. Faculties

Paris

Titled professors

Paul Broca (1824–80), surgery, neurology, anthropology. Sénateur inamovible, 1880

Victor Cornil (1837–1908), pathology, histology. Deputy (Allier), 1876–82; senator, 1885–1903

Odilon Lannelongue (1840–1911), surgery. Deputy (Gers), 1893–8; senator, 1906–11

Samuel Pozzi (1846–1918), gynecological surgery. Senator (Dordogne), 1898–1903

Charles Robin (1821–85), histology. Senator (Ain), 1876–85

Adolphe Wurtz (1817–84), chemistry. Sénateur inamovible, 1881–4

Agrégés

Armand Després (1834–96), surgery. Deputy (Seine), 1889–93

Léon Labbé (1832–1916), surgery. Senator (Orne), 1892–1916

J. M. de Lanessan (1843–1919), natural history. Deputy (Seine), 1881–91; (Rhône), 1898–1906; (Charente-Inférieure), 1910–14

Henry Liouville (1837–87), pathology, anatomy. Deputy (Meuse), 1876–87

Alfred Naquet (1834–1916), chemistry. Deputy (Vaucluse), 1876–83, 1893–8; senator (Vaucluse), 1883–90; deputy (Seine), 1890–3

Jean Peyrot (1843–1917), surgery. Senator (Dordogne), 1903–17

Eugène Villejean (1850–1930), chemistry, toxicology. Deputy (Yonne), 1895–1910

Montpellier

Titled professors

Etienne Bouisson (1813–84), surgery, pathology. Deputy (Hérault), 1871–6

Agrégés

Louis Amagat (1848–90), natural history. Deputy (Cantal), 1881–90
Germain Dupré (1811–93), internal medicine. Deputy (Hautes–Pyrénées), 1882–91
Lucien Penières (1840–1922), anatomy. Deputy (Corrèze), 1881–5

Lille

Titled professors

Théodore Barrois (1857–1920), zoology, parasitology. Deputy (Nord), 1898–1906
Charles Debierre (1853–1932), anatomy, physiology. Senator (Nord), 1911–32
Alfred Giard (1846–1911), zoology. Deputy (Nord), 1882–5

Lyon

Titled professors

Victor Augagneur (1855–1931), pathology, venereology. Deputy (Rhône), 1904–5, 1910–19, 1928–31
Georges Beauvisage (1852–1925), botany, abnormal children. Senator (Rhône), 1909–20
Paul Cazeneuve (1852–1934), chemistry. Deputy (Rhône), 1902–9; senator (Rhône), 1909–20

Nancy

Titled professors
Albin Saillard (1842–1925), surgery. Senator (Doubs), 1897–1912

2. Preparatory schools

Angers

Jean Guignard (1829–1901), anatomy, obstetrics. Deputy (Maine-et-Loire), 1893–8
Ambroise Monprofit (1857–1922), surgery. Deputy (Maine-et-Loire), 1910–14, 1919–22

Clérmont-Ferrand

Antoine Blatin (1841–1911), physiology. Deputy (Puy-de-Dôme), 1885–9

Marseille

Hector Bartoli (1822–83), dermatology. Deputy (Corsica), 1876–83

Reims

Jean Langlet (1841–1927), physiology *(professeur suppléant)*. Deputy (Marne), 1889–93

Adrien Pozzi (1860–1939), surgery. Deputy (Marne), 1906–10

Alfred Thomas (1826–99), anatomy, physiology, chemistry. Deputy (Marne), 1876–7, 1878–86, 1889–93

APPENDIX B: THE DOCTORS' LEGISLATIVE RECORD

Between 1871 and 1914, physicians in both houses served as committee reporters for a total of sixty-eight major bills that touched on public health and hygiene, reform of the medical and allied health professions, and social welfare. Of these, twenty-eight eventually made their way into law, though usually after having undergone modifications at the hands of several committees over the course of two or more legislatures. Although medical men could not claim sole credit for any ultimate success, their reports were often among the most significant in the long legislative process. The laws in question are as follows:

> Law of 8 December 1874 on the creation of new medical faculties
> Law of 23 December 1874 on the regulation of wet nursing
> Law of 21 July 1881 on the animal sanitary police
> Law of 10 December 1887 to award a prize to the person finding a means to determine substances other than chemical or ordinary alcohol in commercial spirits or alcoholic beverages
> Law of 15 November 1887 on the liberty of funerals
> Law of 1 July 1889 on the administration of the army health service (two reporters)
> Law of 24 July 1889 on the protection of mistreated and abandoned children
> Law of 11 July 1891 on the repression of fraud in the sale of wine
> Law of 30 November 1892 on the practice of medicine
> Law of 15 July 1893 on free medical assistance
> Law of 10 July 1894 on the cleaning up of Paris and the Seine (two reporters)
> Law of 24 July 1894 on fraud in the sale of wine (two reporters)
> Law of 25 April 1895 on the preparation and distribution of therapeutic serums
> Law of 16 April 1897 concerning the repression of fraud in the manufacture and sale of butter and margarine
> Law of 19 April 1898 on the practice of pharmacy
> Law of 30 June 1899 concerning agricultural accidents involving machines
> Law of 8 July 1901 concerning the incompatibility of public assistance physicians

Law of 15 February 1902 concerning the protection of public health (two reporters)

Law of 14 July 1905 on assistance to the old, infirm, and incurable

Law of 8 January 1908 concerning slaughterhouses

Law of 21 March 1908 approving an international office of hygiene

Law of 5 August 1908 on the repression of food fraud

Law of 20 July 1909 on the use of lead in paints

Law of 17 November 1909 on the guarantee of jobs for pregnant women in industry

Law of 6 April 1910 on the prohibition of selling or importing infant feeders known as *biberons à tube*

Law of 13 April 1910 on the creation of hydrothermal stations

Law of 28 July 1912 on the modification and completion of the law of 1 August 1905 on fraud in wine

Law of 16 July 1913 on an autonomous disinfection service for towns under twenty thousand population

APPENDIX C: MEDICAL MEMBERSHIP OF THE CHAMBER'S COMMITTEE ON PUBLIC HYGIENE

The following is a list of individuals on the Committee of Public Hygiene after 1898 who held doctorates in medicine. An additional number of pharmacists (three to four per legislature) also sat on the committee, which initially numbered thirty-three members.

Legislature of 1898–1902

Emile Dubois, *chairman,* Seine, socialist Left★
Laurent Amodru, Seine-et-Oise, center Right
François Bachimont, Aube, radical Left★
Charles Borne, Doubs, radical Left
Gustave Chopinet, Oise, radical Left★
Ernest Delbet, Seine-et-Marne, radical Left★
Ernest Ferroul, Aube, socialist Left
Jules Gacon, Allier, center Left
Hippolyte Herbet, Ain, center Right
Paul Pourteyron, Dordogne, center Left★
Henri Ricard, Côte-d'Or, radical Left
Edouard Vaillant, Seine, socialist Left★
Albert Vazeille, Loiret, radical Left
Eugène Villejean, Yonne, radical Left★

Legislature of 1902–6

Eugène Villejean, *chairman,* Yonne, radical Left★
François Bachimont, Aube, radical Left★
Pierre Bichon, Maine-et-Loire, center Left
Paul Bourgeois, Vendée, Right
Auguste Baudon, Oise, radical Left
Emile Chautemps, Seine, radical Left
Clément Clament, Dordogne, center Left★
Ernest Delbet, Seine-et-Marne, radical Left★
Emile Dubois, Seine, socialist Left★

★Served two or more terms on the committee.

Pierre Hugon, Cantal, radical Left★
Léonce Levraud, Seine, radical Left★
Paul Pourteyron, Dordogne, center Left★
Hippolyte Rouby, Corrèze, radical Left
Henri Vacherie, Haute-Vienne, radical Left★

Legislature of 1906–10
Eugène Villejean, *chairman,* Yonne, radical Left★
François Bachimont, Aube, radical Left★
Paul Cazeneuve, Rhône, radical Left
Léon Chambige, Puy-de-Dôme, radical Left★
Gustave Chapuis, Meurthe-et-Moselle, radical Left
Oscar Cibiel, Vienne, center Left
Clément Clament, Dordogne, center Left★
Ernest Delbet, Seine-et-Marne, radical Left★
François Délelis-Fanien, Pas-de-Calais, center Left
Pierre Dudouyt, Manche, center Right
Jean Durand, Aude, radical Left
Pierre Hugon, Cantal, radical Left★
Edouard Lachaud, Corrèze, radical Left★
Léonce Levraud, Seine, radical Left★
Adrien Meslier, Seine, socialist Left★
Paul Pourteyron, Dordogne, center Left★
Henri Vacherie, Haute-Vienne, radical Left★
Edouard Vaillant, Seine, socialist Left★

Legislature of 1910–14
Edouard Lachaud, *chairman,* Corrèze, radical Left
Pierre Archambaud, Réunion, center Right
Louis Augé, Aveyron, Right
François Bachimont, Aube, radical Left★
Eugène Chassaing, Puy-de-Dôme, radical Left
Gustave Chopinet, Oise, radical Left★
Clément Clament, Dordogne, center Left★
Paul Defontaine, Nord, radical Left
Henri Doizy, Ardennes, socialist Left
Paulin Dupuy, Tarn-et-Garonne, radical Left
Pierre Even, Côtes-du-Nord, radical Left
François Fesq, Cantal, center Left
Adrien Meslier, Seine, socialist Left★
Aman Périer, Vendée, radical Left
Paul Pujade, Pyrénées-Orientales, radical Left
Edouard Vaillant, Seine, socialist Left★
Aristide Samalens, Gers, radical Left

★Served two or more terms on the committee.

NOTES

ABBREVIATIONS

AN	Archives nationales
BAM	Bulletin de l'académie de médecine
JO, assemb. nat.	*Journal officiel de la république française (Debates and documents of the National Assembly, 1871–5)*
JOCD	*Journal officiel de la république française, débats, chambre*
JOCD, doc. parl.	*Journal officiel de la république française, documents, chambre*
JOS	*Journal officiel de la république française, débats, sénat*

The place of publication for all French works that are cited is Paris, unless otherwise indicated. Translations from French sources are my own.

INTRODUCTION

1 *AN, Programmes électoraux*, C5506, 1889 (Finistère).

2 *Le Concours médical*, 21 August 1897.

3 *L'Union médicale*, 30 September 1871.

4 See George Rosen, *From Medical Police to Social Medicine: Essays on the History of Health Care* (New York: Science History Publications, 1974), p. 2; Paul Starr, *The Social Transformation of American Medicine* (New York: Basic Books, 1982), p. 4; and John Woodward and David Richards, eds., *Health Care and Popular Medicine in Nineteenth Century England: Essays in the Social History of Medicine* (New York: Holmes and Meier, 1977), pp. 15–55.

5 The census of 1891 divided the judicial professions into *avocats* and *agréés* (7,472); magistrates (8,559); *officiers ministériels*, including *notaires, avoués*, and *huissiers* (18,450); and *agents d'affaires* (6,214). The total number of architects and civil engineers was 12,490. Primary and secondary teachers numbered 143,526. See *Annuaire statistique de la France*, 1892–93–94, p. 19.

6 Yves-Henri Gaudemet, *Les Juristes et la vie politique de la IIIe république* (Presses universitaires de France, 1970), p. 11. Gaudemet provides a detailed breakdown of the numbers, region of representation, and political affiliations of jurists (including *avocats, avoués*, and notaries) in the Chambers of 1881, 1906, 1924, and 1936.

7 Erwin H. Ackerknecht, "Paul Bert's Triumph," in Henry E. Sigerist, ed., *Essays in the History of Medicine* (Baltimore: Johns Hopkins University Press, 1944), pp. 16–31.

8 William A. Glaser, "Doctors and Politics," *American Journal of Sociology* 66 (November 1960): 230–45.

9 I have used a variety of sources in determining medicopolitical representation outside France. Professor Ackerknecht provided me with copies of three unpublished essays on doctors as statesmen and politicians before, during, and after

the eighteenth century. Further information (on England, Italy, Spain, Belgium, and Germany) was taken from Louis Picard's "Les Médecins dans l'état: les médecins parlementaires," *La Gazette médicale de Paris,* 11 January, 22 February, 1 March, 3 March, 12 April, and 19 April 1902; and from the survey published on 3 June 1905 by the *British Medical Journal* ("The Medical Profession Abroad, in Its Educational, Social, and Economic Aspects"), which focuses on France, Germany, Austria, Hungary, Italy, Spain, Portugal, Belgium, Serbia, Romania, Canada, South Africa, and New Zealand; additional details are available in the issues of 30 June and 10 December 1904; 14 January, 4 and 18 March, 22 April, 12 and 19 August, 4 November, and 9 December 1905. On the doctor-politician in Latin America, see Aristides A. Moll, *Aesculapius in Latin America* (New York: Argosy-Antiquarian, 1969), pp. 383–400. On prerevolutionary Russia, see Nancy Mandelker Frieden, *Russian Physicians in an Era of Reform and Revolution, 1856–1905* (Princeton, NJ: Princeton University Press, 1981), especially pp. 77–104 and 179–99.

10   William Coleman, "Health and Hygiene in the *Encylopédie:* A Medical Doctrine for the Bourgeoisie," *Journal of the History of Medicine and Allied Sciences* 24 (October 1974): 399–421. See also Martin S. Staum, *Cabanis: Enlightenment and Medical Philosophy in the French Revolution* (Princeton, NJ: Princeton University Press, 1980), pp. 119–21 and 161–4; Louis S. Greenbaum, " 'Measure of Civilization': The Hospital Thought of Jacques Tenon on the Eve of the French Revolution," *Bulletin of the History of Medicine* 49 (Spring 1975): 43–56; and Caroline C. Hannaway, "Medicine, Public Welfare and the State in Eighteenth Century France: The Société Royale de Médecine de Paris (1776–1793)" (Ph.D. diss., Johns Hopkins University, 1974), especially pp. 146–227 on the investigation of disease.

11   Dominique Lorillot, "1789: Les Médecins ont la parole," *Historical Reflections/ Réflexions historiques* 9 (1980): 103–29

12   Information on the medical men in these assemblies can be found in Constant Saucerotte, *Les Médecins pendant la révolution, 1789–99* (Périn, 1887), and especially in the more accurate series of articles by Miquel-Dalton, "Les Médecins dans l'histoire de la révolution," which ran in *La Chronique médicale* between 15 October 1901 and 15 September 1904. See also Louis Picard, "Les Médecins dans l'état: les médecins parlementaires," *La Gazette médicale de Paris,* 22 February and 1 March 1902, which contains an alphabetical listing of all medical men in the legislatures of France after 1789.

13   See George Rosen, "Hospitals, Medical Care and Social Policy in the French Revolution," *Bulletin of the History of Medicine* 30 (March–April 1956): 124–44; Dora B. Weiner, "Le Droit de l'homme à la santé – une belle idée devant l'assemblée constituante: 1790–91," *Clio Medica* 5 (September 1970): 209–23; and Toby Gelfand, "Medical Professionals and Charlatans. The Comité de Salubrité of 1790–91," *Histoire sociale/Social History* 11 (May 1978): 62–97. More information can be found in David Vess, *Medical Revolution in France, 1789–1796* (Gainseville: University Presses of Florida, 1975), particularly chap. 1.

14   André-Jean Tudesq, *Les Conseillers généraux en France au temps de Guizot, 1840–1848* (Armand Colin, 1967), pp. 112–13, 123–4, 157. On the financial status and political participation of doctors in Paris, see Adeline Daumard, *La Bourgeoisie parisienne de 1815 à 1848* (Ecole pratique des hautes études, 1963), pp. 32, 38, 79, 126.

15   Jean Maitron, *Dictionnaire biographique du mouvement ouvrier français,* vols. 1–3: *1789–1864. De la Révolution française à la fondation de la première internationale* (Les Editions ouvrières, 1964–6); vols. 4–9: *1864–1871. De la Fondation de la première internationale à la commune* (Les Editions ouvrières, 1967–71); and vols. 10–15: *1871–1914. De la Commune à la grande guerre* (Les Editions ouvrières, 1973–7).

16   The idea that the lower social orders had to be educated and socialized according to bourgeois notions of health if the doctor's status were to rise is stressed by

Terence D. Murphy in "The French Medical Profession's Perception of Its Social Function Between 1776 and 1830," *Medical History* 23 (1979): 259–73.

17 *De L'Intervention du corps médical dans la situation actuelle; programme de médecine sociale* (Fain et Thunot, 1848), pp. 4–8.

18 See the doctors' election manifestos in Charles Boutin, ed., *Les Murailles révolutionnaires de 1848* (E. Picard, n.d.), especially vol. 1, pp. 444, 463, 477–9, and vol. 2, pp. 91–2, 103, 122, 153–5, 175–6, 184–5, 212–15, 232, 327–8, 390. On the role of doctors in 1848, see Pierre Astruc, "1848 et le médecin," *Le Progrès médical*, 24 June and 10 July 1946.

19 Statistics on the repression of 1851 can be found in Maurice Agulhon, *1848 ou l'apprentissage de la république 1848–1852* (Editions du Seuil, 1973), pp. 235–7.

20 Louis Girard, A. Prost, and R. Gossez, *Les Conseillers généraux en 1870. Etude statistique d'une personnel politique* (Presses universitaires de France, 1967), pp. 63, 194–7.

21 The revolt of Paris against the authority of the National Assembly led most of those in the capital to withdraw from public affairs. Among those who stayed to the bitter end were Edouard Vaillant, who sat on the Commune's executive committee; François Parisel, who directed its scientific activities; and Paul Rastoul, who became inspector general of ambulances. Further information can be found in Jules Clère, *Les Hommes de la commune* (E. Dentu, 1871); and in *La Chronique médicale*, 1 April 1897, 1 December 1899, and 15 June 1900.

22 Theodore Zeldin, *France 1848–1945*, vol. 1: *Ambition, Love and Politics* (London: Oxford University Press, 1973), pp. 23, 571–604. Jacqueline Pincemin and Alain Laughier have made similar points in "Les Médecins," *Revue française de science politique* 9 (December 1959): 881–900. See also Erwin H. Ackerknecht, "Hygiene in France, 1815–1848," *Bulletin of the History of Medicine* 22 (March–April 1948): 117–55, and *Medicine at the Paris Hospital 1794–1848* (Baltimore: Johns Hopkins University Press, 1967), especially pp. 149–56 and 183–6. The views of contemporaries are reflected in Petre Trisca's *Les Médecins sociologues et hommes d'état* (Félix Alcan, 1923).

23 Quoted in Ackerknecht, *Medicine at the Paris Hospital*, p. 154.

24 Glaser, "Doctors and Politics." See also S. M. Lipset and Mildred A. Schwartz, "The Politics of Professionals," in Howard M. Vollmer and Donald L. Mills, eds., *Professionalization* (Englewood Cliffs, NJ: Prentice-Hall, 1966), pp. 299–310.

25 Christophe Charle, *Les Hauts fonctionnaires en France au XIXe siècle* (Editions Gallimard/Julliard, 1980), pp. 110–11.

26 Thomas R. Osborne, *A Grand Ecole for the Grands Corps: The Recruitment and Training of the French Administrative Elite in the Nineteenth Century* (New York: Social Science Monographs, 1983), pp. 91–103; and Terry Shinn, *Savoir scientifique et pouvoir social: l'école polytechnique, 1794–1914* (Presses de la fondation nationale des sciences polytechniques, 1980), pp. 52–7.

27 *Le Concours médical*, 25 December 1880.

28 Ernest Greenwood summarizes these as a systematic body of theory, professional authority, community sanction, a regulative code of conduct, and a professional culture. See his "Attributes of a Profession," in Vollmer and Mills, eds., *Professionalization*, pp. 10–19.

29 Philip Elliot notes that "it is only a slight exaggeration to argue that a professional will come closer to centres of power and authority the more he relinquishes his specific professional function." *The Sociology of the Professions* (New York: Herder and Herder, 1972), p. 149.

30 See Malcolm G. Taylor, "The Role of the Medical Profession in the Formulation and Execution of Public Policy," *Canadian Journal of Economics and Political Science* 26 (February 1960): 108–27. See also Dietrich Rueschemeyer, "Doctors and Lawyers: A Comment on the Theory of the Professions," in Eliot Freidson and Judith Lorber, eds., *Medical Men and Their Work* (Chicago: Aldine Atherton, 1972), pp. 5–19; and Elliot, *The Sociology of the Professions*, p. 145.

31 In addition to the work of Christophe Charle, Terry Shinn, and Thomas R. Osborne, cited earlier, see Jeanne Siwek-Pouydesseau, *Le Corps préfectoral sous la troisième et la quatrième république* (Armand Colin, 1969); Ezra N. Suleiman, *Politics, Power and Bureaucracy in France: The Administrative Elite* (Princeton, NJ: Princeton University Press, 1974; Guy Thuillier, *Bureaucratie et bureaucrates en France au XIX* siècle (Geneva: Droz, 1980); and Jolyon Howorth and Philip G. Cerny, eds., *Elites in France: Origins, Reproduction and Power* (London: Frances Pinter, 1981). For a more complete bibliography, see Centre national de la recherche scientifique, Institut d'histoire moderne et contemporaine, *Prosopographie des élites (XVI*–*XX* siècles). Guide de recherche* (1980).

32 Gerald L. Geison, ed., *Professions and the French State, 1700–1900* (Philadelphia: University of Pennsylvania Press, 1984), pp. 1–4. See also George Weisz, *The Emergence of Modern Universities in France, 1863–1914* (Princeton, NJ: Princeton University Press, 1983); and Patrick J. Harrigan, *Mobility, Elites, and Education in French Society of the Second Empire* (Waterloo, Ontario: Wilfrid Laurier University Press, 1980).

33 Thomas D. Beck, *French Legislators, 1800–1834: A Study in Quantitative History* (Berkeley and Los Angeles: University of California Press, 1974); Patrick-Bernard Higonnet, "La Composition de la Chambre des Députés de 1827 à 1831," *Revue historique* 239 (April–June 1968): 351–78; and Patrick L. R. Higonnet and Trevor B. Higonnet, "Class, Corruption, and Politics in the French Chamber of Deputies," *French Historical Studies* 5 (Fall 1967): 104–24. For departmental assemblies, see Tudesq, *Les Conseillers généraux en France;* and Girard, Prost, and Gossez, *Les Conseillers généraux en 1870.*

34 "Political Ascent in a Class Society: French Deputies 1870–1958," in Dwaine Marvick, ed., *Political Decision-Makers* (Glencoe, NY: Free Press, 1961), pp. 57–90; "Les Filières de la carrière politique," *Revue française de science politique* 8 (October–December 1967): 468–92; and "La Stabilité du personnel parlementaire sous la troisième république," *Revue française de science politique* 3 (April–June 1953): 319–47. Another useful work is the unpublished study by Michel Bisault, "La Composition socio-professionnelle de la chambre des députés de la IIIᵉᵐᵉ république" (thesis for the diplôme de science politique de la faculté de droit de Paris, 1960), which concentrates on the legislatures of 1876, 1898, 1919, and 1936. A good overview can be found in Jean Charlot, "Les Elites politiques en France de la IIIᵉ à la Vᵉ république," *Archives européenes de sociologie* 14 (1973): 78–92. A popular treatment can be found in Pierre Guiral and Guy Thuillier, *La Vie quotidienne des députés en France de 1871 à 1914* (Hachette, 1980).

35 *Les Ministres de la république, 1871–1914* (Presses de la fondation nationale des sciences politiques, 1982).

36 Jeanne L. Brand, *Doctors and the State: The British Medical Profession and Government Action in Public Health, 1870–1912* (Baltimore: Johns Hopkins University Press, 1965), p. vi.

37 Jacques Léonard, "Les Médecins de l'ouest au XIXᵉᵐᵉ siècle. Thèse presentée devant l'université de Paris IV le 10 janvier 1976." 3 vols. (Lille: Atelier reproduction des thèses, université de Lille III; Diffusion, Paris: Honoré Champion, 1978), especially part 4 of vol. 3, pp. 1127–1452, which deals with the attitudes of doctors in the western departments toward hygiene, politics, religion, the courts, and public education. Table 18 in the appendix of the same volume provides the names and departments of all physician–legislators between 1814 and 1893. Subsequent published works by Léonard, based largely on this study, include *La Médecine entre les savoirs et les pouvoirs* (Mayenne: L'Imprimerie Floch, 1981); *La Vie quotidienne du médecin de province au XIXᵉ siècle* (Hachette, 1977); *La France médicale au XIXᵉ siècle* (Editions Gallimard/Julliard, 1978), which consists primarily of documents; and numerous articles. Of the latter, see "Les Etudes médicales en France entre 1815 et 1848," *Revue d'histoire moderne et contemporaine* 13 (January–March 1966): 87–94, and "Les Femmes, religion et médecine. Les Religieuses qui soignent, en France au XIXᵉ siècle," *Annales. Economies. Sociétés. Civilisations* (September–October 1977): 887–907.

38 See "The Politics of Medical Professionalization in France 1845–1848," *Journal of Social History* 12 (Fall 1978): 3–30; "Reform and Conflict in French Medical Education, 1870–1914," in Robert Fox and George Weisz, eds., *The Organization of Science and Technology in France 1808–1914* (Cambridge, England: Cambridge University Press, 1980), pp. 61–84; "Construction of the Medical Elite in France: The Creation of the Royal Academy of Medicine 1814–20," *Medical History* 30 (1986): 419–43; and "The Medical Elite in France in the Early Nineteenth Century," *Minerva* 25 (Spring–Summer 1987): 150–70.

39 See George D. Sussman, "The Glut of Doctors in Mid-Nineteenth-Century France," *Comparative Studies in Society and History* 19 (July 1977): 287–304; "Enlightened Health Reform, Professional Medicine and Traditional Society: The Cantonal Physicians of the Bas-Rhin," *Bulletin of the History of Medicine* 51 (1977): 565–70; and "Etienne Pariset: A Medical Career in Government Under the Restoration," *Journal of the History of Medicine* 26 (1971): 52–75. See also William Coleman, *Death Is a Social Disease: Public Health and Political Economy in Early Industrial France* (Madison: University of Wisconsin Press, 1982); Matthew Ramsey, "Medical Power and Popular Medicine; Illegal Healers in 19th Century France," *Journal of Social History* 10 (Summer 1977): 560–87, and his *Professional and Popular Medicine in France, 1770–1830: The Social World of Medical Practice* (Cambridge, England: Cambridge University Press, 1988); Robert Nye, *Crime, Madness and Politics in Modern France: The Medical Concept of National Decline* (Princeton, NJ: Princeton University Press, 1984); and Toby Gelfand, *Professionalizing Modern Medicine: Paris Surgeons and Institutions in the 18th Century* (Westport, CT: Greenwood Press, 1980).

40 *Doctors, Bureaucrats and Public Health in France 1888–1902* (New York: Garland Press, 1987).

41 Adolphe Robert and Gaston Cougny, *Dictionnaire des parlementaires français, 1789–1899* (Bourloton, 1891); and Jean Jolly, ed., *Dictionnaire des parlementaires français; notices biographiques sur les ministres, sénateurs et députés français de 1889 à 1940* (Presses universitaires de France, 1960–77). On individual legislatures, see Jules Clère, *Biographie des députés avec leurs principaux votes, depuis le 8 février 1871 jusqu'au 15 juin 1875* (Garnier frères, 1875), along with his *Biographie des députés* (Garnier frères, 1880); Alphonse Bertrand, *La Chambre de 1889* (L. Michaud, 1889), plus additional books by Bertrand on the Chambers of 1893 and 1898 and the Senate of 1894; A. S. Grenier, *Nos sénateurs* (E. Flammarion, 1899), and *Nos députés, 1893–1898* (Berger–Levrault, 1898–1902), plus others on the legislatures of 1898 and 1902; and René Samuel and Georges Bonet-Maury, *Les Parlementaires français (1900–1914)*, 2 vols. (G. Rouston, 1914).

CHAPTER 1. THE SOCIAL FORMATION OF THE PHYSICIAN-LEGISLATORS

1 In Table 1.1 (and in others throughout the book) I have adopted the regional organization of departments used by Jacques Gouault in *Comment la France est devenue républicaine: les élections générales et partielles a l'assemblée nationale 1870–1875* (Armand Colin, 1954), pp. 77–101. In cases in which it has been useful to define a general region by reference to its provinces, I have followed George D. Sussman's idea of using the "natural regions" described by the French historian Charles Pouthas. These can be found in George D. Sussman, "The Glut of Doctors in Mid-Nineteenth-Century France," *Comparative Studies in Society and History* 19 (July 1977): 287–304.

2 André Jardin and André-Jean Tudesq, *La France des notables*, vol. 2: *La Vie de la nation, 1815–1848* (Editions du Seuil, 1973), pp. 63–66 and 114–15.

3 Many of these were "without wealth and probably without clientele." See Adeline Daumard, *La Bourgeoisie parisienne de 1815 à 1848* (Ecole pratique des hautes études, 1963), p. 126.

4 For a discussion of this point, see Toby Gelfand's "Public Medicine and Medical

Table N1.1. *Regional proportion of medical students and doctors, 1866*

Region	Medical students enrolled in one of the three faculties (%)	Medical doctors (%)
North	8.1	5.0
East	15.7	11.9
Paris region and Center	21.3	24.5
West	17.2	17.3
Southwest	15.5	14.6
Massif Central	7.5	7.2
Lyon region, Savoy, and Dauphiné	5.6	8.3
Mediterranean region	8.4	11.1

Careers in France During the Reign of Louis XV," In Andrew W. Russell, ed., *The Town and State Physician in Europe from the Middle Ages to the Enlightenment* (Wolfenbuttel: Herzog August Bibliothek, 1981), pp. 99–122. Gelfand notes the high proportion of medical professionals originating in the Midi during the eighteenth century, and his survey of the origins of students at the Paris College of Surgery shows high proportions coming from the southwest. See also Jacques Léonard, *La Vie quotidienne du médecin de province au XIXe siècle* (Hachette, 1977), pp. 47–51.

5 In the 1840s the medical corps in the department of the Nord was composed of 39% doctors and 61% health officers. In Pas-de-Calais, the respective figures were 26% and 74%. The national average was 60% doctors and 40% health officers. See Sussman, "The Glut of Doctors."

6 Patrick J. Harrigan, *Mobility, Elites, and Education in French Society of the Second Empire* (Waterloo, Ontario: Wilfrid Laurier University Press, 1980), pp. 41–42 and 50–51.

7 Extracting the regional proportions of medical students and physicians for 1866 from Paul Bert's *Rapport sur la création de nouvelles facultés de médecine, presenté à l'assemblée nationale* (Librairie Ch. Delagrave, 1874) yields the percentages shown in Table N1.1.

8 In grouping these occupations, I have used some of Harrigan's categories in *Mobility, Elites, and Education*, pp. 8–9.

9 Ibid., pp. 11–12.

10 Jean Martet, *M. Clemenceau peint par lui-même* (Albin Michel, 1929), pp. 189–90.

11 Examples in which the practice of medicine went back at least two generations included the families of Gabriel Maunoury of Eure-et-Loire; Auguste Baudon of Oise; Clemenceau of the Vendée; Achille Coillot of Haute-Saône; Pierre Even of Côtes-du-Nord; Mathurin Legal-Lasalle of Côtes-du-Nord; and Adolphe Pedebidou of Hautes-Pyrénées.

12 Combes's father, a weaver at Roquecourbe in the Tarn, made barely enough money to support a family of ten children. See the introduction by Maurice Dorre in Emile Combes's *Mon Ministère, memoires 1902–1905* (Plon, 1956), pp. i–xv.

13 These figures are taken from George Weisz, *The Emergence of Modern Universities in France, 1863–1914* (Princeton, NJ: Princeton University Press, 1983), p. 24.

14 Ibid. See also Christophe Charle, *Les Hauts fonctionnaires en France au XIXe siècle* (Editions Gallimard/Julliard, 1980), p. 28; and Terry Shinn, *Savoir scientifique et pouvoir social: l'école polytechnique, 1794–1914* (Presses de la fondation nationale des sciences polytechniques, 1980), pp. 65–80.

15 Jean Estèbe, *Les Ministres de la république, 1871–1914* (Presses de la fondation nationale des sciences politique, 1982), pp. 20–27.
16 *JOS*, 8 March 1892, pp. 217–30.
17 On the cost of medical education, see Jacques Léonard, "Les Etudes médicales en France entre 1815 et 1848," *Revue d'histoire moderne et contemporaine* 13 (January–March 1966): 87–94; along with his "Les Médecins de l'ouest au XIXème siècle" (thesis, University of Paris, 1976), vol. 2, pp. 638–46; and his *La Vie quotidienne du médecin de province*, pp. 22–29. Bert's estimates can be found in *JO, assemb. nat.*, 18 May 1874, pp. 3333–36; and Richet's in "La Médecine, les médecins et les facultés de médecine," *Revue des deux mondes* 45 (1 June 1908): 641–75.
18 Weisz, *Emergence of Modern Universities in France*, pp. 24–25.
19 In a speech to the Senate in 1894, Dr. Labbé indicated that the average age of medical students on leaving the *lycée* was between 18.5 and 19. *JOS*, 9 May 1894, pp. 355–69. According to Harrigan, *Mobility, Elites, and Education in French Society*, p. 75, the proportion of *lycée* graduates among medical students during the 1860s was around 59%.
20 Edouard Charton, *Dictionnaire des professions ou guide pour le choix d'un état* (Hachette, 1880), p. 343.
21 *Le Concours médical*, 10 March 1900.
22 Paul Bert of Yonne, Léopold Dasque of Hautes-Pyrénées, Charles Delarue of Allier, and Louis Devins of Haute-Loire. Dasque, who came from a landed family at Tarbes, returned home to practice both professions.
23 Letter from Dean Wurtz to the rector, dated 29 November 1869, in Naquet file, faculty dossiers, archives of Faculty of Medicine of Paris.
24 *Le Concours médical*, 9 December 1893. Henri Ricard, physician-senator for Côte-d'Or, likened agriculture to medicine, in that both joined theory to practice and had as their prime goals the maintenance of life. Emile Rey, physician-deputy of Lot, argued that agriculture was the most difficult of the sciences and required the broadest knowledge of all fields, from chemistry and botany to physics and mathematics. *JOS*, 13 April 1905, pp. 1304–6, and 27 December 1907, pp. 751–6. See also "L'Agriculture et la médecine," *L'Union médicale*, 22 June 1869.
25 Combes, *Mon ministère*, pp. 32–44.
26 The schools at Lillie, Lyon, and Bordeaux became "mixed" faculties of medicine and pharmacy during the 1870s, followed by those at Toulouse (1890) and Algiers (1909). Another innovation was the Ecoles de plein exercice de médecine et de pharmacie, which offered a full program of instruction but awarded no doctoral degree. These were established at Marseille (1875), Nantes (1876), and Rennes (1895).
27 According to Bouisson, vitalism incorporated *"les idées spiritualistes"* of medicine and, unlike Paris teaching, was consistent with religious faith. See his comments in *JO, assemb. nat.* 29 March 1873, pp. 2193–94; 26 June 1874, pp. 4348–50; and 8 December 1874, pp. 8088–95.
28 The socialist Siméon Flaissières had worked as an intern in the preparatory school of Avignon, where he observed the effects of typhoid. Paulin Dupuy, later deputy for Tarn-et-Garonne, had similar experiences at Alger studying malaria. See Flaissières, *De Quelques genres de mort dans la fièvre typhoide* (Montpellier: Imprimerie centrale du midi, 1877); and Dupuy, *Essai sur quelques troubles d'origine paludéenne dans les fonctions génitales de la femme* (Montpellier: Imprimerie centrale du midi, 1879).
29 *JOS*, 9 May 1894, pp. 355–69.
30 *JO, assemb. nat.*, 19 May 1874, pp. 3362–65.
31 *JOS*, 9 May 1894, pp. 355–69.
32 After examining the statistics for the period between 1830 and 1892, the surgeon and deputy Odilon Lannelongue concluded that most students entered medical school between the ages of nineteen and twenty and finished between twenty-six and twenty-seven. *JOCD*, 18 June 1895, pp. 1746–56.
33 *JO, assemb. nat.*, 17 December 1871, pp. 5041–42.
34 Bourneville's own thesis was a study of temperatures of stroke victims. See his

obituary on Charcot in *Le Progrès médical*, 26 August 1893, and the obituary for Bourneville in *Le Progrès médical*, 5 June 1909.

35 See the *éloge* for Maunoury in *BAM* 95 (Masson, 1926), pp. 58–63; for Pozzi in *BAM* 79 (Masson, 1918), pp. 448–52; and for Monprofit, *BAM* 90 (Masson, 1923), pp. 262–5

36 *Le Progrès médical*, 29 October 1904.

37 See Table E in Bert's *Rapport sur la création de nouvelles facultés de médecine*, p. 143, and his comments in *JO, assemb. nat.*, 18 May 1874, pp. 3333–36.

38 O.-M. Lannelongue, *Un Tour du monde (October 1908–July 1909)* (Larousse, 1910), pp. 207–9.

39 *Du Hachisch, étude clinique, physiologique et thérapeutique* (Imprimerie Simon Raçon, 1872).

40 *La Chronique médicale*, 1 November 1906.

41 *Le Temps*, 28 May 1868. See Owsei Temkin, "The Philosophical Background of Magendie's Physiology," *Bulletin of the History of Medicine* 20 (June 1946) 10–35; and his "Materialism in French and German Physiology of the Early Nineteenth Century," *Bulletin of the History of Medicine* 20 (July 1946): 322–7. See also George Rosen, "The Philosophy of Ideology and the Emergence of Modern Medicine in France," *Bulletin of the History of Medicine* 20 (July 1946): 328–39.

42 The petition bore the signatures of two thousand political and religious leaders from across the country. The full debates are in *Le Moniteur* of 1868, 28 March, pp. 455–6; 20 May, pp. 689–91; 21 May, pp. 701–4; 22 May, p. 709; 23 May, p. 712; and 24 May, pp. 718–21.

43 *Le Mouvement médical*, 12 July 1868.

44 The professors who actually directed the greatest number were Léon Gosselin (7.5%), Auguste Tardieu (6.3%), Alfred Vulpian (5.0%), and Louis-Jules Béhier (4.4%). Apollinaire Bouchardet and Alfred Richet were tied at 3.7%, and Benjamin Ball, Jean-Baptiste Bouillaud, Paul Broca, Paul Brouardel, Jean Depaul, Louis Gavarret, and Aristide Verneuil had 3.1% each.

45 By denying the need for anterior life in the creation of new life, Clemenceau was able to dispense with the necessity for an original creator. He also denied the physiological possibility of a human soul. See *De la Génération des éléments anatomiques* (J. B. Baillière, 1865), pp. 104–9, 221.

46 *Essai sur l'histoire philosophique de la médecine dans l'antiquité* (Bonaventure et Decessois, 1865); and *Du Merveilleux en médecine* (A. Parent, 1869).

47 *Le Progrès médical*, 12 March 1904; and *JOS*, 9 May 1894, pp. 355–69.

48 *JOS*, 18 March 1892, pp. 225–8.

49 T.-B. Paul Lacombe, *De la Méningo-encéphalite tuberculeuse des enfants* (Rignoux, 1860), p. 1; and Pierre-Yves Even, *Etude médicale sur Edmond et Jules de Goncourt* (Bibliothèque cooperative, 1908), p. 83.

50 P.-G.-Ernest Delbet, *Des Vomissements opiniâtres pendant la grossesse; des indications qu'ils presentent, et spécialement de l'avortement provoqué* (Rignoux, 1854).

51 Gustave Gauthier, *Deux années de pratique médicale à Canton (Chine)* (A. Parent, 1863), pp. 16–17, 24. Le Borgne's thesis was entitled *Géographie médicale de l'archipel des iles Gambier (Océanie)* (A. Parent, 1872).

52 *Considérations contre l'hérédité des maladies* (A. Parent, 1868), p. 6.

53 C. Ducher, *Parallèle du typhus et de la fièvre typhoïde* (Rignoux, 1858), pp. 29–30; Paul-L.-H. Frézoul, *Des Vaccinations précoces et de la syphilis vaccinale* (Rignoux, 1862); and Louis Charles Aimé Dubuisson, *Des Effets de l'introduction dans l'économie des produits septiques et tuberculeux* (A. Parent, 1869).

54 Achille Testelin, *Un Mot sur la grippe épidémique de 1837* (Rignoux, 1837), pp. 19–20; Alexis Chavanne, *Relation d'une épidémie de diphthérite gangréneuse des parties génitales, survenu chez des nouvelles accouchées à l'hôspice de la Charité de Lyon, en 1850* (Rignoux, 1851), pp. 30–31; Casimir-Laurent Michou, *De la Congestion pulmonaire dans la fièvre typhoïde, principalement du point de vue du traitement* (Rignoux, 1860), p. 8; Joseph-Nelson Soye, *Des Ulcérations du col de l'utérus* (Rignoux, 1851); and Maximilien Lesage, *De la Scarlatine chez les femmes en couches* (A. Parent, 1877).

55 Joseph-Prosper André, *Essai sur l'hémorrhagie cérébrale (apoplexie)* (Rignoux, 1853), p. 28; Paul Bourgeois, *Considérations physiologiques et thérapeutiques sur l'abstinence et l'alimentation dans les maladies* (Rignoux, 1853), p. 6; and Emile Rey, *L'Exercice musculaire dans ses applications à la médecine* (Rignoux, 1862), pp. 35, 39.

56 H. G. Martin, *De la Circoncision, avec un nouvel appareil inventé par l'auteur* (A. Parent, 1870), p. 37.

57 *Le Progrès médical*, 5 November 1881.

58 François-C. de Mahy, *Essai sur les lésions traumatiques que la femme peut éprouver pendant l'accouchement* (Rignoux, 1855). p. 5.

59 An example is the thesis by Antoine Mas, which attributed miscarriages to such "predisposing causes" as temperament and "an exaggerated nervous sensibility." See his *Du Traitement de l'avortement* (Rignoux, 1856), p. 8. Similar themes appear in Henri Ricard, *Etude sur les troubles de la sensibilité génésique à l'époque de la ménopause* (Alphonse Derenne, 1879); and François-Charles Bachimont, *Documents pour servir à l'histoire de la puériculture intra-utérine* (G. Steinhall, 1898).

60 Charles-Louis Le Bretton, *Considérations sur l'hygiène des enfans pendant l'allaitement* (Didot le Jeune, 1834), p. 7; Jean-Zacharie-Albert Garrigat, *Considérations pratiques sur l'alimentation, les vêtements, la gymnastique de l'enfance* (A. Parent, 1864), pp. 7, 21, 32; and that of his father, Elie-Armand Garrigat, *Considérations générales sur les avantages de l'allaitement étranger pour les enfans nés dans les classes élevées de la société* (Didot le Jeune, 1829), pp. 5–6, 9. See also Louis Laussedat, *Considérations sur les avantages de l'allaitement maternel* (Didot le Jeune, 1832), pp. 5–6, which argues that nature imposed breast feeding on the mother.

61 Maurice Bourrillon, *Etude sur quelques causes de diarrhée et de vomissements chez les enfants du premier âge* (A. Parent, 1879), pp. 2, 12–13, 21–24.

62 Lucien Guillemaut, *Considérations sur l'angine couenneuse ou diphthérique d'après une épidémie observée à Louhans* (A. Parent, 1866), pp. 8–15.

63 *JOS*, 14 March 1893, pp. 278–90.

64 *Le Mouvement médical*, 21 February 1869.

65 Paul Brouardel, *La Profession médicale au commencement du XXᵉ siècle* (J.-B. Baillière, 1903), p. 56. See also Erwin H. Ackerknecht, *Medicine at the Paris Hospital, 1794–1848* (Baltimore: Johns Hopkins University Press, 1967), pp. 15–22; and Jules Rochard, *Traité d'hygiène sociale* (Adrien Delahaye et Emile Lecrosnier, 1888), pp. 152–61.

66 Especially to the dominance of moldy corn in their diet. See Roussel's thesis, *De la Pellagre* (Rignoux, 1845), as well as Daphne A. Roe's *A Plague of Corn: The Social History of Pellagra* (Ithaca, NY: Cornell University Press, 1973), pp. 33–36, 52–54, 66–68.

67 *Etude sur le tremblement saturnin* (Adrien Delahaye, 1869), pp. 8, 17.

68 *De l'Alimentation des nouveau-nés et du rachitisme* (A. Parent, 1871), pp. 2, 10–11, 14, 16, 20–26.

69 *Le Concours médical*, 11 January 1890.

CHAPTER 2. EARLY MEDICAL CAREERS

1 *JOS*, 30 November 1904, p. 972.

2 *JO*, assem. nat., 8 December 1874, p. 8090.

3 Henry Bérenger, *Les Prolétaires intellectuels en France* (Editions de *La Revue*, 1901), p. 8.

4 Never managing to rise in the profession, he passed his life watching people die "from the great and incurable wound of poverty." See Blanchard Livingstone Rideout, "The Medical Practitioner in the French Novel 1850–1900" (Ph.D. diss., Cornell University, 1936), pp. 104–8.

5 Based on figures appearing in *Le Concours médical*, 10 November 1900. The proportion of physician-legislators living in large cities was as follows (in percentages): Paris (9.2), Marseille (1.6), Lille (1.1), Reims (0.8), Limoges (0.8), Angers (0.8), Montpellier (0.5), and Clérmont-Ferrand (0.5)

Table N2.1. *Income levels for doctors and lawyers in* conseils généraux *of 1870*

Doctors' incomes (francs)	(%)	Lawyers' incomes (francs)	(%)
Under 2,500	4.3	Under 2,500	3.5
2,500–5,000	20.9	2,500–5,000	8.7
5,000–10,000	36.5	5,000–10,000	26.3
10,000–15,000	15.5	10,000–15,000	18.8
15,000–20,000	7.5	15,000–20,000	12.0
20,000–30,000	8.0	20,000–30,000	15.6
30,000–50,000	3.7	30,000–50,000	7.8
50,000–100,000	2.1	50,000–100,000	5.5
Over 100,000	1.0	Over 100,000	1.4

Source: see note 8.

6 Only within the last few years, through a study of wills and inheritances, have French scholars begun to describe the range of bourgeois wealth during that era. Examples include the work of Adeline Daumard, *La Bourgeoisie parisienne de 1815 à 1848* (Ecole pratique des hautes études, 1963), and her *Les Fortunes françaises au XIXe siècle* (Mouton, 1973).

7 More than half had private fortunes of over 100,000 francs, and a third of over 1 million francs. See Jean Estèbe, *Les Ministres de la république, 1871–1914* (Presses de la fondation nationale des sciences politiques, 1982), pp. 150–1. See also Guy Thuillier's comments on the cost of seeking office in *La Vie quotidienne des députés en France de 1871 à 1914* (Hachette, 1980), pp. 71–73, 79–114.

8. Louis Girard, A. Prost, and R. Gossez, *Les Conseillers généraux en 1870. Etude statistique d'une personnel politique* (Presses universitaires de France, 1967), pp. 63, 194–7. Income levels (in francs) for doctors compared with those of lawyers are shown in Table N2.1.

9 *Le Progrès médical*, 6 August 1892 and 5 February 1898.

10 *JOCD*, 23 November 1906, p. 2630.

11 André Gorgues, *Les Elections législatives et sénatoriales en Indre et Loire de 1871 à 1879*. Memoire de maîtrise, université de Poitiers (Microeditions Hachette, 1969), pp. 141–50; and Pierre Barral, *Le Département de l'Isère sous la troisième république 1870–1940* (Armand Colin, 1962), p. 356.

12 Dr. Gabriel Maurange, *Livre de raison d'un médecin parisien 1865–1938* (Plon, 1938), pp. 104–6.

13 *La Chronique médicale*, 1 February 1910.

14 *JOCD*, 20 January 1909, p. 63. Emile Combes, whose practice at Pons grew "with an extraordinary rapidity," earned only three thousand francs during his first year. See *Mon ministère, memoires 1902–1905* (Plon, 1956), p. 42; and *La Chronique médicale*, 1 February 1905.

15 *Le Concours médical*, 9 July 1881. A total of 44% of the respondents indicated that their income from practice alone was too small to meet their expenses, and 58% claimed that it was insufficient to cover the cost of caring for their families.

16 Based on five hundred responses in its 1901 survey, *Le Concours médical* (7 September) estimated the incomes of doctors as shown in Table N2.2.

17 *L'Union médicale*, 13 January 1872.

18 See Estèbe, *Les Ministres de la république*, p. 161, for figures on the amounts brought by wives to the marriages of future cabinet ministers.

19 *Le Progrès médical*, 18 May 1889; *La Tribune médicale*, 5 May 1897; and *La Chronique médicale*, 1 July 1911.

20 See Lannelongue's dossier in *AN*, AJ^16 6499–6537, *Académie de Paris, dossiers de personnel*, no. 6514, as well as that for Robin (no. 6521) and Pozzi (no. 6519).

21 *Le Progrès médical*, 30 November 1895; and *La Presse médicale*, 27 December 1911.

Table N2.2. *Doctors' estimated incomes (by region) in 1901*

Region	Inscribed on books (francs)	Collected (francs)
North	12,100	10,000
East	9,500	8,000
Lyon region	9,400	7,800
Southeast	8,800	7,000
Parisian basin	14,000	11,600
Center	10,500	8,700
Massif Central	7,500	6,100
Normandy	13,000	11,300
Northeast	7,700	6,200
West	10,500	8,000
Southwest	6,600	5,100

Source: see note 16.

22 See Labbé's *éloge* in *BAM* 107 (Masson, 1932), pp. 1527–51. See also *La Chronique médicale*, 15 February 1903.
23 His most famous book, *Entre aveugles; conseils à l'usage des personnes qui viennent de perdre la vue* (Masson, 1903), provided advice to those who shared his fate. See the *éloges* in *BAM* 57 (Masson, 1907), pp. 141–4, and *BAM* 122 (Masson, 1939), pp. 531–9. See also the obituary in *Le Progrès médical*, 26 January 1907.
24 *Le Progrès médical*, 8 August 1900. See the biographies of Roussel in *Le Progrès médical*, 2 January 1897 and 3 October 1903 and the *éloge* in *BAM* 50 (Masson, 1903), pp. 119–23.
25 *Le Progrès médical*, 6 January 1906.
26 "All of you know me," he told the voters in 1906, "as the son of cultivators in the canton of Charroux, where I own agrarian and viticultural interests. I am interested in everything that concerns agriculture." AN, *Programmes électoraux*, C7416, 1906 (Vienne).
27 *Union médicale et scientifique du nord-est* 20 (15 October 1896): 312.
28 *Le Progrès médical*, 25 June 1887 and 18 November 1893.
29 Marcel Gillet, *Les Charbonnages du nord de la France au XIX siècle* (Mouton, 1973), pp. 99, 110, 158, 164, 193, 211. At least two others in our group had ties with northern industrial interests. Jules Leurent, deputy for the Nord between 1871 and 1877, owned spinning mills near Tourcoing. Henri Marmottan, a native of Valenciennes who later established himself in Paris, sat on the governing board of the Bruay Coal Company, of which his brother Jules was president.
30 Deputy to the Legislative Assembly, Testelin found himself powerless to stem the tide of reaction in 1851 and was forced to take refuge in Belgium, where he lived for eight years. See his obituary in *Le Progrès médical*, 29 August 1891, and the biographical sketch in Jean Maitron's *Dictionnaire biographique du mouvement ouvrier français*, vol. 9 (Les Editions ouvrières, 1971), pp. 184–5.
31 When Bert presented a report to the Chamber in 1883 favoring a pension for Pasteur, Emile Vernhes, who had practiced at Béziers since 1848, objected that Pasteur was not the only person to have served the country, that he himself had invented a measles vaccine in 1854. "You file our work away in boxes," he said, "and later, at the end of ten, fifteen and twenty years, you seize on the idea as if it belonged to you." *JOCD*, 13 July 1883, p. 1704.
32 9 July 1881 and 7 September 1901.
33 See his *profession de foi* in AN, *Programmes électoraux*, C7333–7335, 1902 (Puy-de-Dôme).
34 *Le Progrès médical*, scorning its bad taste, published the card on 29 March 1890. Its owner was unnamed, but the description could fit only Dr. Haynaut.

35 Dr. Gadaud, mayor of Périgieux, had been a railroad doctor for the Compagnie d'Orléans. Dr. Perréal, mayor of Béziers in Hérault, had worked as both a railroad doctor and a tax collector. Among those who had worked as physicians for insurance companies were Jean Peyrot, Félix Martin, and Victor Petitjean.

36 *AN, Programmes électoraux*, C5610, 1893 (Puy-de-Dôme).

37 *Le Concours médical*, 8 October 1911.

38 *Le Concours médical*, 5 October 1913, essay by Dr. Edouard Duchemin, "Souvenirs d'un médecin de campagne."

39 *Le Concours médical*, 25 July 1891.

40 *AN, Programmes électoraux*, C7416, 1906 (Cher).

41 *JOS*, 30 March 1905, p. 495.

42 Léon Sireyjol, a schoolteacher's son from rural Dordogne, described himself to voters in this way: "I belong to a very modest family of agriculturalists. My father is a native of Cognac, near Thiviers where he owns a little property; he lives at St-Priest-les Fongères in the canton of Jumilhac, where I was born. I myself live at St-Pardoux, and my family has interests at Abjat in the canton of Nontron." *AN, Programmes électoraux*, C7334, 1902 (Dordogne).

43 "In his functions as a doctor," *Le Sarthois illustré* wrote of his early days, "everyone learned to appreciate both the science of the practitioner and the inexhaustible charity of the man." *AN, Programmes électoraux*, C5422, 1885 (Sarthe).

44 These percentages are calculated on the basis of 294 known cases, or about 82% of the total. Information on the physician-legislators' AGMF activities comes from membership lists published in the *Annuaires* of the AGMF and from accounts of the association's meetings in the medical press.

45 In a report in 1876 (*L'Union médicale*, 2 and 4 May), Brouardel noted that although membership levels normally averaged around 50% of all doctors and health officers in a department, there were great variations. Allier had a rate of 92% for example, and Gers had only 13%. A breakdown by department can be found in the *Annuaire de l'association générale de prévoyance et de secours mutuels des médecins de France* (J.-B. Baillière, 1879).

46 Local presidents included Blatin (Puy-de-Dôme), Dufay (Loir-et-Cher), Souchu-Servinière (Mayenne), Mougeot (Haute-Marne), Dufraigne (Seine-et-Marne), Bourcy (Charente-Inférieure), and Turgis (Calvados).

47 The early history of the medical syndicates, with membership lists by department, can be found in *Le Concours médical*, 1 October 1881, 6 May 1882, 6 January and 25 August 1883, 28 June 1884, 18 July 1885, and 24 June 1906. Annual assemblies of the Civil Society were held jointly with those of the Union of Medical Syndicates of France, which Cézilly also founded in 1881. A list of members of the Civil Society, also by department, can be found in *Le Concours médical*, 11 December 1886.

48 *Le Concours médical*, 14 April 1888.

49 "Les Débuts dans la vie médicale," *Le Progrès médical*, 8 November 1902.

50 "Lettre à un jeune médecin," *L'Union médicale*, 9 January 1872.

51 *JOS*, 5 April 1892, pp. 368–80; and *Le Concours médical*, 24 August 1901.

52 A report to parliament in 1872 by two physician-deputies, Théophile Roussel and Auguste Morvan, concluded that it was "better to be operated on in the country by an ordinary surgeon than in a hospital of a large city by a prince of science." *JO, assemb. nat.*, 10 August 1872, pp. 5464–65.

53 Quoted by Charles Monod in *JOS*, 14 March 1893, pp. 278–90.

54 Letter from a Dr. Max to *Le Concours médical*, 22 May 1880. See also Matthew Ramsey's discussion of itinerants, empirics, and folk healers in *Professional and Popular Medicine in France, 1770–1830: The Social World of Medical Practice* (Cambridge, England: Cambridge University Press, 1988), pp. 129–276.

55 *JOCD*, 27 March 1910, p. 1683.

56 Alexandre Layet, *Hygiène et maladies des paysans, étude sur la vie matérielle des campagnards en Europe* (Masson, 1882), pp. 112–13, 354–65.

57 *JOS*, 21 December 1900, pp. 984–98.

58 *JOS*, 5 April 1892, pp. 368–80.

59 Report by Brouardel and du Mesnil in *Annales d'hygiène publique et de médecine légale* 20 (1888): 46–49.
60 *JOS*, 5 April 1886, pp. 536–9; and *JOCD*, 11 April 1895, p. 1305.
61 *Le Progrès médical*, 9 July 1881. In Paris, Bourneville helped create a publishing project known as the *Bibliothèque diabolique*, which examined reported cases of miracles, demonic possession, and other manifestations of the spirit world in light of modern science. *Le Progrès médical*, 5 March 1892.
62 *Le Concours médical*, 6 December 1879.
63 JOS, 19 March 1892, pp. 238–49.
64 Paul Parfait, *L'Arsenal de la dévotion* (Alcan-Lévy, 1877), pp. 1–12, 45–70, 113–40, 219–30, 275–92; and *Le Dossier des pèlerinages. Suite de l'arsenal de la dévotion*, 3rd ed. (Félix Alcan, 1877), pp. 138–86.
65 *Le Progrès médical*, 20 December 1890; and *Le Concours médical*, 2 May 1891.
66 *Le Concours médical*, 24 March 1883, 6 December 1879, and 22 June 1889; and *L'Union médicale*, 19 October 1872.
67 See Peinard Nöel Raynaud, *La Profession médicale en France* (Société d'éditions scientifiques, 1894), p. 43; and *Le Progrès médical*, 6 July 1895. See also Jacques Léonard, "Les Femmes, religion et médecine. Les Religieuses qui soignent, en France au XIXe siècle," *Annales. Economies. Sociétés. Civilisations* (September–October 1977): 887–907.
68 For examples of these allegations, see *Le Progrès médical*, 13 May 1876, 23 February 1878, 6 March 1881, 20 May 1882, 16 June 1883, 23 August 1884, 11 June 1887, and 28 April 1900.
69 *Le Progrès médical*, 21 May, 16 and 23 July 1887.
70 *Le Concours médical*, 21 November 1885, and the comments by Lourties and Turgis in *JOS*, 5 April 1892, pp. 368–80.
71 *Union médical et scientifique du nord-est* 7 (1882): 281–93; *JO, assemb. nat.*, 29 May 1872, pp. 3491–93; and *Le Concours médical*, 25 October 1908.
72 Léonard notes in this regard the parallel paths traveled by the movements for obligatory education and obligatory smallpox vaccination. See his *La France médicale au XIXe siècle* (Editions Gallimard/Julliard, 1978), pp. 25–30; and Bourneville's comments on public education in *Le Progrès médical*, 6 June 1874 and 22 November 1884.
73 *JO, assemb. nat.*, 8 December 1874, pp. 8088–95.
74 *JO, assemb. nat.*, 23 July 1874, pp. 5146–47.
75 Descriptions of this visit were published in Clemenceau's *La Justice*, 25, 28, 29, 30, and 31 July and 4 August, 1884.
76 *AN, Programmes électoraux*, C5420 1885 (Jura).
77 *La Chronique médicale*, 6 September 1870.
78 *AN, Programmes électoraux*, C5422, 1885 (Sarthe).
79 E.-A. Ancelon, *Manuel d'hygiène* (Nancy: Grimblot et veuve Raybois, 1852), pp. 8–9, 11–12, 16–39, 45–47, 94–98, 116, 154–5.
80 Dr. Lucien Guillemaut, *Histoire de la Bresse Louhannaise*, 2 vols. (Louhans: Auguste Roland, 1892).
81 See H. Doizy, "La 'Schistose' ou 'maladie des ardoisiers'," *Le Concours médical*, 1 October 1911.
82 *JOCD*, 25 February 1890, pp. 333–4.
83 *JOS*, 11 December 1912, pp. 1457–71.
84 Julien Noir, "L'Avenir de la profession médicale," *Le Progrès médical*, 9 November 1907. See also the comments by Dr. Aymard in *Le Concours médical*, 16 March 1901, and those by Dr. Courgey ("Le Médecin prêtre laïque") in *Le Concours médical*, 3 June 1905.
85 *Le Concours médical*, 5 December 1891.
86 *Le Progrès médical*, 16 December 1893; and *JOS*, 22 March 1892, pp. 252–65.
87 *JOCD*, 30 June 1901, pp. 1698–1700.
88 A writer for *Le Concours médical* on 8 October 1911 complained of certain doctors: "It's even worse if they're bitten by the tarantula of politics, for then they practice free of charge and overexert themselves in order to enhance their popularity."

89 *L'Union médicale*, 9 January 1872; and *La Chronique médicale*, 1 May 1896.
90 *Revue internationale des sciences biologiques* 1, no. 12 (1878): 382; and 1, no. 23 (1878): 766–77.
91 *Le Concours médical*, 23 July 1898.

CHAPTER 3. EARLY POLITICAL CAREERS

1 AN, *Programmes électoraux*, C7333–7335, 1902 (Lot-et-Garonne).
2 Dr. Gabriel Maurange, *Livre de raison d'un médecin parisien 1865–1938* (Plon, 1938), p. 104.
3 *Le Concours médical*, 17 April and 28 August 1910.
4 Dr. Ruelle, "La Médecine et la politique," reprinted in *Journal de médecine de Bordeaux*, 18 September 1898.
5 *Union médicale et scientifique du nord-est* 21, no. 21 (1897): 322–6.
6 AN, *Programmes électoraux*, C7334, 1902 (Savoie); C5513, 1889 (Dordogne and Cantal).
7 This compromise was incorporated into the Municipal Law of April 1884, but subsequent rulings by the Council of State rendered the issue more ambiguous than ever. Doctors argued that there was little comparison between themselves and civil servants, noting that lawyers and notaries often earned money performing services for local governments. After passage of the Medical Assistance Act of 1893, they could also argue that physicians who received pay for implementing its provisions had been explicitly ruled eligible for membership in the *conseils généraux*. Many thus did as they pleased. In 1901, parliament finally recognized the right of physicians who worked for public assistance to sit on the *conseils généraux*. See *JOS*, 23 February 1901, pp. 389–94; and *JOCD*, 30 June 1901, pp. 1698–1700.
8 Oliver H. Woshinsky, *The French Deputy: Incentives and Behavior in the National Assembly* (Lexington, MA: Heath, 1973). Another useful work, focusing on the backgrounds of 487 deputies elected in June 1968, is by Roland Cayrol, Jean-Luc Parodi, and Colette Ysmal, *Le Député français* (Armand Colin, 1973).
9 See the table in Woshinsky, *The French Deputy*, pp. 4–5, which ennumerates incentive types, the characteristics of each, and the countries in which they have been observed.
10 Ibid., pp. 81–96.
11 *Le Concours médical*, 26 October 1901.
12 Edouard Duchemin, "Souvenirs d'un médecin de campagne," *Le Concours médical*, 5 October 1913.
13 Quoted in Ruelle, "La Médecine et la politique."
14 *Le Progrès médical*, 8 November 1902.
15 *Le Concours médical*, 9 November 1901.
16 In 1904, the republican-dominated hospice commission at Cholet, in the Vendée, fired its chief physician, a Catholic, because he was president of a group that had opposed republicans during the last municipal elections. Four years later, a conservative at Manche, who for ten years had been physician to customs officials at Genets, was fired because his political attitudes had been judged "incompatible" with the job. See *Le Concours médical*, 8 October 1904 and 4 October 1908.
17 "Souvenirs d'un médecin de campagne," *Le Concours médical*, 5 October 1913.
18 In the Chamber of 1876, 42.6% of the deputies had served as municipal councillors and mayors; 23.4% had been elected as mayors alone; and 57.5% had been *conseillers généraux*. See Michel Bisault, "La Composition socio-professionnelle de la chambre des députés de la IIIᵉᵐᵉ république" (thesis, University of Paris, 1960), p. 11.
19 Paul Vigné d'Octon, *Les Grands et les petits mystères du Palais Bourbon. Scènes vécues de la vie parlementaire* (Editions Radot, 1928), pp. 13–14.
20 Following the Massif Central and the southwest were the departments of the southeast, where physicians made up around 15 percent of the winners. Those of the east had close to 12 percent. The weakest showing came in the four departments of the north (Nord, Pas-de-Calais, Somme, and Aisne), where

medical men made up only 3.2 percent of the successful candidates. In identifying the doctors, I used reports appearing in the medical press, along with the departmental lists of candidates published by *Le Temps* on 30 July 1895. Paris and the Seine are not included in these figures.

21 Using the lists appearing in *Le Progrès médical* for the partial elections of 1880, I was able to identify 137 doctors who won election. According to a report published by *La Chronique médicale* (1 August 1909), 169 practictioners were elected in 1887.

22 *La Chronique médicale*, 1 April 1902; and *Le Temps*, 1 August 1912.

23 See obituaries for Michou in *La Chronique médicale*, 15 August 1901; and in *La Tribune médicale*, 28 August 1901. For Grenier, see "Le Député musulman" in *La Chronique médicale*, 1 January 1897. Information on Treille can be found in *La Chronique médicale*, 1 February 1899 and 1 March 1910.

24 *AN, Programmes électoraux*, C7416, 1906 (Cher).

25 In 1906, Dr. Adhémar Pecharde, president of the *conseil général* of the Marne, was chosen by the "Congress of Republicans of the Left of the Arrondissement of Epernay." Adrien Pozzi, mayor of Reims, was chosen by the "Congress of Democratic Associations of the First District of Reims." Victor Delpierre, mayor of Ansauvillers in Oise, was nominated by a congress of republican committees representing eight cantons; leaders of the *conseil général* also urged him to run, and he was assured of the personal support of the three senators for Oise.

26 Jules Clère, *Biographie des députés* (Garnier frères, 1880), p. 679; *AN, Programmes électoraux*, C7333–7335, 1902 (Puy-de-Dôme and Maine-et-Loire) and C7416, 1906 (Drôme).

27 Chambre des députes, troisième legislature, *Professions de foi*, vol. 13 (Imprimerie de la Chambre des députés, n.d.), p. 537.

28 *AN, Programmes électoraux*, C5610, 1893 (Puy-de-Dôme) and C7333–7335, 1902, (Puy-de-Dôme).

29 *Le Concours médical*, 1 December 1894.

30 *Journal de médecine de Bordeaux*, 6 February 1898.

31 *Le Concours médical*, 2 and 23 April 1898. The same strategy was attempted in 1906 and again in 1910. See *Le Concours médical*, 13 May 1906; 24 April; and 1, 8, and 15 May 1910.

32 *Le Concours médical*, 14 July 1912.

33 *La Tribune médicale*, 3 May 1899.

34 Mattei Dogan, "Political Ascent in a Class Society: French Deputies 1870–1958," in Dwaine Marvick, ed., *Political Decision-Makers* (Glencoe, NY: Free Press, 1961), pp. 57–90.

35 In a rematch, the doctor won by eighty-eight votes. Information on this election can be found in *AN, Programmes électoraux*, C7333–7335, 1902 (Cantal). Further details were taken from the invalidation debate in *JOCD*, 10 July 1902, pp. 2209–14.

36 *JOCD*, 11 February 1878, pp. 1398–1404.

37 *JOCD*, 11 March 1890, pp. 508–18.

38 As in challenges to doctors Joseph Soye of Aisne and Jacques Even of Côtes-du-Nord, both republicans. See *JOCD*, 14 May and 4 June, 1878, pp. 5147–48 and 6220–23, respectively.

39 *AN, Programmes électoraux*, C7333–7335, 1902, and C7416, 1906 (Dordogne).

40 This article, from an unnamed conservative journal, was reprinted in *Gazette obstétricale de Paris*, 5 August 1876.

41 According to Dogan, in 1871 the representatives of the *petite* bourgeoisie constituted only 8% of parliament, and those of the *moyenne*, only 19%. By 1919, the respective figures had increased to 15 and 35%. See Dogan, "Les Filières de la carrière politique en France," *Revue française de science politique* 8 (October–December 1967): 468–92; and Jean Charlot, "Les Elites politiques en France de la IIIᵉ à la Vᵉ république," *Archives européenes de sociologie* 14 (1973); 78–92.

42 Yves-Henri Gaudemet, *Les Juristes et la vie politique de la IIIᵉ republique* (Presses universitaires de France, 1970), p. 32.

43 See Table 47 ("Ancienneté de l'orientation à gauche") in François Goguel, *Géo-

graphie des élections françaises sous la troisième et la quatrième république (Armand Colin, 1970), p. 117.

44 The north's attachment to conservative traditions weakened over time, while by 1900 the moderate republicanism of the east was slowly ceding to more rightist attitudes. See Goguel's discussion in ibid., pp. 166–7, as well as that of Jacques Gouault in *Comment la France est devenue républicaine: les élections générales et partielles à l'assemblée nationale 1870–1875* (Armand Colin, 1954), pp. 77–101.

45 *L'Evolution sociale* (Librairie Fischbacher, 1893), pp. 227–43.

46 *AN, Programmes électoraux*, C5512, 1889 (Basses-Pyrénées); C7333–7335, 1902 (Haute-Loire); and C7416, 1906 (Corsica). On Daniel, see Jacques Léonard, "Les Médecins de l'ouest au XIXème siècle" (thesis, University of Paris, 1976), vol. 3, pp. 1260, 1268.

47 *La Morale républicaine* (Félix Alcan, 1912), pp. 117–23.

48 *AN, Programmes électoraux*, C5610, 1893 (Puy-du-Dôme); C7333–7335, 1902 (Côtes-du-Nord and Dordogne).

49 *Revue internationale des sciences biologiques* 1, nos. 1 and 5 (1878): 61–63 and 158–9, respectively. See also Alfred Naquet, *Religion, propriété-famille* (Chez tous les librairies, 1869); and Paul Bert, *Le Clericalisme. Questions d'éducation nationale* (Armand Colin, 1900).

50 *JOS*, 15 March 1912, pp. 623–38.

51 On the Amagat affair, see *Le Progrès médical*, 29 May; 5, 12, and 19 June; and 21 August 1880.

52 Dr. Jules Carret, *Demonstration de l'inexistence de Dieu* (Alphonse Lemerre, 1912), especially pp. 8, 32, 53–54, 114–17, 480–2.

53 *AN, Programmes électoraux*, C7333–7335, 1902 (Gironde and Finistère). Le Monnier's comment can be found in Chambre des députés, troisième législature, *Professions de foi*, vol. 13, p. 267.

54 Data on Masonic membership were taken from Pierre Saint-Charles, *La Franc-maçonnerie au parlement* (Librairie française, 1956).

55 Comment by Debierre in *JOS*, 4 July 1911, p. 1066.

56 Mildred J. Headings, *French Freemasonry Under the Third Republic* (Baltimore: Johns Hopkins University Press, 1949), pp. 68–9.

57 *Le Temps*, 23 August 1891.

58 The rumor that Bernard experienced a death-bed conversion outraged De Lanessan, who rejected the possibility that the beliefs of Bernard's childhood could suddenly return to "take the place of the solid reasoning that made Claude Bernard the greatest physiologist of our epoch." *Revue internationale des sciences biologiques* 1, no. 7 (1878): 255.

59 *Le Temps*, 1 August 1878.

60 *La Chronique médicale*, 15 November 1897.

61 The fifty-two cases in which the form of burial is known for certain include eighteen religious and thirty-four civil. Additional probable cases include eighteen religious and thirty-two civil. Whichever figures are used, the proportions remain almost identical – around 35% religious and 65% civil.

62 *Le Progrès médical*, 27 November 1880 and 18 June 1892.

63 Martin, *La Morale républicaine*, pp. 137–43, 147, and 152, note 1.

64 Bernard Lavergne, *L'Evolution sociale*, pp. 115–17.

65 *AN, Programmes électoraux*, C7416, 1906 (Marne).

66 *AN, Programmes électoraux*, C7333–7335, 1902 (Dordogne).

67 *AN, Programmes électoraux*, C7333–7335, 1902 (Nord).

68 *AN, Programmes électoraux*, C7416, 1906 (Oise); C5610, 1893 (Côte-d'Or); C7333–7335, 1902 (Saône-et-Loire, Puy-de-Dôme).

69 *AN, Programmes électoraux*, C5610, 1893 (Gers); C7416, 1906 (Haute-Vienne); and C5506, 1889 (Haute-Garonne).

70 *AN, Programmes électoraux*, C5506, 1889 (Lot).

71 *AN, Programmes électoraux*, 1889 and C5610, 1893 (Creuse).

72 "Caught up in this movement that concentrates in the big cities all the hands that are lacking in agriculture, they left their land of origin healthy in body and

spirit but, under the influence of existing conditions that I don't have to describe but in which so many causes of physical alteration are added to so many deceptions, mental equilibrium is lost." *JOS*, 17 February 1887, pp. 165–79.

73 AN, *Programmes électoraux*, C5504, 1889 (Basses-Alpes).

74 *L'Héritage de Jacques Farreul* (Hachette, 1885).

75 AN, *Programmes électoraux*, C5610, 1893 (Hérault) and C7416, 1906 (Loire).

76 AN, *Programmes électoraux*, C7333–7335, 1902 (Nord) and C7416, 1906 (Pas-de-Calais).

77 AN, *Programmes électoraux*, C5610, 1893 (Charente-Inférieure, Gers, and Hérault) and C5504, 1889 (Aude).

78 AN, *Programmes électoraux*, C7333–7335, 1902 (Orne); C7416, 1906 (Jura and Meurthe-et-Moselle).

79 AN, *Programmes électoraux*, C7333–7335, 1902 (Seine); C5420, 1885 (Corrèze).

80 AN, *Programmes électoraux*, C5513, 1892 (Haute-Savoie).

81 AN, *Programmes électoraux*, C7333–7335, 1902. (Examples include Basses-Alpes, Corrèze, Côtes-du-Nord, Dordogne, Lot-et-Garonne, Savoie, Seine-et-Oise, and Yonne.)

82 AN, *Programmes électoraux*, C7333–7335, 1902 (Seine-et-Oise); C5505, 1889 (Lot, Dordogne).

83 AN, *Programmes électoraux*, C7333–7335, 1902 (Dordogne).

84 AN, *Programmes électoraux*, C5512, 1889 (Yonne) and C7333–7335, 1902 (Maine-et-Loire and Haute-Loire).

85 AN, *Programmes électoraux*, C5610, 1893 (Meurthe-et-Moselle and Puy-de-Dôme) and C7333–7335, 1902 (Corrèze).

86 AN, *Programmes électoraux*, C5420, 1885 (Corrèze); C5610, 1893 (Lozère, Charente-Inférieure); C7333–7335, 1902 (Côtes-du-Nord, Puy-de-Dôme).

CHAPTER 4. PATTERNS OF MEDICOPOLITICAL CAREERS IN PARLIAMENT

1 "French Deputies 1870–1958." Research by Mattei Dogan on the academic backgrounds of all deputies between 1898 and 1940 shows that among intellectuals, law dominated with 33%, medicine and pharmacy with 11%, and science with 8%. Letters and training colleges had 3% each. For a complete breakdown of the social composition of French legislatures between 1871 and 1893 and between 1919 and 1936, see Table IV of his "Les Filières de la carrière politique," *Revue française de science politique* 8 (October–December 1967): 468–92; along with his "La Stabilité du personnel parlementaire sous la troisième république;" *Revue française de science politique* 3 (April–June 1953): 319–47.

2 Edmond Demolins's celebrated tribute to the "superiority of the Anglo-Saxons," translated into English in 1898, argues that England's parliament was more representative of the real economic interests of the country than was that of France, primarily because wealthy French landowners seldom lived on their estates. The latter "have only themselves to thank for the discredit into which they have fallen in the eyes of the country electors, who in preference to them vote for physicians or lawyers." *Anglo-Saxon Superiority: To What It Is Due*, trans. Louis Bert. Lavigne (London: Leadenhall Press, 1898), pp. 204–35.

3 *La Profession parlementaire* (Ernest Flammarion, 1937), p. 14.

4 Figures for the ages of all deputies are taken from Dogan, "French Deputies 1870–1958," and, for the legislature of 1898, from Michel Bisault, "La Composition socio-professionnelle de la chambre des députés de la IIIème république" (thesis, University of Paris, 1960).

5 André Tardieu, *La Profession parlementaire*, p. 41, and Paul Vigné d'Octon, *Les Grands et les petits mystères du Palais Bourbon. Scènes vécues de la vie parlementaire* (Editions Radot, 1928), pp. 134–40. See also Pierre Guiral and Guy Thuillier, *La Vie quotidienne des députés en France, 1871 à 1914.* (Hachette, 1980), pp. 116–30, particularly the complaints of the fictional physician-deputy Denisot.

6 Yves-Henri Gaudemet, *Les Juristes et la vie politique de la IIIe république* (Presses universitaires de France, 1970), pp. 24, 27–30; and Jean Estèbe, *Les Ministres de la république, 1871–1914* (Presses de la fondation nationale des sciences politiques, 1982), pp. 24–27. See also Guiral and Thuillier, *La Vie quotidienne des députés*, pp. 259–64, on the difficulty of achieving ministerial rank.

7 *Journal de Bernard Lavergne* (Bibliothèque nationale, manuscrits N.A.F. 15906–15910.

8 Vigné d'Octon, *Les Grands et les petits mystères du palais bourbon*, pp. 141–7.

9 See the concluding comments of Leo A. Loubère's "The French Left-Wing Radicals: Their Economic and Social Program Since 1870," *American Journal of Economics and Sociology* 26 (April 1967): 189–203.

10 See the analysis of Antoine Prost and Christian Rosenzveig in "La Chambre des députés (1881–1885). Analyse factorielle des scrutins," *Revue française de science politique* 21 (February 1971): 5–50.

11 The motion was passed by 307 to 218, with 39 abstaining. A little under 28% of the doctors voted in favor, and 7.5% abstained. *JOCD*, 15 February 1889, p. 404.

12 See the Barodet committee's analysis of campaign platforms for 1893 in *JOCD*, doc. parl., 15 March 1894, no. 532, pp. 1250–93.

13 Judith F. Stone, *The Search for Social Peace. Reform Legislation in France 1890–1914* (Albany: State University of New York Press, 1985), pp. 22–23.

14 See the comments by Ricard in *JOCD*, 9 June 1895, pp. 1624–5; by Vazeille, *JOCD*, 14 April 1905, p. 1370; and by Sireyjol, *JOCD*, 24 October 1905, pp. 1865–67.

15 As noted earlier, the fall of Casimir-Périer's cabinet in May 1894 was occasioned more by his policy toward the church than toward the railroads, which was the subject that had initiated the debate. Nevertheless, after refusing the government its confidence, the Chamber followed with a vote on Millerand's motion urging the government to force the railroad companies to honor union rights. This was defeated by 240 to 224. The vote of doctors was 52% in favor, 27% opposed, and 21% abstaining.

16 The confidence motion passed by 288 to 190. A separate order of the day approving government actions while urging the passage of new laws to improve the lot of the miners failed by 377 to 133. The vote among doctors on the latter was 43.9% in favor, 46.3% opposed, and 9.7% abstaining. *JOCD*, 11 February 1886, pp. 202–3.

17 *JOCD*, doc. parl., 22 February 1897, no. 2299, p. 319.

18 *L'Union médicale*, 17 April 1877. Dubuisson of Finistère complained in 1898 that he and his colleagues in parliament were often "viewed with defiance." *Le Concours médical*, 3 December 1898.

19 *JOCD*, 17 December 1904, pp. 3091–3103.

20 *JOS*, 2 April 1892, pp. 353–65.

21 *JO, assemb. nat.*, 24 January 1873, p. 516; *JOCD*, 8 March 1881, pp. 437–42, and 25 July 1884, pp. 1830–43; and *JOS*, 14 and 16 December 1888, pp. 1546–59 and 1577–89; respectively.

22 R. K. Gooch, *The French Parliamentary Committee System* (Hamden, Conn.: Archon books 1969). pp. 32-42.

23 For example, doctors made up over half the membership of a committee formed in December 1876 to consider the proposals of Richard Waddington and Roussel on medical assistance in the countryside. Another, created in 1892 to study a Chamber-approved bill on the protection of public health (the future public health law of 1902), included 44%, besides the chemist Berthelot, who was the president. The various committees that sat throughout the period to consider proposals dealing with the mentally ill (the *commission des aliénés*) generally had a proportion of 35 to 40 percent physicians.

24 *L'Union médicale*, 1 August 1871; 8 and 16 July and 24 August 1872; and 30 January and 25 February 1873.

25 *JO, assemb. nat.*, 29 May 1872, pp. 3490–94.

26 *L'Union médicale* 9, 16, and 20 June 1874.
27 *L'Union médicale*, 29 April 1873.
28 *L'Union médicale*, 2 and 4 May 1876.
29 *L'Union médicale*, 10 and 17 April 1877.
30 Because the parliamentary medical group functioned as an informal caucus, no official minutes were published. I thus used the membership lists, debate summaries, and resolutions published in the medical press, in this case *Le Progrès médical*, 17 June, 22 July, 18 and 25 November, 2 and 9 December, 1876; and 20 and 27 January, 1877.
31 *L'Union médicale*, 9 and 13 January, 13 and 27 February, 1877.
32 *Le Concours médical*, 10 July 1880.
33 *Le Concours médical*, 30 June 1894.
34 One finds physicians in almost all these groups, an indication of the diversity of interests that each represented. Examples include the *groupe agricole, groupe forestier, groupe des députés maires, groupe de la mutualité, groupe de politique extérieure et coloniale, groupe viticole,* and *groupe de défense des intérêts économiques de la région du Nord.* A complete list appears in René Samuel and Georges Bonet-Maury, *Les Parlementaires français, 1900–1914,* 2 vols. (G. Rouston, 1914), pp. 421–61.
35 Labbé served as president for most of the post-1902 period. Others among the most active were Cornil, Dubuisson, Pédebidou, Lachaud, Laurent, Reymond, Devins, Piettre, Gauthier (Haute-Sâone), and Treille.
36 *Le Concours médical,* 2 April 1898. See also the "Lettre aux médecins-législateurs membres du Concours" in the 18 June 1898 issue, and the comments by Dr. Coillot to the medical syndicate of Haute-Sâone in the 23 August 1890 issue.

CHAPTER 5. REFORM OF THE MEDICAL PROFESSION

1 Michelle Perrot, *Les Ouvriers en grève: France, 1871–1890,* 2 vols. (Mouton, 1974), p. 90.
2 Emile Combes likewise extolled the doctor as having been the most "persevering defender of ideas of liberty" among the rural masses for the duration of the Second Empire. On the arrests of Bavoux and Le Monnier, see Chambre des députés, troisième legislature, *Professions de foi,* vol. 13 (Imprimerie de la Chambre des députés, n.d.), p. 537; and *Le Progrès médical,* 12 January 1895. For the comments by Turgis and Combes, see *JOS,* 5 April 1892, pp. 368–80, and 23 February, 1901, p. 393.
3 See Jacques Léonard, "Les Médecins de l'ouest au XIXème siècle" (thesis, University of Paris, 1976), vol. 2, pp. 787–822, 1086–94; and George Weisz, "The Politics of Medical Professionalization in France 1845–1848," *Journal of Social History* 12 (Fall 1978): 3–30.
4 Most critics ridiculed the notion of making Paris the sole center of instruction, and a vocal minority believed the time had come to end state control over medical education entirely. See *L'Union médicale,* 23 December 1871; and *Le Mouvement médical,* 24 and 31 December 1871, and 7 January, 5, and 11 February 1872. Naquet's proposal is found in *JO, assemb. nat.,* 17 and 20 December 1871, Annex 672, pp. 5041–42.
5 Minutes of the committee can be found in *AN,* C-3132, dossiers 1326–27.
6 *Rapport sur le projet de révision de la législation de l'an XI en ce qui concerne l'exercice de la médecine et de la pharmacie (août 1872),* in *AN AD XIX D,* t. 2, *Recueil des travaux du comité consultatif d'hygiène,* pp. 319–38.
7 Paul Brouardel, *De L'Exercice et de l'enseignement de la médecine* (Félix Malteste, 1873)), pp. 6–7, 10–18.
8 See *Procès-verbaux de la commission relative à la création de cinq facultés de médecine, AN,* C-3102; and the comments by Naquet and Bouisson in *JO, assemb. nat.,* 6 June 1874, pp. 3787–89, 4348–53.
9 Assorted publications on the propaganda campaigns of these cities can be found in *AN,* C-3102.
10 Paul Bert, *Rapport sur la création de nouvelles facultés de médecine, presenté à l'assemblée*

nationale (Librairie Ch. Delagrave, 1874). See especially the maps detailing the distribution of doctors, health officers, and medical students, pp. 23, 27, 30, 41, and 44, and the graphs and tables on ratios of practitioners to populations, pp. 80, 83, 85, and 137–45.

11 For the debates, see *JO, assemb. nat.*, 6 and 26 June and 8 and 9 December 1874, pp. 3782–90, 4348–55, 8088–95, and 8119–30, respectively. The most active participants were Bert, Naquet, Bouisson, and Testelin, with Testelin making a special plea that his home city of Lille be included among those receiving a full-fledged faculty. Partly as a result of his efforts, Lille offered a mixed faculty of medicine and pharmacy in 1875.

12 *L'Union médicale*, 9, 16, 20, and 23 June 1874.

13 *Le Concours médical*, 13 May 1882. On foreign practitioners, see the bill presented by the deputy Roger-Marvaise in *JO, assemb. nat.*, 9 May 1878, Annex 612, pp. 4884–86; and the analysis by Dr. Valery Meunier of the AGMF, in *AN*, C362, dossier 425.

14 *Le Concours médical*, 3 November 1883.

15 *JOCD, doc. parl.*, January 1884, Annex 2336, pp. 2010–21.

16 Minutes of the committee's meetings can be found in *AN*, C3383, dossier 1623. The full report is in *JOCD, doc. parl.*, October 1885, Annex 3828, pp. 790–802.

17 At first, the committee itself contained a minority inclined toward this view, which *Le Concours médical* accused of playing into the hands of the Right. See *Le Concours médical*, 13 February 1886.

18 The Brouardel report is included as an appendix in the government bill presented by Edouard Lockroy, minister of commerce and industry, in *JOCD, doc. parl.*, April 1887, Annex 1164, pp. 935–50.

19 *JOCD, doc. parl.*, 1888, Annex 2327, pp. 143–61.

20 *JOCD, doc. parl.*, 1889, Annex 15, pp. 35–51 and Annex 99, pp. 222–26; and 1890, Annex 360, pp. 280–1 and Annex 620, pp. 913–19. The full committee report can be found in *JOCD doc. parl.*, 1890, Annex 951, pp. 344–57. Minutes of committee meetings are in *AN*, C5492, dossier 1923.

21 *Le Concours médical*, 19 April and 17 May 1890; 5 December 1891; 10 December 1892; and 2 December 1893.

22 *JOCD*, 18 and 20 March 1891, pp. 651–60 and 674–83, respectively.

23 Minutes of the committee can be found in *Archives du sénat*, (1891), *Commission chargée d'examiner le projet de loi, adopté par la chambre, sur l'exercice de la médecine.*

24 For the first, see *JOS*, 18, 19, 22, and 23 March, pp. 217–38, 238–49, 252–65, and 268–74, respectively; and for the second, 2, 5, 6, and 9 April, pp. 353–65, 368–80, 385–93, and 402–12, respectively. The Chevandier bill had needed only one reading in the lower house, because at the outset of debate the deputies had voted *urgence*, which meant that a single reading sufficed.

25 *Le Concours médical*, 26 March 1892.

26 Three doctors voted against it, among them Combes, who protested the next day that he had actually voted in favor. *JOS*, 22 March 1892, pp. 252–65.

27 *Le Concours médical*, 2 April 1892.

28 See chap. 3 ("The Loi Chevandier") of Martha L. Hildreth, *Doctors, Bureaucrats and Public Health in France 1888–1902* (New York: Garland Press, 1987), pp. 164–214.

29 Léonard, "Les Médecins de l'ouest au XIXème siècle," vol. 2, p. 1124.

30 *Le Concours médical*, 24 December 1892; and *Le Progrès médical*, 28 January 1893.

31 Other physician-deputies belonging to the Civil Society were Amodru, Bourgeois, Cosmao-Dumenez, Dron, Gacon, Isambard, Legludic, Signard, and Viger. Among physician-senators were Cornil, Dufay, Dellestable, Paul Gérente, Laurens, Taulier, Lourties, and Pitti-Ferrandi. See *Le Concours médical*, 2 and 9 December 1893, and 13 January and 21 July 1894.

32 *La Tribune médicale*, 3 May, 7 and 21 June 1899; and *Le Progrès médical*, 23 December 1899.

33 On 13 May 1906, *Le Concours médical* cited the names of fourteen who had been helpful during the previous legislature. They were Amodru, Cazeneuve, Gustave

Chapuis, Dêche, Defontaine, Devins, Dron, Dubief, Dubuisson, Empereur, Lachaud, Marot, Simyan, and Vaillant. Mentioned on other occasions were Laurent, Dudouyt, Gustave Gauthier, Héritier, Piettre, Pujade, Sireyjol, and Vazeille.

34 *Le Concours médical*, 4 February 1888, 27 April and 18 May 1889.
35 Cornil pointed out that the fee scales, established in 1811, provided only five francs for an autopsy, whereas German physicians received the equivalent of fifteen (and twice this for a body exhumed after a month), plus an additional twenty-two for paperwork. *JOS*, 10 December 1889, pp. 1184–90.
36 *Le Concours médical*, 27 October 1894.
37 *La Tribune médicale*, 7 and 21 June 1899.
38 George Weisz, *The Emergence of Modern Universities in France, 1863–1914* (Princeton, NJ: Princeton University Press, 1983), pp. 356–68.
39 *JOS*, 6 July 1894, pp. 620–22; and *JOCD*, 18 June 1895, pp. 1746–56.
40 *JOS*, 9 May 1894, pp. 355–69.
41 *Le Concours médical*, 15 April 1904.
42 *Le Concours médical*, 10 March 1907.
43 See the criticism by Emile Goy, Debierre, and Reymond in *JOS*, 2 and 4 July 1911, pp. 1031–36 and 1060–68; and by Augagneur, Vaillant, Monprofit, and Laurent in *JOCD*, 10 February 1912, pp. 255–73.
44 See his testimony on 10 February 1894 before the committee considering the reform of pharmacy, in *Archives du sénat*, session 1893, no. 249.
45 Bert, *Rapport sur la création de nouvelles facultés de médecine*, pp. 3333–36.
46 *JOCD, doc. parl.*, 1882, Annex 918, pp. 1575–80.
47 Naquet's report is found in *JOCD, doc. parl.*, 1883, Annex 1969, pp. 894–902. For minutes of committee meetings, see *AN*, C3386, dossier 1880.
48 In the words of one petition addressed to Duval's committee, the diploma was "the most sacred of properties because it is personal and because it dies out with the individual." See *Pétition aux pouvoirs publics sur l'exercise simultané de la médecine et de la pharmacie* (A. Quelquejeu, 1890), in *AN*, C5492, dossier 1921.
49 *AN*, C5786, dossier 1279.
50 Debates for the first reading can be found in *JOCD*, 22 March 1891, pp. 694–98; and for the second, in *JOCD*, 28 June and 1 July 1893, pp. 1863–67 and 1891–94, respectively.
51 *Le Concours médical*, 29 July and 30 September 1893. Minutes of the Cornil committee can be found in *Archives du sénat*, session 1893, no. 249.
52 For the first reading, see *JOS*, 21, 23, and 27 November 1894, pp. 875–84, 886–93, 897–906, and 912–18, respectively; and for the second, 19, 21, and 22 December 1894, pp. 1013–24, 1029–33, 1034–39, and 1042–57, respectively.
53 *Le Concours médical*, 17 August 1895, and the comments by Dr. Gassot, 23 March 1895.
54 *Le Concours médical*, 25 January 1896.
55 *JOCD, doc. parl.*, 1898, Annex 3126, pp. 870–1. One more law derived from these efforts. In 1894, Cornil's committee had added a new article, specifying that all therapeutic serums, whether antitoxins or attenuated viruses, could be sold only by pharmacists, after approval of the Academy of Medicine and the Consultative Committee of Public Hygiene. The Senate approved the addition, which was separated out from the main bill and became law in 1895. See *JOCD, doc. parl.*, 1895, Annex 1245, pp. 313–16.
56 In 1899 and again in 1902, the pharmacist-deputy of Ardèche, Alexandre Astier, submitted essentially the same bill that the Senate had passed in 1894, but without results. See *Le Concours médical*, 15 August and 5 September 1903, and 19 March and 30 April 1904.
57 *JOCD, doc. parl.*, 1895, Annex 1486, pp. 869–72; *JOCD, doc. parl.*, 1908, Annex 1661, pp. 305–6; and *JOS*, 17 December 1898, 1011–17.
58 The Seine, with 259, had nearly three times the number found in all the Massif Central. A breakdown of the totals in each department can be found in *JOCD, doc. parl.*, 1894, Annex 723, pp. 951–3.

59 *JOCD, doc. parl.*, 1886, Annex 1027, pp. 459–61.
60 *JOCD, doc. parl.*, 1890, Annex 850, pp. 1604–6.
61 Medical men constituted a majority on the committee reporting out this bill. See *JOCD, doc., parl.*, 1881, Annex 3315, pp. 160–7. For the debates, see *JOCD*, 9 March 1881, pp. 454–63; and *JOS*, 9 July 1881, pp. 1072–80.
62 *JOCD, doc. parl.*, 1895, Annex 1486, pp. 869–72.
63 Especially Vaillant and Cazeneuve. See *JOCD, doc. parl.*, 1906, Annexes 2885 and 3094, pp. 1–2 and 285–87, respectively; and 1907, Annexes 643 and 898, pp. 30–31 and 327–29, respectively. For the debates, see *JOCD*, 16 June 1908, pp. 1191–1208; and *JOS*, 24 December 1908, pp. 1386–87.
64 *JOCD, doc. parl.*, 1914, Annex 3618, pp. 1319–24.
65 *Le Progrès médical*, 23 and 30 March 1878, and 24 November 1888.
66 *Le Progrès médical*, 10 January 1890, and also 24 October 1885.
67 Bourneville describes the founding of these schools in *Le Progrès médical*, 21 August 1880 and 4 June 1881.
68 A third of all hospital physicians and surgeons signed petitions opposing the laicizing campaign. See *Le Progrès médical*, 19 March 1881; *L'Union médicale*, 24 March 1881; and *Le Temps*, 4 December 1885.
69 For examples of the Bourneville–Després dispute, see *Le Progrès médical*, 26 March 1881, 2 October 1882, 17 February 1883, 7 February 1885, and 7 May 1887.
70 *JOS*, 31 May 1881, pp. 736–45.
71 *JOCD*, 19 and 21 January 1887, pp. 49–50 and 63–64, respectively.
72 *JOCD*, 19 December 1890, pp. 2567–77.
73 *Le Progrès médical*, 20 May and 3 June 1893.
74 *Le Progrès médical*, 19 February 1898.
75 *Le Progrès médical*, 30 June 1900.
76 *Le Progrès médical*, 21 November 1903, and 27 February and 21 May 1904.
77 *La Tribune médicale*, 11 March 1903.
78 *Le Concours médical*, 23 May 1903.
79 *Le Concours médical*, 19 March 1911.
80 *Le Concours médical*, 17 December 1911 and 21 January 1912.
81 This resolution is included in Doizy's bill to create new nursing schools, in *JOCD, doc. parl.*, 1912, Annex 2244, pp. 51–54.
82 *Le Concours médical*, 16 March 1913.

CHAPTER 6. DEFENSE OF THE PEOPLE'S HEALTH

1 In England, the most important laws were the Local Government Board Act of 1871, which created a central mechanism for overseeing hygienic matters, and the Public Health Acts of 1872 and 1875, which divided the country into sanitary districts and placed poor-law medical officers in charge of enforcing existing legislation. In Germany, the same era saw the creation of the Reich Health Office, which built on poor-law and public medical services available in Prussia and other states and which marked the beginnings of a unified health system for the Empire. Charles Chamberland praised the Reich Health Office in 1887 as "one of the most important central sanitary services that exists in Europe" and compared it with the Local Government Board in England. For a discussion of its membership and functions, see Chamberland's report in *JOCD, doc. parl.*, 1887, Annex 2152, p. 586. On the development of public medicine in England, Belgium, and Germany, see George Rosen, *From Medical Police to Social Medicine: Essays on the History of Health Care* (New York: Science History Publications, 1974), pp. 71–116. On England's sanitary laws, see Jeanne L. Brand, *Doctors and the State: the British Medical Profession and Government Action in Public Health, 1870–1912* (Baltimore: Johns Hopkins University Press. 1965), pp. 14–21. Alfred Fillasier's *De la Determination des pouvoirs publics en matière d'hygiène* (Jules Roussel, 1902), pp. 393–441, contains a detailed comparison of the public health laws and systems existing in most European countries at the turn of the century.

2 See the graph contained in Claire Salomon-Bayet, *Pasteur et la révolution pastorienne* (Payot, 1986), p. 396.
3 Paul Strauss, *La Croisade sanitaire* (Charpentier, 1902).
4 *JOCD*, 6 March 1896, pp. 388–97.
5 *L'Anarchie et le collectivisme* (Bibliothèque internationale d'édition, 1904), p. 120.
6 *JOS*, 30 November 1906, pp. 1045–56.
7 *JOS*, 11 March 1903, pp. 388–93.
8 *JOCD*, 15 June 1907, pp. 1371–73.
9 *JOCD*, doc. parl., 1892, Annex 2334, pp. 2162–90.
10 *JOCD*, doc. parl., Annex 2464, 21 June 1901, pp. 782–93; and *JOS*, 3 February 1897, pp. 73–79.
11 Robert Nye, *Crime, Madness, and Politics in Modern France: The Medical Concept of National Decline* (Princeton, NJ: Princeton University Press, 1984), pp. xi–xii.
12 *JOS*, 19 December 1900, pp. 968–79.
13 *JO, assemb. nat.*, 26 and 17 July 1874, pp. 5250–54 and 5268–72, respectively.
14 *BAM*, 24 (1890), sessions of 16 and 23 September, pp. 332–44 and 355–67, and 36 (1896), session of 25 August, pp. 224–29.
15 *JOCD*, doc. parl., 1892, Annex 2334, pp. 2162–90.
16 Salomon-Bayet, *Pasteur et la révolution pastorienne*, pp. 11, 277, 300.
17 *JOS*, 19 December 1900, pp. 968–79, and *JOCD*, 23 February 1890, pp. 323–7.
18 *JOCD*, 25 February 1890, pp. 333–4.
19 *JOCD*, 12 June 1896, pp. 916–25.
20 *JOCD*, 7 April 1895, pp. 1226–30.
21 Jean-Pierre Goubert, *La Conquête de l'eau: l'avènement de la santé à l'âge industriel* (Robert Laffont, 1986), pp. 29, 75.
22 *JOCD*, doc. parl., 1892, Annex 2334, pp. 2162–90.
23 *JOS*, 13 February 1897, pp. 154–63.
24 See the comments by the economist Léon Say in *JOS*, 14 December 1888, pp. 1551–88.
25 *JOCD*, doc. parl., Annex 2464, 21 June 1901, pp. 782–93.
26 *JOS*, 19 November 1898, pp. 878–86.
27 *JOCD*, doc. parl., 1887, Annex 2152, pp. 573–8.
28 *JOS*, 3 February 1897, pp. 73–79.
29 *JOCD*, 27 June 1893, pp. 1834–42.
30 *BAM* 55, session of 13 February 1906, pp. 234–7.
31 The titled members of the Academy of Medicine were Bourgoin, Cornil, Javal, Labbé, Lannelongue, Larrey, Samuel Pozzi, Robin, Roussel, and Wurtz. Those on the Consultative Committee of Public Hygiene were Borne, Bourneville, Cornil, Levraud, Liouville, Villejean, and Wurtz. The Superior Council of Public Assistance had Borne, Bourneville, Blatin, Chautemps, Dron, Dubief, Goujon, Labrousse, Lafont, Georges Martin, Pedebidou, Petitjean, Emile Rey, Roussel, and Villeneuve. On the Superior Council for the Protection of Infants were Roussel, Soye, and Laussedat, and the Superior Council of Labor had Dron, Dubief, and Lourties.
32 See Ricard's speech on agriculture, medicine, and nutrition in *JOS*, 13 April 1905, pp. 751–6.
33 On the organization of this congress, see *AN*, F^{17} 3097^5, Congrès d'hygiène, nationale et internationale, Paris, 1878. See also *Le Progrès médical*, 16 March, 6 April, and 10 August 1878.
34 *AN*, F^{17} 3097^5, Congrès d'hygiène internationale, Turin, 1880. See also *Le Progrès médical*, 11 and 23 September and 20 October 1880.
35 At Geneva (1882), the Hague (1884), Vienna (1887), Paris (1889), London (1891), Budapest (1894), Madrid (1898), Paris (1900), Brussels (1903), and Berlin (1907). Those whose names most often appear in these proceedings are Liouville, Bourneville, Cornil, Roussel, Langlet, Chautemps, Levraud, Brousse, Vaillant, and Dron.
36 Minutes of the Committee of Public Hygiene can be found in *AN*, C7324, dossier

1492 (1902–6); C7398, dossier 1452 (1906–10); and C7470, dossier 1787 (1910–14).

37 Martha L. Hildreth, *Doctors, Bureaucrats and Public Health in France, 1888–1902* (New York: Garland Press, 1987), pp. 140–53.

38 Marcel Peschaud, *De L'intervention de l'état en matière d'hygiène publique* (Lamulle et Poisson, 1898), pp. 96–105, 198–209; and Fillassier, *De La Determination des pouvoirs publics en matière d'hygiène*, pp. 115–32. On the Consultative Committee of Public Hygiene, see *Recueil des travaux du comité consultatif d'hygiène publique de France*, vol. 1 (J.-B. Baillière, 1872), pp. v–xxiv.

39 Pierre Darmon, *La Longue traque de la variole: les pionniers de la médecine préventive* (Perrin, 1986), pp. 16–17.

40 Jules Rochard, *Traité d'hygiène sociale* (Adrien Delahaye et Emile Lecrosnier, 1888), pp. 157–8, 530–1; and *JOCD, doc. parl.*, 1887, Annex 1417, pp. 13–17.

41 Le Maguet's report is in *JOCD, doc. parl.*, 1881, Annex 3908, pp. 136–8; and the debates are in *JOCD*, 8 March 1881, pp. 437–42.

42 The government had earlier solicited the advice of the Academy of Medicine, as had Liouville. In the spring of 1881, it voted forty-six to nineteen in favor of obligatory vaccination. See *BAM* 10, sessions of 29 March, 5, 12, 19, and 26 April, and 3 May 1881, pp. 397–418, 429–53, 463–81, 492–505, and 523–70, respectively.

43 *JOCD, doc. parl.*, 1882, Annex 324, pp. 195–6.

44 *JOCD*, 25 July, 1884, pp. 1830–43. Afterwards, Clemenceau formed his own committee to visit the south and on August 2 presented to the Chamber an account of his trip. See *JOCD*, 3 August 1884, pp. 1965–6.

45 *JOCD, doc. parl.*, 1886, Annex 864, pp. 135–8.

46 *JOCD, doc. parl.*, 1887, Annex 2152, pp. 573–8. Socialist doctors formed an exception on the issue of a ministry of health. In 1893, Vaillant presented a bill to create a ministry of labor that would have included hygiene and welfare under its jurisdiction. The bill got a favorable report, but it never arrived on the floor. *JOCD, doc. parl.*, 1897, Annex 2498, pp. 1365–66; and *JOCD, doc. parl.*, 1898, Annex 120, pp. 1287–88.

47 *JOCD, doc. parl.*, 1892, Annex 2334, pp. 2162–90. Minutes of the committee's deliberations are in *AN*, C5492, dossier 1608.

48 *JOCD*, 27 and 28 June 1893, pp. 1834–42 and 1859–63, respectively.

49 For the minutes of this committee, see *Archives du sénat*, Commission relative à la protection de la santé publique, no. 267, session 1893.

50 *JOS*, 17 December 1897, pp. 1431–34. For the other debates of the first reading see *JOS*, 3, 5, 6, 10, and 13 February 1897, pp. 73–79, 86–91, 93–96, 108–12, 124–35, and 154–63, respectively.

51 *JOS*, 12, 19, and 21 December 1900, pp. 950–6, 968–79, 984–98; and 22, 24, and 25 May and 29 June 1901, pp. 660–72, 675–83, 685–90, and 1117, respectively.

52 *JOCD, doc. parl.*, 1910, Annex 3305, p. 440.

53 *Le Concours médical*, 4 June 1911.

54 Rejecting the *"esprit centralisateur à outrance"* that had influenced this arrangement, Cazeneuve urged including all professors of hygiene at provincial medical faculties. His bill, which attracted over a hundred cosponsors (a fifth of them medical men), got a favorable review and was passed in April 1905. *JOCD, doc. parl.*, 1904, Annex 1450, pp. 41–43.

55 *JOCD, doc., parl.*, 1912, Annex 2226, pp. 30–35.

56 *Le Concours médical*, 2 and 9 August 1902.

57 Hildreth, *Doctors, Bureaucrats, and Public Health in France*, p. 312.

58 The official list included typhoid fever, typhus, smallpox, scarlet fever, diphtheria, miliary fever, cholera, bubonic plague, yellow fever, dysentery, puerperal fever, infant ophthalmia, measles, pneumonia, bronchial pneumonia, and cerebrospinal meningitis. Several others, including pulmonary tuberculosis, were attached as part of another group for which notification was voluntary. See the debates in *BAM* 30, sessions of 10 and 17 October 1893, pp. 354–66 and 397–

402, respectively; *BAM* 40, session of 19 July 1898, pp. 38–46; and *BAM* 49, sessions of 13 and 20 January 1903, pp. 34–56 and 64–78, respectively.

59 *Archives du sénat,* Commission chargée de l'examen de la proposition de loi, adopté par la chambre des députés, tendant à modifier les articles 20 et 25 de la loi du 15 février 1902 (sessions of 30 June and 25 November 1909).

60 *JOCD, doc. parl.,* 1912, Annex 2258, pp. 67–69.

61 Rochard, *Traité d'hygiène sociale,* p. 48.

62 *JOCD, doc. parl.,* 1886, Annex 1303, pp. 1116–57; and *JOS,* 14 December 1888, pp. 1546–59.

63 At that time, the houses of Paris used one of several methods, of which the most common was that of fixed tanks *(fosses fixes),* which often leaked into the soil. Another method was by means of portable soil tubs *(tinettes mobiles),* which were made of wood or zinc and were emptied every eight to ten days. Around eleven thousand houses had a direct flow into the sewers and from there into the river. See Bourneville's detailed treatment in *JOCD, doc. parl.,* 1886, Annex 1303, pp. 1116–57. See also Gérard Jacquemet, "Urbanisme parisien: la bataille du *tout-à-l'égout* à la fin du XIXe siècle," *Revue d'histoire moderne et contemporaine* 26 (October–December 1979): 505–48.

64 At the request of the Consultative Committee of Arts and Manufactures, Freycinet had gone abroad during the 1860s to study the newest methods of urban hygiene. For his recommendations, see *Emploi des eaux d'égout en agriculture d'après les faits observés en France et à l'étranger* (Dunod, 1869), pp. 1, 37–70, 128–9; and *Principes de l'assainissement des villes, comprenant la description des principaux procédés employés dans les centres de population de l'europe occidentale pour protéger la santé publique* (Dunod, 1870), pp. iii, 4. Published the same year by Dunod was Freycinet's *Traité d'assainissement industriel, comprenant la description des principaux procédés employés dans les centres manufacturiers de l'europe occidentale pour protéger la santé publique et l'agriculture contre les effets des travaux industriels.*

65 An exception was Camille Raspail, who contended that too little land had been set aside for the project and that the undertaking would create an infectious marsh. Both he and Chamberland favored the alternative of a canal to the sea. *JOCD,* 25 and 26 January 1888, pp. 132–46 and 153–63, respectively.

66 *JOS,* 14, 15, 16, 18, and 19 December 1888, pp. 1546–59, 1562–75, 1577–89, 1594–1612, and 1615–19, respectively; and for the second reading, 16 and 18 January 1889, pp. 26–35 and 41–45, respectively. For further debate, following submission of a bill allowing Paris to borrow the money for implementation, see *JOCD,* 25, 27, 28, 1894, pp. 332–44, 351–62, 365–76, respectively; and 25 and 29 April, 1894, pp. 615–29 and 642–58, respectively.

67 Jacquemet, "Urbanisme parisien."

68 Georges Martin, physician-senator of Paris, was a leader in the drive to create mortuaries in the capital. It was essential, he argued, that corpses be removed from apartments and houses as quickly as possible and that the clothing of the deceased be disinfected. See *Annales d'hygiène publique et de médecine legale* 5 (January 1881): 61–79, along with his comments on the dangers of local burial practices in *JOS,* 20 and 29 November 1885, pp. 1181–88 and 1193–1201, respectively, and 22 January 1886, pp. 13–21.

69 *JOCD, doc. parl.,* 1881, Annex 3982, pp. 1406–10.

70 *JOCD,* 25 February 1894, pp. 336–44.

71 *La Progrès médical,* 27 November 1880 and 2 February 1884.

72 *JOCD,* 31 March 1886, pp. 609–24.

73 *JOCD, doc. parl.,* 1892, Annex 2444, p. 2349.

74 *JOCD, doc. parl.,* 1898, Annex 575, pp. 582–3; *JOCD, doc. parl.,* 1899, Annex 835, pp. 939–40; and *JOCD, doc. parl.,* 1900, Annex 1460, p. 660.

75 *La Presse médicale,* 30 April 1902; and *JOCD,* 11 November and 2 December 1904, pp. 2364–65 and 2785–96, respectively.

76 *JOCD,* 18 November 1904, pp. 2485–87.

77 *JOCD, doc. parl.,* 1888, Annex 2946, p. 995.

78 *JOCD,* 17 and 23 June, 1896, pp. 948–65 and 1019–30, respectively.

79 *JOCD*, 4 and 8 April, 1908, pp. 872–8 and 916–31, respectively.
80 *JOCD, doc. parl.*, 1905, Annex 2224, p. 47.
81 *JOCD, doc. parl.*, 21 June 1882, pp. 665–76.
82 *JOCD, doc. parl.*, 1882, Annex 590, pp. 823–7. The debates can be found in *JOCD*, 28 and 29 March 1882, pp. 404–9 and 418–28, respectively.
83 *JOCD*, 22 and 23 December 1883, pp. 2948–49 and 2963–68, respectively. In the end, the government reimposed the ban, which stayed on the books until 1891, when a presidential decree repealed it.
84 *JOS*, 7 February 1887, pp. 97–102; and *JOCD*, 31 January and 2, 3, 4, and 6 February 1896, pp. 114–24, 137–46, 341–56, 367–79, and 384–8, respectively.
85 *JOCD*, 11, 18, 25 November and 2, 9, 16, 17, and 23 December 1904, pp. 2355–67, 2485–97, 2625–35, 2785–96, 2929–41, 3055–68, 3091–3103, 3227–34, and 3235–38, respectively.
86 *JOCD*, 15 June 1907, pp. 1371–73; and *JOS*, 12 and 19 June 1903, pp. 979–82 and 1034–44, respectively.
87 *JOCD*, 12 June 1880, pp. 1694–98.
88 *Le Progrès médical*, 23 December 1876. Supporting these ideas was Baron Larrey, director of army health services in 1856 and 1870. See *JOCD*, 15 June 1880, pp. 6497–6505.
89 *JOCD*, 11, 14, and 17 June, 1880, pp. 6394–98, 6497–6505, and 6643, respectively.
90 *JOCD, doc. parl.*, 1881, Annex 3809, pp. 115–36.
91 *JOCD, doc. parl.*, 1889, Annex 3808, pp. 1909–10. See also *Le Progrès médical*, 13 July 1889.
92 By the turn of the century, French military mortality rates stood at 4.5 per 1,000 (2.3 for Germany), down from 10.5 in 1875. Statistics assembled by Brouardel reveal that between 1872 and 1884, the French army recorded 151,319 cases of typhoid, of which 17,642 ended in death. See "Répartition de la fièvre tyhpoïde en France," *Annales d'hygiène publique et de médecine légale* 21 (1889): 5–35.
93 *JOS*, 26 November 1902, 1161–64.
94 As an example, see Labbé's speech on a typhoid outbreak at the garrison of Eure, in *JOS*, 19 November 1898, pp. 878–86.
95 *JOS*, 6, 7, 11, and 13 March 1903, pp. 354–64, 370–81, 386–93, and 405–23, respectively.
96 *JOS*, 15 June 1912, pp. 1489–98; and *JOCD, doc. parl.*, 1914, Annex 3533, pp. 1153–54. Labbé's bill was approved by voice vote on 19 December 1913 and went on to the Chamber, where it had no opposition. It became law on 27 March 1914.
97 *JOCD*, 27 January and 14, 21, and 24 February 1914, pp. 231, 742–58, 962–81, and 991–5, respectively.
98 *JOCD, doc. parl.*, 1914, Annex 3758, pp. 1617–1732.
99 *JOCD, doc. parl.*, 1899, Annex 622, pp. 447–8.
100 Pierre Guillaume, *Du Désespoir au salut: les tuberculeux aux XIXe et XXe siècles* (Aubier, 1986), p. 147–8.
101 *BAM* 68, session of 8 October 1912, pp. 158–229.
102 Ann-Louise Shapiro, *Housing and the Poor of Paris, 1850–1902* (Madison: University of Wisconsin Press, 1985), p. 82. See also *JOCD, doc. parl.*, 1901, Annex 2464, pp. 782–93; and *BAM* 54, session of 10 October 1905, pp. 213–14.
103 See the comments by Dr. Pedebidou in *JOS*, 7 March 1903, pp. 370–81.
104 *JOCD*, 4 June 1901, pp. 1218–33.
105 *BAM* 22, session of 30 July and 26 November 1889, pp. 104–7 and 549–55, respectively. Dr. Roussel chaired another committee of the Academy of Medicine that presented a report in May 1898. Among its recommendations were isolation of tuberculosis patients in the hospitals, distribution of pocket spittoons containing an antiseptic solution, the disinfection of rooms where a tuberculosis death had occurred, and new measures regulating the slaughter of animals destined for consumption. *BAM* 39, session of 3 May 1898, pp. 470–528.
106 Participants in the Paris congress of 1905, for example, included Amodru, Vail-

lant, Villejean, Lannelongue, Augagneur, Jean Peyrot, Labbé, Lachaud, Langlet, Lesage, Meslier, Adrien Pozzi, Ricard, Monprofit, and Borne. See *La Presse médicale*, 22 April 1905.

107 *JOCD, doc. parl.*, 1913, Annex 2484, pp. 31–33.

108 *JOCD, doc. parl.*, 1901, Annex 2464, pp. 782–93.

109 Nicholas Bullock and James Read, *The Movement for Housing Reform in Germany and France 1840–1914* (Cambridge, England: Cambridge University Press, 1985), pp. 474–8.

110 *BAM* 46, session of 2 July 1901, p. 5. See also *Le Progrès médical*, 1 December 1900; and Guillaume, *Du Désespoir au salut*, p. 178.

CHAPTER 7. THE SOCIAL QUESTION

1 Judith F. Stone, *The Search for Social Peace. Reform Legislation in France 1890–1914* (Albany: State University of New York Press, 1985), pp. xiii–xiv, 22–23.

2 *BAM* 19, session of 13 March 1888, pp. 383–94.

3 *BAM* 39, session of 25 January 1898, pp. 87–88.

4 *BAM* 68, session of 24 December 1912, pp. 587–8.

5 *La Tribune médicale*, 2 May 1900; and *Le Concours médical*, 3 November 1912.

6 *JOCD, doc. parl.*, 1887, Annex 1952, pp. 1019–33. See also the comments by Roussel in *JOS*, 17 February 1887, pp. 165–79.

7 *JOS*, 18 January 1911, pp. 17–18.

8 *JOCD*, 7 June 1895, pp. 1602–11.

9 Dr. Moinet argued in the Senate that the "street politics" of 1871 grew out of excessive drinking among the National Guard, which explained why such episodes as the Commune, like other revolutions in French history, were produced "in volcaniclike movements, after which all is forgotten." *JOS*, 27 June 1893, pp. 955–63. The notion that the Commune could be traced to alcohol was the subject of an impassioned exchange of letters in *La Chronique médicale* in 1902. See the issues dated 15 December 1901, and 15 January, 1 February, 15 March, and 15 May 1902.

10 *JOCD*, 11 December 1900, pp. 2584–2602.

11 For a regional breakdown of the largest alcohol-producing departments, see *JOCD, doc. parl.*, 1892, Annex 2291, pp. 2105–40.

12 *Le Progrès médical*, 19 September 1896. On his speech to the Chamber, see *Le Concours médical*, 15 June 1895.

13 See the comments of Dr. Félix-Martin to the Senate in *JOS*, 26 November 1910, pp. 1792–1801.

14 *JOCD*, 31 January 1888, pp. 213–19.

15 *JO, assemb. nat.*, 24 January 1873, p. 516.

16 *JOCD*, 2 July 1895, pp. 1933–44. For Guesde's views, see *JOCD*, 14 December 1898, pp. 2425–36.

17 The 1886 report came in response to an inquiry from Dr. Roussel, who, with four other physicians, was part of a Senate committee studying alcoholism "from the viewpoint of health and morality as well as from the viewpoint of the treasury." Its conclusions, which incorporated those approved by the Academy of Medicine in July 1886, can be found in *JOS*, 2 and 25 June 1887, pp. 602 and 669–78, respectively. For the 1886 report of the Academy of Medicine itself, see *BAM* 16, session of 6 July 1886, pp. 10–18.

18 *BAM* 14, session of 17 November 1885, pp. 1524–34.

19 *JOS*, 27 June 1893, pp. 955–63. See also the comments by Treille in *JOS*, 19 December 1900, pp. 968–79; by Amagat in *JOCD*, 31 January 1888, pp. 213–19; by Lannelongue in *JOCD*, 7 June 1895, pp. 1602–11; and by Michou in *JOCD*, 14 November 1896, pp. 1517–35.

20 *JOCD, doc. parl.*, 1887, Annex 1952, pp. 1019–33.

21 *JOS*, 16 June 1896, pp. 466–75.

22 JOCD, 11 June 1883, pp. 1238–40.

23 *JO, assemb. nat.*, 17 and 24 March, pp. 2080–82 and 2160–63, respectively.

24 *JOCD*, 11 December 1900, pp. 2584–2602.
25 *JOS*, 23 June 1893, pp. 917–30.
26 *JOCD, doc. parl.*, 1887, Annex 1952, pp. 1019–33.
27 *JOCD, doc. parl.*, 1910, Annex 440, pp. 78–79.
28 *AN*, C7398, dossier 1452; sessions of 17 and 25 June 1907.
29 *Archives du sénat*, Commission chargée de l'examen de la proposition de loi de M. de Lamarzelle . . . à interdire la fabrication et la vente de l'absinthe, nommée le 19 novembre 1908. Vol. 1: 26 November 1908 to 17 February 1909; vol. 2: 20 February 1909 to 3 March 1909; and vol. 3: 17 March 1909 to 22 March 1912. For Borne's ideas, see *JOS*, 11 July 1908, pp. 969–70.
30 P. E. Prestwich suggests that the antiabsinthe campaign may even have distracted the antialcohol forces from the real enemy at hand, which was the power of the wine and alcohol industries. See her "Temperance in France: The Curious Case of Absinthe," *Historical Reflections/Réflexions historiques* 6 (Winter 1979): 301–19.
31 *JOCD, doc. parl.*, 1894, Annex 474, pp. 298–300.
32 *JOS*, 23 and 28 December, 1900, pp. 1019–36 and 1087–1100, respectively.
33 *JOCD*, 14 December 1898, pp. 2425–36; and 27 and 28 October 1903, pp. 2357–59 and 2373–91, respectively.
34 *JOCD*, 1, 7, and 14 November 1896, pp. 1327–42, 1397–1413, and 1517–35, respectively. The big winegrowing departments produced numerous supporters for the bill, including Cot and Vigné of Hérault; Clament, Pourteyron, and Theulier of Dordogne; Chambige of Puy-de-Dôme; Mandeville of Haute-Garonne, and Marfan of Aude. Besides Defontaine and Lesage of the north, opponents included all five physician-deputies of Paris (Vaillant, Paulin-Méry, Frébault, Chautemps, and Chassaing).
35 *JOCD*, 30 July 1884, pp. 1892–93.
36 *JOCD*, 7 November 1896, pp. 1397–1413.
37 *JOS*, 16 June 1896, pp. 466–75.
38 These included Haute-Saône, Yonne, Eure, Orne, Sarthe, Vosges, and Calvados. See *JOS*, 20 June 1896, pp. 509–17.
39 In almost every case, doctors who voted against the *bouilleurs de cru* represented departments in which the *bouilleurs* were weak as a political force. *JOCD*, November 20 and 21, 1900, pp. 2159–65 and 2185–95, respectively.
40 *JOS*, 18 January 1911, pp. 17–18.
41 Jan Goldstein, *Console and Classify: The French Psychiatric Profession in the Nineteenth Century* (Cambridge, England: Cambridge University Press, 1987), pp. 361–77.
42 *JOS*, 25 November 1886, pp. 1307–10.
43 *JOS*, 30 November 1886, pp. 1333–48.
44 For a description of his work, see Bourneville's *Assistance, traitement et éducation des enfants idiots et dégénérés. Rapport fait au congrès national d'assistance publique (session de Lyon, juin 1894)* (Félix Alcan, 1895).
45 *Le Progrès médical*, 12 January 1889.
46 Robert Nye, *Crime, Madness, and Politics in Modern France: The Medical Concept of National Decline* (Princeton, NJ: Princeton University Press, 1984), pp. 29–34. For further treatment of the 1838 law, see Goldstein, *Console and Classify*, pp. 276–321.
47 *JOCD, doc. parl.*, 1889, Annex 3934, pp. 425–54; and *JOS*, 25 November 1886, pp. 1310–13.
48 The minutes of this committee can be found in *Archives du sénat*, Commission chargé de l'examen du projet de loi portant revision de la loi du 30 juin 1838 sur les aliénés, no. 37, 4 vols.
49 Responding to a request from Dr. Dupré, committee chairman, the Academy of Medicine drew up its own report, which was approved in March 1884. The report accepted the principle of judicial intervention in determining the fate of patients and endorsed the idea of requiring two medical certificates, rather than one, to commit a person to an asylum. *BAM* 13, sessions of 22 January and 18 March 1884, pp. 133–68 and 390–402, respectively.

50 Debates on the first reading can be found in *JOS*, 25, 27, and 30 November and 2, 4, 6, 7, 9, 11, and 14 December, 1886 pp. 1307–16, 1319–30, 1333–48, 1352–56, 1368–81, 1383–91, 1395–1407, 1409–20, 1422–34, and 1442–48, respectively. For the second, see *JOS*, 11, 15, 17, and 26 February and 7 and 11 March 1887, pp. 124–34, 151–63, 165–79, 351–5, 378–82, and 385–90, respectively. For Combes's remarks, see *JOS*, 4 December 1886, pp. 1370–74, and 15 February 1887, pp. 151–63.

51 Bourneville's report is in *JOCD, doc. parl.*, 1889, Annex 3934, pp. 425–54.

52 Goldstein, *Console and Classify*, pp. 366–7, stresses that differences concerning the status of clerical asylums were especially crucial to undermining the reform movement.

53 Lafont's report can be found in *JOCD, doc. parl.*, 1891, Annex 1829, pp. 2970–3018. Dubief's report is in *JOCD, doc. parl.*, 1898, Annex 579, pp. 737–66. Minutes of the 1898 committee, chaired by the deputy Jean Cruppi, can be found in *AN*, C5617, dossier 129.

54 *JOCD*, 15, 18, 22, and 23 January 1907, pp. 19–33, 52–66, 99–112, and 122–42, respectively. See also the analysis in Nye, *Crime, Madness, and Politics in Modern France*, pp. 236–43.

55 The minutes of the Senate committee between 1909 and 1913 can be found in *Archives du sénat*, Commission sur les aliénés, 1909–13. For the debates, see *JOS*, 20 and 24 December 1913, pp. 1565–78 and 1603–9, respectively.

56 *JOCD, doc. parl.*, 1900, Annex 1350, pp. 184–92. A good expression of these views can be found in Dr. J.-L. De Lanessan's *La Concurrence sociale et les devoirs sociaux* (Félix Alcan, 1904), pp. 143–61.

57 Dr. A. Balestre and A. Gilleta de Saint-Joseph, *Etude sur la mortalité de la première enfance dans la population urbaine de France de 1892 à 1897* (Octave Doin, 1901), pp. 2–7, 17–27. For Lagneau's analysis, see *BAM* 24, session of 15 July 1890, pp. 62–77. See also the tables on mortality rates in Rachel Fuchs, *Abandoned Children: Foundlings and Child Welfare in Nineteenth-Century France* (Albany: State University of New York Press, 1984), pp. 194–204.

58 See George D. Sussman, *Selling Mothers' Milk: The Wet-nursing Business in France, 1715–1914* (Urbana: University of Illinois Press, 1982), especially pp. 121–9 on the background of the Roussel bill.

59 Roussel's report can be found in *JO, assemb. nat.*, 26 and 27 July 1874, pp. 5250–54 and 5268–72, respectively. See also Fuchs, *Abandoned Children*, pp. 206–34, on hygienic conditions among wet nurses.

60 *BAM* 14, session of 10 March 1885, pp. 348–62; and *BAM* 24, session of 9 December 1890, pp. 745–61.

61 See Sussman's conclusions in *Selling Mothers' Milk*, pp. 182–5, and in "The Wet-nursing Business in Nineteenth-Century France," *French Historical Studies* 9 (Fall 1975): 304–28.

62 *BAM* 24, session of 9 December 1891, pp. 745–61.

63 *BAM* 47, session of 30 December 1902, pp. 668–73, 680–700, and 712–13; and *BAM* 60, session of 8 December 1908, pp. 473–4.

64 A Senate bill by Labbé in 1901 adopted most of Roussel's revisions, but it was never reported out of committee. See *BAM* 47, session of 30 December 1902, pp. 668–73, 680–700, 712–13. In May 1913, a committee of the Academy of Medicine again urged revisions, including expanding the number and categories of infants who were covered. *BAM* 69, session of 6 May 1913, pp. 358–71.

65 See the comments by Dr. Cazeneuve in *JOS*, 12 June 1909, pp. 424–6; and his report to the Academy of Medicine on his research on milk sterilization, in *BAM* 33, session of 19 March 1895, pp. 313–21.

66 *JOCD, doc. parl.*, 1913, Annex 2499, p. 53.

67 *JOS*, 12 June and 27 October 1909, pp. 424–6 and 828, respectively; and *JOCD*, 2 April 1910, p. 1881. For deliberations by the Committee of Public Hygiene, see *AN*, C7398, dossier 1452, sessions of 17 and 22 December 1909 and 27 February 1910. Durand's report can be found in *JOCD, doc. parl.*, 1910, Annexe 3143, pp. 190–1.

68 *JOS*, 7 February 1913, pp. 44–45. See also the discussion in Angus McLaren, *Sexuality and Social Order: The Debate over the Fertility of Women and Workers in France, 1770–1920* (New York: Holmes and Meier, 1983), pp. 136–53.

69 *AN*, C3228, dossier 1212; and *JOCD, doc. parl.*, 1885, Annex 3548, pp. 466–73.

70 *BAM* 25 (1891), session of 21 April, pp. 637–49.

71 See the Senate debates in *JOS*, 2 December 1903, pp. 1447–55; and *JOS*, 27 February and 2 March 1904, pp. 229–39 and 242–7.

72 The bill became law in 1889. See *JOS*, 1, 11, 18, 20, 22, and 25 May; 3 and 13 June; and 3, 6, 8, and 11 July 1883, pp. 422–5, 461–7, 483–94, 499–510, 517–27, 529–42, 552–5, 558–73, 618–29, 676–8, 807–12, 824–30, 834–49, and 854–5, respectively. The debates in the Chamber, where Dr. Couturier was the reporter, can be found in *JOCD*, 26 May 1889, pp. 1122–28; and *JOS*, 11 and 14 July 1889, pp. 901–3 and 995–7.

73 *JO, assemb. nat.*, 24 and 31 January and 5 February 1873, pp. 485–6, 675–8, and 872–3, respectively, and 30 May 1874, pp. 3382–83. See also the comments by Drs. Ferroul, Chautemps, and Dron in *JOCD*, 28 January and 1 February 1891, pp. 131 and 170–8; respectively.

74 *JOS*, 14 March 1893, pp. 278–90. Information on departments having programs of medical assistance can be found in Henri Monod, *L'Assistance médicale obligatoire en France (premières applications de la loi du 15 juillet 1893)* (Melun: Imprimerie administrative, 1897), pp. 9, 14–17.

75 For the Roussel–Morvan plan, see *JO, assemb. nat.*, 7, 8, 9, 10, and 11 August 1872, pp. 5417–18, 5419–20, 5448–50, 5463–65, and 5480, respectively. For the committee report, see *Enquête parlementaire sur l'organisation de l'assistance publique dans les campagnes*, in *JO, assemb. nat.*, 29 June 1874, pp. 4461–65. The questionnaire and responses can be found in *AN*, C3078.

76 Discussions in the budget committee can be found in *AN*, C3173, dossier 230, sessions of 31 January and 17 February 1877. For the debates, see *JOCD*, 20 and 23 February 1877, pp. 1324–37 and 1374–75, respectively.

77 As examples, see the platforms of Dellestable (Corrèze), Denoix (Dordogne), Guillemaut (Saône-et-Loire), Lafont (Basse-Pyrénées), Merlou (Yonne), Rey (Lot), and Vacherie (Haute-Vienne), in *AN*, C5504–5512, *Programmes électoraux* (1889).

78 Others were Blatin, Labrousse, Georges Martin, and Chautemps. By 1908, seven of the twenty-two members from parliament were doctors. See *Le Progrès médical*, 21 April 1888.

79 Martha L. Hildreth, "Medical Rivalries and Medical Politics in France: The Physicians' Union Movement and the Medical Assistance Law of 1893," *Journal of the History of Medicine and Allied Sciences* 42 (January 1987): 5–29. See also Martha L. Hildreth, *Doctors, Bureaucrats, and Public Health in France, 1888–1902* (New York: Garland Press, 1987), pp. 215–69. For the proposal, see *JOCD, doc. parl.*, 1890, Annex 621, pp. 919–44.

80 *JOCD, doc. parl.*, 1892, Annex 1899, pp. 185–93. Committee minutes are in *AN*, C5437, dossier 220. For the debates, see *JOCD*, 12 June and 13 December 1892, pp. 774–7 and 1784–87, respectively.

81 *JOS*, 11 and 14 March and 12 July 1893, pp. 272–4, 278–90, and 1109–24, respectively.

82 Hildreth, *Doctors, Bureaucrats, and Public Health in France*, pp. 253–4, and 270–313.

83 Peter N. Stearns, *Old Age in European Society: The Case of France* (New York: Holmes and Meier, 1976), pp. 125–7.

84 Ibid., pp. 51–52. See also Henri Hatzfeld, *Du Paupérisme à la sécurité sociale en France, 1850–1940* (Armand Colin, 1971), pp. 56–64. Doctors voted overwhelmingly in favor of obligatory pension plans, which many wished to extend to both farm and factory workers. The issue occupies an especially prominent place in their platform of 1906.

85 These had required the state to provide greater amounts of aid to poorer de-

partments and had imposed the same obligations on departments in regard to the poorest communes. For the Rey–Lachièze bill, see *JOCD, doc. parl.*, 1895, Annex 1193, pp. 218–22.

86 *JOCD, doc. parl.*, 1900, Annex 1434, pp. 535–48; and *JOCD, doc. parl.*, 1903, Annex 889, pp. 447–9.

87 Because urgency was declared, there was only one reading. See *JOCD*, 28, 30, and 31 May 1903, pp. 1741–60, 1777–96, and 1799–1818, respectively, and 5, 9, 10, 12, 13, and 16 June, 1903, pp. 1826–43, 1866–83, 1910–22, 1930–45, and 1956–77, respectively.

88 For the minutes of the committee, see *Archives du sénat*, no. 186 (1903), Commission chargée de la proposition de loi, adoptée par la chambre, créant un service public de solidarité sociale sous forme d'assistance obligatoire aux vieillards, infirmes et incurables, nommée le 2 juillet 1903. For the debates, see *JOS*, 9, 10, and 16 June and 7 and 8 July 1905, pp. 972–86, 989–99, 1006–13, 1148–56, and 1161–72, respectively.

89 Stearns, *Old Age in European Society*, p. 76, n. 30.

90 Charles de Freycinet, *Traité d'assainissement industriel*... (Dunod, 1870), pp. 1–4, 69–169.

91 *JOCD*, 1 February 1891, pp. 170–8.

92 Other doctors on the Committee of Labor before 1914 were Denoix (Dordogne), Delpierre (Oise), Dubief (Saône-et-Loire), Cazeneuve (Rhône), Cosmao-Dumenez (Finistère), Isambard (Eure), Lacôte (Creuse), Le Borgne (Finistère), Lesage (Oise), Reybert (Jura), and Sarrazin (Dordogne).

93 Other doctors on the Committee of Social Insurance before 1914 were Amodru (Seine-et-Oise), Lannelongue (Gers), Isoard (Basses-Alpes), Rey (Lot), Ricard (Côte-d'Or), Pourteyron (Dordogne), Laurent (Loire), De Lanessan (Charente-Inférieure), and Samalens (Gers).

94 At its initial meeting following the elections of 1906, Levraud, Cazeneuve, and Lachaud stressed that the role of the committee needed to be clarified and the scope of its authority to be recognized by the Chamber. See *AN*, C7398, dossier 1452. Minutes of the Committee of Public Hygiene, 1906–1910, session of 3 July 1906.

95 *JOCD*, 5 February 1902, pp. 419–24.

96 *JOCD*, 17 and 22 June 1888, pp. 1787 and 1876, respectively.

97 See Dr. Thivrier's comments on disease in the extractive industries in *JOCD*, 31 March 1912, pp. 1061–80. See also Dr. Augagneur's *La Prostitution des filles mineurs* (Lyon: A. Storck, 1888). After entering the Chamber in 1904, Augagneur, already a member of the special extraparliamentary commission on prostitution, inveighed against repressive laws to control it, arguing that the vice police did far less to contain its hygienic dangers than did competent and humane hospital treatment. See *La Province médicale*, 4 and 11 November 1899. A summary of the commission of which he was a member can be found in *Le Progrès médical*, 21 November 1903; 26 March, 16 and 30 April, 2 July, and 3 December 1904; and 8 December 1906.

98 *JOCD*, 23 June 1896, pp. 1019–30.

99 *JOCD*, 29 June 1888, pp. 1925–26.

100 *JOCD*, 12 March 1912, pp. 678–84.

101 *JOS*, 22 May 1909, pp. 307–21.

102 *JOCD, doc. parl.*, 1904, Annex. 1159, pp. 2032–53; and *JOCD, doc. parl.*, 1905, Annex 2447, pp. 532–9.

103 For deliberations of the Committee of Social Insurance on this issue, see *AN*, C 7343 dossier 214, vol. 7 (1906–10); and *AN*, C7422, dossier 416–17, vol. 3 (1910–14).

104 *JOCD*, 13, 20, and 27 June and 4 July 1913, pp. 1877–79, 2035–49, 2211–21, and 2395–2414, respectively.

105 *JOS*, 24, 28, and 30 November and 1 and 5 December 1906, pp. 1013–26, 1027–41, 1045–56, 1059–66, and 1072–85, respectively.

106 *JOCD, doc. parl.*, 1901, Annex 2134, p. 34; and *JOCD*, 31 May 1901, p. 1183.

107 *Le Concours médical,* 25 June 1904; and *JOS,* 17 June 1904, pp. 551–61.
108 *Le Concours médical,* 25 February 1905.
109 Agricultural societies, like the Central Union of Agricultural Syndicats of France, warned that if rural workers came under protection of the law, doctors' fees would have to be set carefully. See the letter on this issue by Gabriel Peschaud, former physician-deputy of Cantal, in *Le Concours médical,* 31 March 1907.
110 *AN,* C7422, dossiers 416–17, session 8 July 1913. See also the comments in *Le Concours médical* (20 April 1913) on Augagneur's ideas.
111 *Le Concours médical,* 6 and 20 July 1913 and 4 January 1914.
112 *JOCD,* 4 November 1892, pp. 1387–95.

BIBLIOGRAPHY

A work attempting to portray the physician's role in public life must rely on a variety of sources drawn from both the history of medicine and the history of politics. What follows is a general description of those that have proved to be most useful for my study; further citations pertaining to particular themes or events may be found in the footnotes. There is an abundance of works by the physician-legislators themselves in the form of books, pamphlets, articles in the medical and political press, and parliamentary reports. The most important have already been cited, including their medical theses, which I was able to consult at the Paris faculty and at the National Library of Medicine in Bethesda, Maryland.

Archival sources

Parliamentary archives

Assemblée nationale. Services des archives. Birth certificates of physician-legislators and biographical dictionaries of all members of parliament.

Sénat. Services des archives. Minutes and records of Senate committees, available by year and topic.

Archives nationales

AD XIX D 231 and AD XIX^1 158. Recueil des travaux du comité consultatif d'hygiène publique de France et des actes officiels de l'administration sanitaire. 1872–1911.

AJ^{16} 6502–24. Professeurs, Faculté de médecine de Paris, 1870–1914. Biographical information for doctors in parliament who held teaching positions in Paris.

C2792–C7487. Procès-verbaux des assemblées nationales et pièces annexes, 1871–1914. Legislative proposals, documents and reports, and committee minutes for each legislature.

C5417–C7416. Programmes électoraux, professions de foi. Campaign platforms, biographies, autobiographies, and newspaper clippings, by department.

F Series. Assorted items, ranging from F^{22} 300–4 (Correspondance de la direction et du ministère du travail, 1874–1932) to F^8 208 (Assainissement de Paris, 1880–2). Especially helpful on the role of the physician-legislators in international congresses was F^{17} 3097,[5] Congrès d'hygiène (national et internationaux) 1876–1920; and F^{17} 3097', 3097^2, and 3097^3, Congrès de médecine (national et internationaux) 1867–1913.

Faculté de médecine de Paris

Services des archives. Student dossiers, arranged by year of graduation and normally containing information on personal backgrounds, performance on examinations, composition of examination committees, prizes awarded, and service as extern or intern.

Publications of the French government

Journal officiel de la république française. Debates and documents of the National Assembly, 1871–5, and the Chamber of Deputies, 1876–80.
Journal officiel de la république française, débats parlementaires, Chambre des députés, June 1880 to April 1914.
Journal officiel de la république française, débats parlementaires, sénat, January 1881 to March 1914.
Journal officiel de la république française, documents, chambre, June 1881 to July 1914.
Le Moniteur universel. Journal officiel de l'empire française, Parliamentary debates during the 1860s.

Biographical dictionaries

Bertrand, Alphonse. *La Chambre de 1889.* Paris: L. Michaud, 1889.
Bertrand, Alphonse. *La Chambre de 1893. Biographies des 581 députies.* Paris: Librairies-imprimeries réunies, 1893.
Clère, Jules. *Biographie des députés avec leurs principaux votes, depuis le 8 février 1871 jusqu'au 15 juin 1875.* Paris: Garnier frères, 1875.
Clère, Jules. *Biographie des députés.* Paris: Garnier frères, 1880.
Grenier, A. S. *Nos députés, 1893–1898.* Paris: Berger–Levrault, 1898.
Grenier, A. S. *Nos députés, 1898–1902.* Paris: Berger–Levrault, 1902.
Grenier, A. S. *Nos sénateurs.* Paris: E. Flammarion, 1899.
Jolly, Jean, ed. *Dictionnaire des parlementaires français; notices biographiques sur les ministres, sénateurs et députés français de 1889 à 1940.* Paris: Presses universitaires de France, 1960–77.
Maitron, Jean. *Dictionnaire biographique du mouvement ouvrier français.* Vols. 1–3: *1789–1864. De la Révolution française à la fondation de la première internationale.* Paris: Les Editions ouvrières, 1964–6. Vols. 4–9: *1864–1871. De la Fondation de la première internationale à la commune.* Paris: Les Editions ouvrières, 1967–71. Vols. 10–15: *1871–1914. De la Commune à la grande guerre.* Paris: Les Editions ouvrières, 1973–7.
Nicole-Genty, Geneviève, and Chapuis, Monique. *Index biographique des membres, des associés et des correspondants de l'académie de médecine.* 2nd ed. Paris: Doin, 1972.

Robert, Adolphe, and Cougny, Gaston, *Dictionnaire des parlementaires français, 1789–1899.* Paris: Bourloton, 1891.
Samuel, René, and Bonet-Maury, Georges. *Les Parlementaires français 1900–1914.* 2 vols. Paris: G. Rouston, 1914.

Medical press

The dates following each entry indicate the years that have been researched for that particular journal. Several of the following are available in the United States, especially at the College of Physicians of Philadelphia.

Annales d'hygiène publique et de médecine légale. 1870–93. Published by the Society of Legal Medicine of France.
Bulletin de l'académie de médecine. 1870–1914.
Le Bulletin médical. 1887–98.
La Chronique médicale: revue bi-mensuelle de médecine scientifiques, littéraire et anecdotique. 1894–1914.
Le Concours médical. Journal de médecine et de chirurgie. 1879–1914. A. Cézilly, editor.
Gazette obstétricale de Paris. Journal de l'art des accouchements, des maladies des femmes et des enfants, 1872–8.
Journal de médecine de Bordeaux, 1890–1900.
Le Mouvement médical. Journal de la santé publique. 1867–80.
La Presse médicale. 1896–1912.
Le Progrès médical, journal de médecine, de chirurgie et de pharmacie. 1873–1914. D. M. Bourneville, editor.
La Province médicale. 1887–1914. Victor Augagneur, editor.
Revue internationale des sciences (later *Revue internationale des sciences biologiques*). *1878–83.* Jean de Lanessan, editor.
La Tribune médicale. 1867–1910.
L'Union médicale. Journal des intérêts scientifiques et pratiques, moraux et professionnels du corps médical. 1867–96. Amédée Latour, editor.
Union médicale et scientifique du nord-est. 1877–1914.

Select list of books and articles

Ackerknecht, Erwin H. "Anticontagionism Between 1821 and 1867." *Bulletin of the History of Medicine* 22 (September–October 1948): 562–93.
Ackerknecht, Erwin H. "Hygiene in France, 1815–1848." *Bulletin of the History of Medicine* 22 (March–April 1948): 117–55.
Ackerknecht, Erwin H. *Medicine at the Paris Hospital, 1794–1848.* Baltimore: Johns Hopkins University Press, 1967.
Ackerknecht, Erwin H. "Paul Bert's Triumph." In Henry E. Sigerist, ed. *Essays in the History of Medicine,* pp. 16–31. Baltimore: Johns Hopkins University Press, 1944.
Beck, Thomas D. *French Legislators, 1800–1834: A Study in Quantitative History.* Berkeley and Los Angeles: University of California Press, 1974.

Bon, Henri. *Précis de médecine catholique*. Paris: Félix Alcan, 1935.

Brand, Jeanne L. *Doctors and the State: The British Medical Profession and Government Action in Public Health, 1870–1912*. Baltimore: Johns Hopkins University Press, 1965.

Brouardel, Paul. *La Profession médicale au commencement du XXe siècle*. Paris: J.-B. Baillière, 1903.

Bullock, Nicholas, and Read, James. *The Movement for Housing Reform in Germany and France 1840–1914*. Cambridge, England: Cambridge University Press, 1985.

Cayrol, Roland, Parodi, Jean-Luc, and Ysmal, Colette. *Le Député français*. Paris: Armand Colin, 1973.

Charle, Christophe. *Les Hauts fonctionnaires en France au XIXe siècle*. Paris: Editions Gallimard/Julliard, 1980.

Coleman, William. *Death Is a Social Disease: Public Health and Political Economy in Early Industrial France*. Madison: University of Wisconsin Press, 1982.

Coleman, William. "Health and Hygiene in the *Encyclopédie*: A Medical Doctrine for the Bourgeoisie." *Journal of the History of Medicine and Allied Sciences* 24 (October 1974): 399–421.

Darmon, Pierre. *La Longue traque de la variole: les pionniers de la médecine préventive*. Paris: Perrin, 1986.

Daumard, Adeline. *La Bourgeoisie parisienne de 1815 à 1848*. Paris: Ecole pratique des hautes études, 1963.

Daumard, Adeline. *Les Fortunes françaises au XIXe siècle*. Paris: Mouton, 1973.

Dechambre, A. *Le Médecin, devoirs privés et publics, leurs rapports avec la jurisprudence et l'organisation médicales*. Paris: G. Masson, 1883.

Dogan, Mattei. "Les Filières de la carrière politique." *Revue française de science politique* 8 (October–December 1967): 468–92.

Dogan, Mattei. "Political Ascent in a Class Society: French Deputies 1870–1958." In Dwaine Marvick, ed. *Political Decision-Makers*, pp. 57–90. Glencoe, NY: Free Press, 1961.

Dogan, Mattei. "La Stabilité du personnel parlementaire sous la troisième république." *Revue française de science politique* 3 (April–June 1953): 319–47.

Elliot, Philip. *The Sociology of the Professions*. New York: Herder and Herder, 1972.

Elwitt, Sanford. *The Making of the Third Republic: Class and Politics in France, 1868–1884*. Baton Rouge: Louisiana State University Press, 1975.

Fillassier, Alfred. *De la Determination des pouvoirs publics en matière d'hygiène*. Paris: Jules Rousset, 1902.

Forster, Robert, and Ranum, Orest, eds. *Medicine and Society in France*, trans. Elborg Forster and Patricia M. Ranum. Baltimore: Johns Hopkins University Press, 1980.

Fox, Robert, and Weisz, George, eds. *The Organization of Science and Technology in France 1808–1914*. Cambridge, England: Cambridge University Press, 1980.

Frieden, Nancy Mandelker. *Russian Physicians in an Era of Reform and Revolution, 1856–1905*. Princeton, NJ: Princeton University Press, 1981.

Fuchs, Rachel. *Abandoned Children: Foundlings and Child Welfare in Nineteenth-Century France*. Albany: State University of New York Press, 1984.

Gaudemet, Yves-Henri. *Les Juristes et la vie politique de la IIIe république.* Paris: Presses universitaires de France, 1970.

Geison, Gerald L., ed. *Professions and the French State, 1700–1900.* Philadelphia: University of Pennsylvania Press, 1984.

Gelfand, Toby. "Medical Professionals and Charlatans. The Comité de Salubrité of 1790–91." *Histoire sociale/Social History* 11 (May 1978): 62–97.

Gelfand, Toby. *Professionalizing Modern Medicine: Paris Surgeons and Institutions in the 18th Century.* Westport, Conn.: Greenwood Press, 1980.

Gelfand, Toby. "Public Medicine and Medical Careers in France During the Reign of Louis XV." In Andrew W. Russell, ed. *The Town and State Physician in Europe from the Middle Ages to the Enlightenment,* pp. 99–122. Wolfenbuttel, West Germany: Herzog August Bibliothek, 1981.

Girard, Louis, Prost, A., and Gossez, R. *Les Conseillers généraux en 1870. Etude statistique d'une personnel politique.* Paris: Presses universitaires de France, 1967.

Glaser, William A. "Doctors and Politics." *American Journal of Sociology* 66 (November 1960): 230–45.

Goguel, François. *Géographie des élections françaises sous la troisième et la quatrième république.* Paris: Armand Colin, 1970.

Goguel, François. *La Politique des partis sous la IIIe république.* Paris: Seuil, 1957.

Goldstein, Jan. *Console and Classify: The French Psychiatric Profession in the Nineteenth Century.* Cambridge, England: Cambridge University Press, 1987.

Gooch, R. K. *The French Parliamentary Committee System.* Hamden, Conn.: Archon Books, 1969.

Greenbaum, Louis S. "'Measure of Civilization': The Hospital Thought of Jacques Tenon on the Eve of the French Revolution." *Bulletin of the History of Medicine* 49 (Spring 1975): 43–56.

Gouault, Jacques. *Comment la France est devenue républicaine: les élections générales et partielles à l'assemblée nationale 1870–1875.* Paris: Armand Colin, 1954.

Goubert, Jean-Pierre. *La Conquête de l'eau: l'avènement de la santé à l'âge industriel* Paris: Robert Laffont, 1986.

Goubert, Jean-Pierre. "1770–1830: la première croisade médicale." *Historical Reflections/Réflexions historiques* 9 (Spring and Summer 1982): 3–13.

Guillaume, Pierre. *Du Désespoir au salut: les tuberculeux aux XIXe et XXe siècles.* Paris: Aubier, 1986.

Guiral, Pierre, and Thuillier, Guy. *La Vie quotidienne dans les ministères au XIXe siècle.* Paris: Hachette, 1976.

Hannaway, Caroline C. "Medicine, Public Welfare and the State in Eighteenth Century France: The Société Royale de Médecine de Paris (1776–1793)." Ph.D. diss., Johns Hopkins University, 1974.

Hannaway, Caroline C. "Veterinary Medicine and Rural Health Care in Pre-Revolutionary France." *Bulletin of the History of Medicine* 51 (Fall 1977): 431–47.

Harrigan, Patrick J. *Mobility, Elites, and Education in French Society of the Second Empire.* Waterloo, Ontario: Wilfrid Laurier University Press, 1980.

Harrigan, Patrick J. "Secondary Education and the Professions in France During the Second Empire." *Comparative Studies in Society and History* 17 (January–October 1975): 349–71.

Hatzfeld, Henri. *Du Paupérisme à la sécurité sociale en France, 1850–1940.* Paris: Armand Colin, 1971.

Headings, Mildred J. *French Freemasonry Under the Third Republic.* Baltimore: Johns Hopkins University Press, 1949.

Higonnet, Patrick-Bernard. "La Composition de la Chambre des députés de 1827 à 1831." *Revue historique* 239 (April–June 1968): 351–78.

Higonnet, Patrick L.-R., and Higonnet, Trevor B. "Class, Corruption, and Politics in the French Chamber of Deputies, 1846–1848." *French Historical Studies* 5 (Fall 1967): 104–24.

Hildreth, Martha L. *Doctors, Bureaucrats and Public Health in France 1888–1902.* New York: Garland Press, 1987.

Hildreth, Martha L. "Medical Rivalries and Medical Politics in France: The Physicians' Union Movement and the Medical Assistance Law of 1893." *Journal of the History of Medicine and Allied Sciences* 42 (January 1987): 5–29.

Howorth, Jolyon, and Cerny, Philip G., eds. *Elites in France: Origins, Reproduction and Power.* London: Frances Pinter, 1981.

Jacquemet, Gérard. "Urbanisme parisien: la bataille du *tout-à-l'égout* à la fin du XIXe siècle." *Revue d'histoire moderne et contemporaine* 26 (October–December 1979): 505–48.

Jardin, André, and Tudesq, André-Jean. *La France des notables.* Vol. 2: *La Vie de la nation, 1815–1848.* Paris: Editions du Seuil, 1973.

Kayser, Jacques. *Les Grandes batailles du radicalisme, 1820–1901.* Paris: Marcel Rivière, 1962.

Knibiehler, Yvonne, Leroux-Hugon, Veronique, Dupont-Hess, Odile, and Tastayre, Yolande. *Cornettes et blouses blanches: les infirmières dans la société française (1880–1980).* Paris: Hachette Litterature, 1984.

La Berge, Ann Fowler. "The Paris Health Council, 1802–1848." *Bulletin of the History of Medicine* 49 (Fall 1975): 339–52.

Layet, Alexandre. *Hygiène des professions et des industries.* Paris: J.-B. Baillière, 1875.

Layet, Alexandre. *Hygiène et maladies des paysans, étude sur la vie matérielle des campagnards en Europe.* Paris: G. Masson, 1882.

Lefranc, Georges. *Les Gauches en France (1789–1972).* Paris: Payot, 1973.

Le Gendre, P., and Lepage, G. *Le Médecin dans la société contemporaine.* Paris: Mason, 1902.

Léonard, Jacques. "Les Etudes médicales en France entre 1815 et 1848." *Revue d'histoire moderne et contemporaine* 13 (January–March 1966): 87–94.

Léonard, Jacques. "Les Femmes, religion et médecine. Les Religieuses qui soignent, en France au XIXe siècle," *Annales. Economies. Sociétés. Civilisations* (September–October 1977): 887–907.

Léonard, Jacques. *La France médicale au XIXe siècle.* Paris: Editions Gallimard/Julliard, 1978.

Léonard, Jacques. *La Médecine entre les savoirs et les pouvoirs.* Mayenne: L'Imprimerie Floch, 1981.

Léonard, Jacques. "Les Médecins de l'ouest au XIXème siècle. Thèse presentée devant l'université de Paris IV le 10 janvier 1976." 3 vols. Lille: Atelier reproduction des thèses, université de Lille III. Diffusion, Paris: Honoré Champion, 1978.

Léonard, Jacques. *La Vie quotidienne du médecin de province au XIXe siècle*. Paris: Hachette, 1977.

Lévy, Michel. *Traité d'hygiène publique et privé*. Paris: J.-B. Baillière, 1862.

Lorillot, Dominique. "1789: Les Médecins ont la parole." *Historical Reflections/Réflexions historiques* 9 (1980): 103–29.

Loubère, Leo A. *Radicalism in Mediterranean France. Its Rise and Decline, 1848–1914*. Albany: State University of New York Press, 1974.

McLaren, Angus. *Sexuality and Social Order: The Debate over the Fertility of Women and Workers in France, 1770–1920*. New York: Holmes and Meier, 1983.

Moll, Aristides A. *Aesculapius in Latin America*. New York: Argosy-Antiquarian, 1969.

Morache, Georges Auguste. *Naissance et mort. Etude de sociobiologie et de médecine légale*. Paris: Félix Alcan, 1904.

Murphy, Terence D. "The French Medical Profession's Perception of Its Social Function Between 1776 and 1830." *Medical History* 23 (1979): 259–73.

Nordman, Jean-Thomas. *Histoire des radicaux 1820–1973*. Paris: Editions de la table ronde, 1974.

Nye, Robert. *Crime, Madness, and Politics in Modern France: The Medical Concept of National Decline*. Princeton, NJ: Princeton University Press, 1984.

O'Boyle, Lenore. "The Problem of an Excess of Educated Men in Western Europe, 1800–1850." *Journal of Modern History* 42 (December 1970): 471–95.

Osborne, Thomas R. *A Grand Ecole for the Grands Corps: The Recruitment and Training of the French Administrative Elite in the Nineteenth Century*. New York: Social Science Monographs, 1983.

Peschaud, Marcel. *De L'intervention de l'état en matière d'hygiène publique*. Paris: Lamulle et Poisson, 1898.

Peter, Jean-Pierre. "Les Mots et les objets de la maladie. Remarques sur les épidémies et la médecine dans la société française de la fin du XVIII siècle." *Revue historique* 246 (July–September 1971): 13–38.

Pincemin, Jacqueline, and Laughier, Alain. "Les Médecins." *Revue française de science politique* 9 (December 1959): 881–900.

Prestwich, P. E. "Temperance in France: The Curious Case of Absinthe." *Historical Reflections/Réflexions historique* 6 (Winter 1979): 301–19.

Ramsey, Matthew. "Medical Power and Popular Medicine: Illegal Healers in 19th Century France" *Journal of Social History* 10 (Summer 1977): 560–87.

Ramsey, Matthew. *Professional and Popular Medicine in France, 1770–1830: The Social World of Medical Practice*. Cambridge, England: Cambridge University Press, 1988.

Rideout, Blanchard L. "The Medical Practitioner in the French Novel 1850–1900." Ph.D. diss., Cornell University, 1936.

Rochard, Jules. *Histoire de la chirurgie française au XIXe siècle*. Paris: J.-B. Baillière, 1875.

Rochard, Jules. *Questions d'hygiène sociale*. Paris: Hachette, 1891.

Rochard, Jules. *Traité d'hygiène sociale*. Paris: Adrien Delahaye et Emile Lecrosnier, 1888.

Rosen, George. *From Medical Police to Social Medicine: Essays on the History of Health Care.* New York: Science History Publications, 1974.

Rosen, George. "Hospitals, Medical Care and Social Policy in the French Revolution." *Bulletin of the History of Medicine* 30 (March–April 1956): 124–44.

Rosen, George. "The Philosophy of Ideology and the Emergence of Modern Medicine in France." *Bulletin of the History of Medicine* 20 (July 1946): 328–39.

Rueschemeyer, Dietrich. "Doctors and Lawyers: A Comment on the Theory of the Professions." In Eliot Freidson and Judith Lorber, eds. *Medical Men and Their Work,* pp. 5–19. Chicago: Aldine Atherton, 1972.

Saint-Charles, Pierre. *La Franc-maçonnerie au parlement.* Paris: Librarie française, 1956.

Salomon-Bayet, Claire. *Pasteur et la révolution pastorienne.* Paris: Payot, 1986.

Saucerotte, Constant. *Les Médecins pendant la révolution, 1789–99* Paris: Périn, 1887.

Schiller, Francis. *Paul Broca, Founder of French Anthropology, Explorer of the Brain.* Berkeley and Los Angeles: University of California Press, 1979.

Shapiro, Anne-Louise. *Housing the Poor of Paris, 1850–1902.* Madison: University of Wisconsin Press, 1985.

Shinn, Terry. *Savoir scientifique et pouvoir social: l'école polytechnique, 1794–1914.* Paris: Presses de la foundation nationale des sciences polytechniques, 1980.

Siwek-Pouydesseau, Jeanne. *Le Corps préfectoral sous la troisième et la quatrième république.* Paris: Armand Colin, 1969.

Smith, Robert J. *The Ecole Normale Supérieure and the Third Republic.* Albany: State University of New York Press, 1982.

Sournia, Jean-Charles. *Histoire de l'alcoolisme.* Paris: Flammarion, 1986.

Starr, Paul. *The Social Transformation of American Medicine.* New York: Basic Books, 1982.

Staum, Martin S. *Cabanis: Enlightenment and Medical Philosophy in the French Revolution.* Princeton, NJ: Princeton University Press, 1980.

Stearns, Peter N. *Old Age in European Society: The Case of France.* New York: Holmes and Meier, 1976.

Stone, Judith F. *The Search for Social Peace. Reform Legislation in France 1890–1914.* Albany: State University of New York Press, 1985.

Suleiman, Ezra N. *Politics, Power and Bureaucracy in France: The Administrative Elite.* Princeton, NJ: Princeton University Press, 1974.

Sussman, George D. "Enlightened Health Reform, Professional Medicine and Traditional Society: The Cantonal Physicians of the Bas-Rhin." *Bulletin of the History of Medicine* 51 (1977): 565–70.

Sussman, George D. "Etienne Pariset: A Medical Career in Government Under the Restoration." *Journal of the History of Medicine* 26 (1971): 52–75.

Sussman, George D. "The Glut of Doctors in Mid-Nineteenth-Century France." *Comparative Studies in Society and History* 19 (July 1977): 287–304.

Sussman, George D. *Selling Mothers' Milk: The Wet-nursing Business in France, 1715–1914.* Urbana: University of Illinois Press, 1982.

Sussman, George D. "The Wet-nursing Business in Nineteenth-Century France." *French Historical Studies* 9 (Fall 1975): 304–28.

Taylor, Malcolm G. "The Role of the Medical Profession in the Formulation and Execution of Public Policy." *Canadian Journal of Economics and Political Science* 26 (February 1960): 108–27.

Temkin, Owsei. "Materialism in French and German Physiology of the Early Nineteenth Century." *Bulletin of the History of Medicine* 20 (July 1946): 322–7.

Temkin, Owsei. "The Philosophical Background of Magendie's Physiology." *Bulletin of the History of Medicine* 20 (June 1946): 10–35.

Thuillier, Guy. *Bureaucratie et bureaucrates en France au XIXe siècle*. Geneva: Droz, 1980.

Thuillier, Guy. *La Vie quotidienne des députés en France de 1871 à 1914*. Paris: Hachette, 1980.

Trisca, Petre. *La Dictature sanitaire*. Paris: Norbert Maloine, 1930.

Trisca, Petre. *Les Médecins sociologues et hommes d'état*. Paris: Félix Alcan, 1923.

Tudesq, André-Jean. *Les Conseillers généraux en France au temps de Guizot, 1840–1848*. Paris: Armand Colin, 1967.

Vess, David. *Medical Revolution in France, 1789–1796*. Gainseville: University Presses of Florida, 1975.

Virtanen, Reino. *Marcelin Berthelot. A Study of a Scientist's Public Role*. Lincoln: University of Nebraska Press, 1965.

Vollmer, Howard M., and Mills, Donald L., eds. *Professionalization*. Englewood Cliffs, NJ: Prentice-Hall, 1966.

Weill, Georges. *Histoire du mouvement sociale en France, 1852–1902*. Paris: Félix Alcan, 1904.

Weiner, Dora B. "Le Droit de l'homme à la santé – une belle idée devant l'assemblée constituante: 1790–91." *Clio Medica* 5 (September 1970): 209–23.

Weisz, George. "Construction of the Medical Elite in France: The Creation of the Royal Academy of Medicine 1814–20." *Medical History* 30 (1986): 419–43.

Weisz, George. *The Emergence of Modern Universities in France, 1863–1914*. Princeton, NJ: Princeton University Press, 1983.

Weisz, George. "The Medical Elite in France in the Early Nineteenth Century." *Minerva* 25 (Spring–Summer 1987): 150–70.

Weisz, George. "The Politics of Medical Professionalization in France 1845–1848." *Journal of Social History* 12 (Fall 1978): 3–30.

Weisz, George. "Reform and Conflict in French Medical Education, 1870–1914." In Robert Fox and George Weisz, eds. *The Organization of Science and Technology in France 1808–1914*, pp. 61–84. Cambridge, England: Cambridge University Press, 1980.

Willard, Claude. *Les Guesdists: le mouvement socialiste en France (1893–1905)*. Paris: Editions sociales, 1965.

Woodward, John, and Richards, David, eds. *Health Care and Popular Medicine in Nineteenth Century England: Essays in the Social History of Medicine*. New York: Holmes and Meier, 1977.

Woshinsky, Oliver H. *The French Deputy: Incentives and Behavior in the National Assembly*. Lexington, MA: Heath, 1973.

Zeldin, Theodore. *France 1848–1945*. Vol. 1: *Ambition, Love and Politics*. London: Oxford University Press, 1973.

GLOSSARY

Medical

Académie de médecine.   An elite body founded in 1820 to offer scientific advice to the government on matters of public health and hygiene.

AGMF (Association générale de prévoyance et de secours mutuels des médecins de France).   A medical mutual-aid society founded in 1858.

Agrégé.   An assistant professor in the medical faculties who was chosen by competitive examination and who aided regular faculty in lectures and examinations.

Concours.   A competitive examination introduced under Napoleon with the goal of opening faculty and other medical posts to the most talented.

Médecin-agriculteur.   A farmer, often a prosperous one, who held a degree in medicine though rarely practiced.

Médecin de campagne.   A country doctor.

Médecin des pauvres.   A term applied to a physician who treated the urban or rural poor for little or no payment.

Officiat.   The institution of health officer.

Officier de santé.   A medical practitioner of the second order, created by the law of 18 ventôse an XI (10 March 1803). In theory, such practitioners were confined to a single department and prohibited from performing major surgery.

Société civile du Concours médical.   As association of physicians founded in 1879 by Auguste Cézilly, editor of *Le Concours médical,* to advance the economic and political interests of the medical profession.

Syndicats médicaux.   Medical unions growing up during the 1880s and gaining legal recognition in 1892.

Union des syndicats médicaux de France.   An association of doctors' unions founded in 1881 by Cézilly.

Political

Comité consultatif d'hygiène publique.   An elite body founded in 1848 under the Ministry of Commerce and Industry to advise the government on practical issues of public health and sanitation.

Commission d'assurance et de prévoyance sociale.   A standing committee of the Chamber of Deputies to handle legislation on social welfare, created in 1893.

Commission d'hygiène publique.   A standing committee of the Chamber of Deputies to handle legislation on health and hygiene, created in 1898.

Conseil supérieur d'assistance publique.   An elite body founded in 1888 under the Ministry of the Interior to advise the government on matters of public welfare.

Conseils généraux.   Departmental legislatures.

Groupe médical parlementaire.   A caucus of physicians in the Chamber and Senate formed during the 1870s and, in theory, committed to professional reform and to the cause of public health and welfare legislation.

Interpellation.   A parliamentary challenge of the cabinet emanating from a deputy or group of deputies and calling into question a particular act or policy, thereby leading to a vote of confidence.

Professions de foi.   Campaign platforms of winning deputies, the publication of which was required by law.

Projet de loi.   A government bill.

Proposition de loi.   A private bill, necessitating approval from a committee of initiative before being sent on to a regular committee of parliament.

Rapporteur.   An individual deputy or senator who prepared and introduced a particular bill and served as its floor manager.

Scrutin d'arrondissement.   Voting according to the method of single-member districts.

Scrutin de liste.   List voting, or voting for departmentwide slates of candidates with the goal of achieving greater party discipline. Used in 1871 and in 1885.

INDEX

Names in italics are those of doctors of medicine having served in parliament between 1871 and 1914. French terms marked with an asterisk are defined in the Glossary. Abbreviations: n = note, t = table